# Disability in Adolescence

# Disability in Adolescence

*Elizabeth M. Anderson*
and *Lynda Clarke*

in collaboration
with *Bernie Spain*

METHUEN

LONDON and NEW YORK

First published in 1982 by
Methuen & Co. Ltd
11 New Fetter Lane, London EC4P 4EE

© 1982 Lynda Clarke and the Estate of Elizabeth M. Anderson

Typeset in Great Britain by
Scarborough Typesetting Services
and printed at the
University Press, Cambridge

British Library Cataloguing in Publication Data
Anderson, Elizabeth M.
    Disability in adolescence.
    1. Cerebral palsied – Great Britain
    2. Spina bifida    3. Social adjustment
    I. Title    II. Clarke Lynda    III. Spain, Bernie
    362.4'3'0914      HV3024.G7

    ISBN 0–416–72730–1
    ISBN 0–416–72740–9 Pbk

Library of Congress Cataloging in Publication Data

Anderson, Elizabeth Marian.
    Disability in adolescence.

    Bibliography: p.
    Includes index.
    1. Cerebral palsy – Psychological aspects.   2. Spina bifida – Psychological
aspects.   3. Physically handicapped youth – Psychology.   4. Cerebral palsy
– Social aspects.   5. Spina bifida – Social aspects.   6. Social adjustment.
7. Physically handicapped youth – Services for.   8. Physically handicapped
youth – Rehabilitation.   I. Clarke, Lynda.   II. Spain, Bernie.   III. Title.
[DNLM:

1. Handicapped – Psychology.   2. Social adjustment – In adolescence.
3. Adaptation, Psychological – In adolescence.   4. Rehabilitation – In
adolescence.   5. Abnormalities – In adolescence.   QS 675 A546d]
RJ496.C4A53   1982   362.4'088055                      82–8181

ISBN 0–416–72730–1                                  AACR2
ISBN 0–416–72740–9 (pbk)

# Contents

# List of tables

# *Authors' note*

The research study on which this book is based was originally conceived by the late Elizabeth Anderson and the research was carried out by her and Lynda Clarke. Elizabeth unfortunately died towards the end of the fieldwork when only part of the study findings were written up. As a consequence the final manuscript was prepared by Lynda Clarke and Bernie Spain, and while we have incorporated Elizabeth's ideas and proposals as far as possible, we must accept full responsibility for the views expressed although we hope and believe that the originator of the study would concur with all our conclusions. We acknowledge that in the final drafting the book will lack the benefit of Elizabeth's great experience and expanse of knowledge, but we hope that the reader will still find it informative and stimulating.

Lynda Clarke
Bernie Spain

# Acknowledgements

We are greatly indebted to the National Fund for Research into Crippling Diseases and the Department of Health and Social Security who provided the financial support for this study, although all the views expressed here are our own.

We are particularly grateful to the late Professor Jack Tizard, Director of the Thomas Coram Research Unit, for his invaluable help in planning the project, his advice concerning the design of the survey, for reading all the earlier drafts of this book and for his very helpful comments, encouragement and unfailing interest.

Next we must thank all those who participated in the study, in particular the school health service departments and the local education authorities who co-operated by giving access to their records and in providing facilities for interviewing the teenagers; the head teachers and all other teachers who so kindly gave us a great deal of time and information; and, above all, the young people themselves and their parents without whom this study could not have been carried out.

Our warm thanks go to Chris Kiernan, David Hutchinson and most especially to Steven Dorner for their helpful advice during the completion of the manuscript and for giving us encouragement at those points when we needed it most.

We would like to thank many other individuals who gave help, including Charlie Owen for his cheerful help with computing the data; Chris Cope, Professor Ron Gulliford and Hazel Brenner for reading and commenting so helpfully on the manuscript; Margaret Morgan of the Spastics Society and Barbara Newman of the Association for Spina Bifida and Hydrocephalus (ASBAH), who showed unfailing interest and concern in this research; and to John Coleman, Jonathan Bradshaw and Alan Brindley for discussions and information which we found useful.

We are most appreciative of the hard work from Ruth Pepper in acting as secretary to the study, typing several drafts of the manuscript and helping in many other ways. Our thanks also to Olwen Davis and Sue Tongue for typing subsequent drafts of the manuscript.

Finally our thanks must be extended to our publishers, especially John Naylor, for their support and patience during the completion of this book.

# *Foreword*

In 1966 a book edited by Paul Hunt was published, entitled *Stigma. The Experience of Disability*. It consists of twelve remarkable essays, written by people with physical handicaps, in which the psychological, philosophic and economic aspects of disability are discussed. Everyone seriously interested in the problems of disabled people *as people* should read this book.

The author of the first of these essays, Louis Battye, is a writer. Like most other contributors, he is especially concerned with the relationship of disabled people to society. He writes bluntly that he prefers ('at the risk of causing offence') the word 'cripple' to disabled person and he sums up thus:

> The cripple is an object of Christian charity, a socio-medical problem, a stumbling nuisance, and an embarrassment to the girl he falls in love with. He is a vocation for saints, a livelihood for the manufacturers of wheelchairs, a target for busybodies, and a means by which prosperous citizens assuage their consciences. He is at the mercy of over-worked doctors and nurses and under-worked bureaucrats and social investigators. He is pitied and ignored, helped and patronized, understood and stared at. But he is hardly ever taken seriously as a *man*.

As social investigators (though not under-worked) we are fully aware that Louis Battye's remarks are entirely true. We are also aware that however hard we have tried to overcome this problem, it will appear that we have, in our book, often treated those who took part in the study as statistics: as numbers and percentages, as 'above and below average', as 'the control group' and 'the handicapped group'. The purpose of this foreword is simply to state that this is not how we have perceived the young people and their parents. Altogether, we have met and talked to over 150 teenagers, most of them disabled, but some able-bodied. Each of them has been for us above all an *individual* boy or girl in their teens. They happen to be encumbered with physical problems, sometimes mild, sometimes very severe. In order to draw attention to their needs, and to the failure of society to meet these, we have been obliged throughout much of the book to focus on their emotional and physical problems and to present these in terms of statistical material. But we remember them as *young people*. We took them seriously as people, we derived, in many cases, great pleasure from talking to them and we are deeply grateful to them for their honesty, their spontaneity, and the ways in which meeting them and their parents has enriched our own lives.

ELIZABETH M. ANDERSON
July 1979

# Introduction

> There is a surprising failure to recognise the acute problems of isolation from their peers that confront many of the more seriously handicapped adolescents, who in fact share, often without the chance to satisfy them, the normal urges of young people, such as companionship, relations with the opposite sex, sport, enjoyment of leisure pursuits, travel, spending money, achievement, and the prospects of their own future home and family. We think it urgent that the needs of adolescents who are handicapped should receive more systematic study and that greater effort should be made to meet them.
>
> (Younghusband *et al.* (1970) *Living with Handicap*)

The idea for the research study on which this book is based came directly from the quotation above. Its impact lay in its complete accuracy: the failure to recognize the needs of handicapped adolescents is surprising, their problems are acute, and the need for research is urgent. It was for these reasons that the present study was initiated early in 1976.

In 1978, while the study was under way, the Warnock Report, *Special Education Needs*, was published. The scope of this report is wide and its influence is likely to be far-reaching. It was encouraging, therefore, to see that one of the three 'areas of first priority' singled out in the report was 'provision for young people over sixteen with special needs'. Our own research, which broadly covers the fifteen to eighteen year old age group and the periods just before and just after leaving school, suggests that it is without doubt the over-sixteens, rather than those still at school, for whom provision is poorest. It also shows, however, that many adolescents have marked psychological and social problems before they leave school, that these are often unrecognized and that, at least in the case of physically handicapped young people, far too little is done both while the young people are still at school and afterwards to ease the transition from school to post-school life.

### Reasons for focusing on adolescents with cerebral palsy and spina bifida

The term 'disabled adolescents' or, in current terminology, adolescents 'with special needs' covers a very wide spectrum of young people in terms of age, handicaps and needs, and our initial task was to decide which young people we should focus on. The decision to investigate the problems of those who were physically rather than substantially intellectually handicapped was easily made, since in the UK at least, the bulk of recent research on the handicapped adolescent has been in the field of mental rather than physical handicap. This includes the National Children's Bureau study of severely mentally handicapped school leavers (Walker, 1977) and the work of Richardson and his colleagues in Aberdeen (Richardson, 1977) while a study of a slightly younger age group, mentally handicapped fourteen year olds, is being carried out at the Hester Adrian Research Unit (Jeffree, 1977). In contrast, apart from a study carried out by Dorner of adolescents with spina bifida (Dorner, 1975; 1976) no comparable work was being done in the field of physical handicap.

### Criteria for inclusion in the study

Young people classified in the UK as physically handicapped are a very heterogeneous group. The majority are congenitally handicapped, although there is a rather neglected minority (in research terms) with disabilities acquired later in life. Earlier epidemiological research (e.g. Rutter *et al.*, 1970a) as well as smaller scale studies (e.g. Anderson, 1973; Seidal *et al.*, 1975) have provided consistent evidence that among children with congenital disabilities it is those with a combination of a physical disability *and* associated neurological abnormalities who are most likely to have emotional, social and behavioural problems. In other words, children with cerebral palsy or spina bifida *accompanied by hydrocephalus* (the two most common conditions involving physical disability *and* neurological involvement) have been generally found (with many individual exceptions) to have more problems in their school work and their peer relationships and a higher incidence of behavioural and emotional problems than do, for example, children with physical disorders which do not involve the brain. They also form the bulk (around two-thirds) of the population in special schools for the physically handicapped. For these reasons we decided to concentrate the study on these two groups. Those with spina bifida and no hydrocephalus were excluded.

The opening quotation referred to the problems of 'more seriously handicapped' adolescents. Research covering comparatively *mildly* handicapped children, as well as the experience of staff at the Spastics Society, indicates that it is not only severely handicapped young people who lack self-confidence, suffer from social isolation and so on (Tew and Laurence, 1975; Dorner, 1975, 1976). We therefore thought it important to include in the study those with mild as well as moderate and severe handicaps. However, since the young people were identified mainly through the AHA Handicap Registers, there is likely to be a sizeable group of young people with very mild cerebral palsy attending ordinary schools in the study area who are not known to the AHAs, and who were therefore not identified in the study.

Many cerebral-palsied teenagers (probably at least half) have moderate or severe intellectual handicaps (that is, have IQs of below about 70) and this is also true for a substantial proportion (probably around 25–30 per cent) of those with spina bifida and hydrocephalus. However, our aim was to concentrate on those whose main problems were physical rather than intellectual. Also, since the data were to be obtained from interviews with the teenagers, to have included those with a considerable degree of intellectual handicap would have meant asking questions different in content and very differently worded. We therefore decided to include only those in the 'normal' or 'borderline normal' range of intelligence, that is, with IQs of around 70 upwards, although many of our findings are applicable for the whole range of intellectual ability. Since many of the mildly handicapped teenagers and even some of those with severe physical handicaps had never had a psychological assessment or at least not a recent one, it was difficult to make decisions about whether or not to include certain 'borderline' cases, and the final sample probably includes a few children whose measured IQ would in fact fall within the 60–70 range.

Finally, the decision to restrict the study to those with cerebral palsy and spina bifida accompanied by hydrocephalus was taken in the knowledge that these conditions frequently give rise to impairment in more than one area of functioning. The teenagers in our study had to contend with a wide range of problems, many of which are very similar to those of teenagers with other disabling conditions. The group included young people with 'invisible' handicaps such as incontinence or epilepsy; those with obvious disabilities including impaired mobility, sometimes very mild and more of a stigma than a physical disability, and sometimes so severe that the teenager could not move unaided at all; hand control problems of all degrees of severity, sometimes resulting in what appeared to be simply 'clumsiness', sometimes affecting only one limb and sometimes making both limbs virtually useless; progressive speech defects, often very severe; physical unattractiveness, in some cases arising from obesity, which was very hard to control, combined with short stature, or from uncontrollable, writhing limbs, or from facial distortions produced by an inability to control the muscles of the face when the young person was trying to speak. Many of those with spina bifida also had frequent bouts of ill-health or hospitalization. These cerebral-palsied and spina bifida young people had, in other words, to cope with most of the problems (apart from the knowledge that their condition was progressive) faced by teenagers disabled in other ways. Thus, most of our findings and recommendations are highly relevant to *all* teenagers with congenital disabilities. In addition to their other problems, many of our group, although not substantially mentally handicapped, had learning difficulties of varying degrees arising from perceptual, visuo-motor and other specific problems, and were often well aware that they were 'not very bright' without knowing why.

## Choice of age group to study

There is no general agreement among writers on adolescence about the duration of the adolescent period. Some define it as the stage from about eleven or twelve years (or biological sexual maturation) to completion of secondary education, others take the pre-pubertal growth spurt as the beginning of adolescence, and yet others full sexual maturity. However, as Tanner (1962) points out, the criteria used to define puberty or sexual maturity are inexact, and Weiner (1970) suggests that 'the duration of adolescence can be reasonably defined only in terms of a psychological process. Within this frame of reference, adolescence begins with a youngster's initial psychological reactions to his pubescent physical changes and extends to a reasonable resolution of his personal identity . . . for the majority of young people . . . these events will occur largely between the ages of eleven and twenty-one.'

The factors determining our choice of age group were as follows. We wanted to look at the young people, at least initially, while they were still at school. There were several reasons for this. Firstly, we hoped to make some comparison with the large-scale Isle of Wight Study of non-handicapped teenagers, in which the age-cohort consisted of fourteen year olds. Secondly, after leaving school, young people's placements are very diverse, and we wanted to look at them while their experiences were still comparatively homogeneous. Thirdly, we wanted to look at the services which the schools were providing or could provide. Fourthly, we hoped, at least in some cases, to look at how the young people coped with the 'transition' year, that is the year immediately after leaving school, and this meant seeing them first whilst still at school. Finally, and not least important, it would have been almost impossible to have traced something approximating to a total population had we not taken those still at school.

We took fifteen years rather than fourteen years as the minimum age for inclusion for two main reasons. One was that among handicapped young people, especially those with brain dysfunction, chronological age cannot always be equated with social or emotional age; in other words, handicapped youngsters are more likely to be functioning in terms of social and emotional maturity at a level two or three years behind that of their peers, particularly those in special schools. Even those in ordinary schools often appeared to us, and to their parents, to be 'young for their age', and this was sometimes reflected in their choice of younger children as friends. Another reason for not going below the age of fifteen was that it was planned to follow up as many as possible of the original sample one year after they had left school. Since the duration of the research study was only three years, and also since many handicapped young people stay on beyond school-leaving age, we had to start with those likely to leave school during the first or second year of the study, that is, who were already near the school-leaving age. Details of the sample and how it was drawn are given in Appendix A.

### Aims and scope of the research study

It must be stated at the outset that it was not the purpose of this study to investigate the validity of any general theory of adolescence as it applied to disabled young people. Any attempt to review theories of adolescence – one example being Coleman's short review (1974, pp. 1–23) of theories put forward by Freud, Piaget, Blos, Elkind, Erikson and others – shows that these are, in Coleman's words, 'scattered and unco-ordinated', with 'remarkable gaps between theory and experimental evidence', and 'enormous variations in the quality and quantity of ideas'.

One issue which is, however, common to most of the theoretical literature and which was of particular interest to us, was whether adolescence is, in Weiner's words (1970) 'a period of basic psychological stability, or an era of crisis, disruption and maladaption'. Recent work carried out by Rutter and his colleagues (1976) with ordinary fourteen year olds, and discussed in more detail in chapter 5, suggests that adolescence is not, generally, nearly as stormy a period as popular mythology suggests. However, the teenagers in this study did experience a considerable degree of anxiety and unhappiness, as one would expect in the case of young people who have the extra burden of coping, both emotionally and physically, with all the social and practical consequences of disability, at the same time as the 'development tasks' which face all adolescents. Havighurst (1951) identified nine such tasks which he saw as central to adolescent adjustment. These included accepting one's physique and sexual role; establishing new peer relationships; attaining emotional independence of parents; achieving assurance of economic independence; choosing and preparing for an occupation; developing the intellectual skills and concepts necessary for civic competence; acquiring responsible behaviour patterns; preparing for marriage and family life; and building conscious values. It is not difficult to see how the presence of a physical disability is likely to interfere with or slow down the mastery of nearly all of these developmental tasks, and to give rise to a much higher level of anxiety and stress than most non-handicapped adolescents experience.

The main aims of the study in general can be summarized as follows:

1  To ascertain the nature and extent of psychological and social problems in adolescents with congenital cerebral palsy or spina bifida and hydrocephalus.

2 To identify some of the factors associated with good or poor 'adjustment' (the term is discussed in chapter 5).

3 To assess the adequacy of the services available to the young people, within and outside the schools prior to and during the transition from school to life afterwards (including pastoral care, social education, careers education, and vocational and placement guidance).

Only so much can be achieved within a three-year research period, and we planned to study the issues described above in the young people *prior* to school leaving (that is, in Phase I). The fact that the study extended over three years did, however, give us the opportunity to follow up nearly half of the teenagers one year after they had left school (that is, Phase II). The main aims of the follow up were:

1 To find out what sort of placements the young people had obtained.

2 To investigate the extent to which the transition year had been experienced by them as stressful, and to see what changes had taken place in the psychological adjustment of the teenagers and in their social lives and aspirations during the transition year.

3 To examine their own satisfaction and that of their parents with the services provided to help them in making the transition to adult life.

## Measures and methods of data collection

In Phase I, data were obtained from a structured interview with the teenager in school, usually of between $1\frac{1}{2}$–2 hours but sometimes longer, an interview of two or more hours in the home with the mother, in most cases, but sometimes with both parents or a substitute for the mother (e.g., father or guardian); and finally, a short interview with selected members of the school staff, in particular those concerned with pastoral care and counselling, with social education, and with careers education and guidance. The interviews were supplemented by the Rutter Teacher Scale, completed for each teenager by the teacher who knew him or her best (usually the class teacher in special schools and the year or house head in large comprehensives), and by a Health Questionnaire (Malaise Inventory) which both the teenager and the mother completed. The teenagers were interviewed before the parents. Although this meant that we lacked prior information about areas of anxiety which might otherwise have been probed in more detail, we felt it more important to meet each teenager with unbiased ideas about him or her.

During the first phase of the study, a control group of non-handicapped teenagers was included for those disabled teenagers attending ordinary schools. Both they and their parents were interviewed, but were only asked some of the questions, questions relating directly to handicap being omitted. The schools were asked to select as a control the boy or girl nearest in age to the disabled teenager from the same class or set, provided that he or she was broadly in the same ability band, and of the same ethnic background.

We must stress that our control group was very small, since only thirty-seven disabled teenagers were in ordinary schools, and in four cases we did not obtain controls (two schools raised difficulties, and two teenagers did not wish this). Also, in some instances, we had the strong impression that the control was selected because he or she was friendly with the disabled pupil. However, our controls appeared to be fairly representative of the normal school population, and the main value in including them was that they provided a good picture of the kind of social life and patterns of peer relationships enjoyed by non-handicapped young people.

In Phase II, the follow up, the data were again collected by somewhat longer interviews with the young people, this time usually in their homes, although occasionally elsewhere (e.g. a day centre), and with their mothers or both parents, supplemented again by completion of the Health Questionnaire by the teenagers and mother. Controls were not included in this phase, as the numbers involved would have been too small to be useful.

# I
# The last years at school

# 1
# Teenagers' disabilities and their schooling

## Section A

The purpose of the first two sections of this chapter is to give an account of the physical and medical problems faced by the young people in our study. Such an account could easily be no more than a depressing and arid catalogue of impairments in which the personalities of the young people and the diversity and extent of their disabilities were totally obscured. For this reason, we begin with descriptions of three cerebral-palsied and two spina bifida teenagers. They were chosen from the total group of 119 to illustrate the range and severity of the disabilities encountered, and the multiplicity of the physical and psychological problems with which some of them had to cope. Following those descriptions is a short account of the two conditions for those readers who are unfamiliar with these handicaps. The intention in beginning this chapter with descriptions rather than with figures (which follow in profusion) is to remind ourselves as well as our readers that behind the anonymous statistics are 119 highly individual young people.

*Three young people with cerebral palsy*

*Anne.*    Anne, who is cerebral-palsied with right hemiplegia, was just fifteen when interviewed and one of the youngest in the study. She attended a mixed sex comprehensive school of over 1300 pupils. The head of her ordinary junior school had suggested special schooling might be necessary at the secondary stage but her physiotherapist and the hospital staff insisted that an ordinary school would be more appropriate.

An attractive girl with a mild speech defect (something like a lisp) Anne's most obvious disability is her spastic right arm. It is very weak, with a greatly restricted range of movement and control and she hardly makes use of it, except as a support. A cosmetic operation had been suggested, but she did not much like the idea of this. In contrast, following an operation on her right leg, her gait appears almost normal. She occasionally finds balance a problem, but she can run and walk long distances and rides a bicycle.

From the age of two to eight years she had physiotherapy twice a week at a special clinic, and once a week from that age till she left primary school. Her parents spoke highly of the practical advice in management they had received there. She still attends the clinic three or four times a year, and at home continues with the exercises she has been taught. She is extremely independent physically, and can dress and undress, wash her own hair under the shower, make herself a snack, make her own bed, helps regularly with the washing up, and so on. Her parents have always been very supportive and from an early age urged her to be physically independent. They described her sister as 'giving her no quarter' in this respect.

Most cerebral-palsied pupils in ordinary schools take little part in sports. Anne is unusual in that she is very interested in all physical activities. She takes a keen part in athletics, can run faster than some of her non-handicapped peers, is a good swimmer and has even had a go at hurdling. She has recently completed a sixteen-mile sponsored walk. Her main interest is in horse riding and although one arm is virtually useless (the reins are looped over it) she has won rosettes at gymkhanas in competition with the non-handicapped, and her family showed the interviewer her various sports trophies with great pride.

Despite her remarkable tenacity in mastering new physical skills, Anne's parents feel they still have to work very hard to build up her self-confidence. At the interview she was shy and giggly, especially about the questions on sex education, and behaved more like a thirteen year old than a fifteen year old. She professes not to be interested in boys, which cuts her off from other fifteen year olds, and she prefers the company of girls a year or two younger. In fact, she is quite self-conscious about her disability but hides this most of the time. She has one close friend, but is something of a loner and has had to cope with several incidents of teasing at school, for example being called 'spas'. She was keen to leave school at sixteen and get a job, although she has no clear idea of what this might be, but her parents insisted that she stay on for an extra year after taking CSEs, in order to become more socially mature.

*John.* John was sixteen when interviewed and in his last term at a day special school. He has the same diagnosis, right hemiplegia, as Anne, although his gait looks much more awkward than Anne's. He can run and walk long distances without tiring, can use the underground, and travels alone to school by bus. As in Anne's case, his arm is more affected than his leg. It is noticeably spastic, and although he *can* do more with it than Anne can (for instance, turn on switches and taps, and hold a knife), he tends to use it very little, and then mainly as a support. Unlike Anne's parents, his mother felt that the physiotherapy he had been given was of poor quality. However, he is independent for all self-care activities and for several years has set his own alarm, got his own breakfast, and left for school often without seeing the family.

He differs from Anne in having the additional problem of epilepsy. When first interviewed he had *petit mal* fits at least weekly: $1\frac{1}{2}$ years later, when interviewed again, he reported that the fits had increased to once or twice a day, preceded by a 'dimness'. When he was particularly anxious or nervous he might have as many as five a day. He said that his fits did not usually worry him and he was completely responsible for taking the drugs and renewing the prescription. Less able intellectually than Anne, he did not take any CSEs and left school at sixteen. He obtained a place in a special residential college taking a general course, and had been there a year at the second interview.

Although John's overt physical disability was very similar to Anne's, he had many more problems to cope with. As well as the extra 'invisible' problems of epilepsy and some special learning difficulties, his parents, particularly his father, have found it difficult to accept his handicap. His mother who was open and honest felt 'Very sorry for him', but made comments such as 'It's not very nice to see him'; 'If we take him on holid    he's    embarrassr                            tter in surroundings
                                                              cated itself to John,
                                                              ; a life unnecessarily
isolated from his non-handicapped peers.

Whereas Anne appeared as a very ordinary though rather giggly and immature teenager, John gave a totally different impression at the first interview, though not so much at the second. He looked pale and sad, had an odd, stilted and old-fashioned turn of speech, was excessively polite and clearly trying very hard to please the interviewer. He was highly self-conscious about his disability and attempted to hide his spastic arm during the first part of the interview, although eventually he relaxed enough to show the interviewer what he could do with it. He did not know the name of his condition ('paralysed I think') and when asked about the cause he blamed himself saying that he had been 'very lazy about using my arm . . . when I was about five'. Further questioning showed that he definitely believed he was spastic *because* 'I didn't use it [my arm] enough'. He frequently referred to his efforts to 'get a bit more life' into his arm.

In contrast to Anne, who would go out walking, cycling or riding in her free time, John's leisure time was mainly spent in his own room, listening to the radio, making tapes, doing crosswords. He said that his greatest worry was his appearance: he was aware of people in the street staring and said that when he went out 'I put my hand in my pocket so as to pretend I'm just limping'. At his special school he had many behavioural problems especially in relationships. He was frequently teased and retaliated with aggression. These problems eased during his year at college which he enjoyed much more than school, although he was still frequently picked on.

*Jackie.* Jackie was fifteen when interviewed and attending a boarding school for cerebral-palsied teenagers. She has the athetoid type of cerebral palsy. She can walk unsupported on a level surface but has great difficulty in keeping her balance, and in trying to do so makes gross involuntary movements of her arms, so that her gait looks extremely odd. Even with adult support she is very slow, and when she goes out with her family it is usually in a wheelchair. Her hand control is very poor. She cannot manage to write, but can type very laboriously. She can take a bath and use the toilet alone, but needs help with dressing and washing her hair. Although she can use a spoon it is only with great difficulty, so that she is a messy eater; usually a member of her family feeds her. Jackie is thoughtful and intelligent (she is taking some O levels and some CSEs) but, because of a severe speech defect, even her family find it difficult at times to understand her. In her efforts to control her speech, her face becomes very contorted.

Jackie was attractively dressed, her hair was done carefully, she had a most delightful and humorous personality and she was very mature for her age. When questioned, she could give a precise and accurate description of her condition and of the benefits she would be entitled to at sixteen.

Unlike many disabled teenagers, she talked freely and honestly about what it felt like to be disabled; she said that she had been greatly helped in this by group discussions with a counsellor who visited the school who 'talked to us about how to overcome feeling fed up and frustrated, and trying to make the best of what we can do'. Through her brothers and sisters (she is the oldest in a close family of eight) she had met non-handicapped teenagers in the holidays and because she is so outgoing and pleasant had made several friends. 'At first,' she commented with absolute frankness, 'they weren't too keen on me, but they got used to me.' This was important to her because although 'I like mixing with my friends here [i.e., at the special school where she is popular and respected], I've got a thing about mixing with normal people; I like the things they talk about – the boys they fancy . . . and the clothes they're going to buy . . . and their teachers.'

She gave the interviewer many insights into what it felt like to be disabled. For instance, in spite of all her efforts to try to feed herself there were certain foods which 'I just can't control . . . then I get irritated with myself . . . I get in a temper and bang the spoon down'. Because of her mobility problem she can't go out alone 'to meet normal children'. At school 'when we go out shopping we go out with house-parents . . . we don't feel like normal children'. At home, when her brothers' friends visit, they chat with her but she is aware that 'they're nervous at first' and described an incident when she had overheard one say 'I thought she was mental'. Like most disabled teenagers she worried about whether she would ever find a boyfriend. She often longs 'to be normal' and wonders why it was her lot to be born disabled; she also worries about whether she is 'a burden to my parents'. When she gets depressed, Jackie usually 'keeps quiet till it goes away', or gets her younger sister to take her out to meet friends, or talks to her mother 'about everything'.

Jackie is, in many ways, a very disadvantaged girl. She is severely multiply-handicapped, with great difficulties in walking unaided, balancing, using her hands and making herself understood. Her involuntary movements mean that she is stared at whenever she meets strangers. As the only black teenager in her school she also had to cope initially with some racial prejudice. Her home is crowded, her parents are not well-off, and the neighbourhood in which she lives offers little in the way of leisure-time facilities. Despite all this she is, at fifteen, a mature, poised and charming girl, able to keep on top of her frustrations although realistic about her problems. She is respected and liked by her peers, and completely integrated into her very warm and accepting family.

## Cerebral palsy: a brief account

The three cerebral-palsied young people described above were chosen not only to give a glimpse of the range of problems covered by this umbrella term, but also to show how those with many similarities in their physical disabilities can, because of differences in physical care in the early years and in their own and their parents' attitudes, actually function very differently.

The term 'cerebral palsy' refers to a group of conditions characterized by disorders in the control of voluntary movement, originating within the brain itself. The disorder may be so mild that, for example, the person affected has only a barely discernible lack of control over one limb, or so severe that the individual is almost completely helpless. The condition is not hereditary and arises either in utero or in the early weeks of life as a result of damage to the brain, which can be produced in a variety of ways including pre- or perinatal factors such as interuterine infection, disturbances in nutrition and oxygen as well as many post-natal causes, such as jaundice, meningitis or trauma. (Gordon, 1976). The incidence has been estimated at around two per 1000 live births, although there is some evidence that it is now dropping. Like most other handicapping conditions, cerebral palsy is found more frequently in boys than in girls.

The range of disorders included in the term 'cerebral palsy' can usually be classified into one of three main types: the spastic, the athetoid and the ataxic forms. By far the most common is spasticity. Although this term is frequently used to refer to any individual with cerebral palsy (hence the name Spastics Society) strictly speaking it refers only to those whose muscles become abnormally stiff and resistant when an attempt is made to move them, resulting in partial or complete paralysis. The individual with spasticity is commonly categorized according to the number of limbs affected.

In monoplegia one limb – usually a leg – is affected; in hemiplegia two limbs on the same side of the body are affected, the arm usually being more paralysed than the leg; the term diplegia (sometimes also known as Little's disease) indicates paralysis of the upper and lower limbs on both sides, and usually the legs are more severely affected than the arms; paraplegia means that both legs are affected, but not the arms; and in triplegia three limbs, usually both legs and one arm; the two terms quadriplegia and tetraplegia are often used interchangeably to mean that all four limbs are affected.

In the athetoid type of cerebral palsy the lower parts of the brain are damaged resulting in abnormal posture or involuntary movements, which may be present continuously or occur only when voluntary movement is attempted. Consequently, it is very difficult for the individual to gain control of movement in the parts of the body affected. Athetosis usually affects a number of different parts of the body, the arms, legs, facial muscles, lips, tongue and throat may all be involved. If the facial muscles are affected then the individual may find it difficult to control the expression on his face or to keep his mouth closed (dribbling being the result) or, most serious of all, to speak unintelligibly.

Ataxia, which is much less common than either spasticity or athetosis, is the third main type. Here, damage to the part of the brain concerned with the control of movement (the cerebellum) is involved, the result being that co-ordination of movement and the ability to balance are affected.

Some cerebral-palsied individuals suffer from a mixture of these conditions. For example, those with spastic hemiplegia may have associated athetoid movements, while ataxic symptoms are also quite common in the spastic forms of cerebral palsy. Almost any combination of separate disabilities can be found. In cerebral palsy the process which caused damage to the motor areas of the brain (resulting in disorders of movement) may have affected other parts of the brain as well.

Many cerebral-palsied children (at least half) are also mentally handicapped as a result of generalized brain damage, and even if someone is functioning within the normal range of intelligence or near to it, as were all those in our group, they may well have specific problems in perception or in visuo-motor ability (Wedell, 1960, 1961, 1973; Abercrombie, 1964; Tyson, 1964). These defects often affect school work, particularly maths, even in a teenager who appears to be of average ability and with little physical handicap. School work in general will also be affected among those with difficulties in speaking or in writing (because of poor hand control). Since it would have been impossible without systematic testing to assess the presence or severity of problems with school work these are not discussed further in this book, but it should be remembered, when we refer to the anxieties of the teenagers about their school work, that many of them undoubtedly had real problems with academic attainments.

Damage to other parts of the brain may cause additional problems for some individuals, the most common ones being epilepsy and defects of hearing or vision, squinting being especially frequent.

*Two teenagers with spina bifida and hydrocephalus*

*Michelle.* Michelle, one of the youngest spina bifida teenagers in the study, was just fifteen when interviewed. A very short girl with a marked bilateral squint, she was extremely talkative with an endearing manner, and made many spontaneous comments throughout the interview. Her physical problems were typical of those with a severe degree of spina bifida. At present she can walk only a few steps with calipers and spends most of the time in her wheelchair. Her mother said that she had been putting on weight for the past three or four years, and although the family keep a careful eye on her diet she looked as if she would soon have a marked obesity problem. This will almost inevitably result in her becoming totally wheelchair-bound in the near future. Her manual dexterity was poor, her mother describing her as 'fumbly'.

Like most of the spina bifida teenagers in the study, Michelle was doubly incontinent. The family had established a satisfactory bowel routine, apart from occasional accidents related to her diet. Michelle had had a urinary diversion at the age of five. She empties her urinary bag but has not yet learned to change it; she said that she wanted to get used to doing this on her own and would sometimes start shouting at her mother when she tried to help her; her mother's version was that Michelle got into such a state about trying that her hands shook. She thought that Michelle became highly embarrassed when her bag leaked. She could usually 'get through a month' without this happening but started getting worried if she was outside home 'for hours on end'.

During the year prior to the interview, Michelle had been largely free from health problems. She had had one small pressure sore behind her knee, and one urinary infection for which she was put on a ten-day course of antibiotics. The special school doctor checks her urine at six-weekly intervals since Michelle had had a near-fatal kidney infection a couple of years previously. She also makes twice-yearly visits to hospital for a general check-up.

Michelle is so severely handicapped that she is heavily dependent on her parents for physical care. She says she finds her impaired mobility by far the greatest problem. She is 'really frustrated' that she can't move on her own and feels badly that her parents and sibs have to do so much for her. She can get into but not out of bed on her own, and needs more help in dressing and undressing than when she was younger. She still needs help in coping with her periods. She can't even make a hot drink for herself, as the only electric sockets are at floor-level so she can't reach them. There is one step outside the house so she can wheel herself out of the house but not back in, and Michelle is therefore totally dependent on the help of an adult or able-bodied peer if she wishes to enter her home. Consequently her mother feels uneasy about leaving her alone at home even for an hour. The local authority has helped this family by re-housing, installing a lift, and putting a hoist in the bathroom, although Michelle said they did not make a great deal of use of the hoist because 'Mum's not very sure of it'.

Although articulate, Michelle has many marked learning probems and intellectually was one of the least able in the study. Emotionally and socially she was only just entering the adolescent stage: her mother said that 'the way she sees the world is about as a twelve year old'. She was just beginning to realize the implications of the severity of her handicap. She said that from time to time, she would become depressed or very irritable usually about 'my handicap and the things I can't do'. The only way in which she could express her feelings physically was, in her words, to 'moan and scream and shout at people', or 'to take the lid off my brother's record player and slam it down', or 'to turn up a record to the highest possible volume'. Major outbursts of this kind usually occurred she said, every two or three months. She was just beginning to worry about boyfriends and about what she would do when she left school, but planned to stay at her special school for an extra year rather than leave at sixteen.

*Patrick.*   Patrick was also just fifteen when first interviewed. Unlike Michelle, Patrick was considered by his special school to be 'slightly above average' in ability. He sat, and passed, five CSEs at school and was accepted at a special college of further education one year earlier than usual on account of his potential. He took five O levels in his first year at college and hoped to go on to take A levels.

Patrick is a tall boy who wears calipers on both legs and uses crutches to swing himself along. Even though he has no feeling from the knee down, he can move around fairly quickly and has no mobility problems indoors. However, he cannot manage to balance on his sticks when there are strong winds or if it is wet and slippery, so tends to use them only in the immediate vicinity of his home and uses his wheelchair if he is going further afield with his brother, who is two years younger. Patrick has normal bowel control, but his bladder incontinence is managed by the use of a penile bag which is typical of most incontinent spina bifida boys. Patrick told us that although he would have preferred an ordinary school for academic reasons, overall he was glad to have gone to a special school because of worries about his penile bag leaking and the other boys finding out about his incontinence. Certainly Patrick's father saw this incontinence as their 'biggest bugbear'. He complained about the bag tearing or falling off, resulting in leaks most days, although he thought this was preferable to wearing nappies (which he had done until he was thirteen). When Patrick is at home he has to share a bedroom with his brother, which his father said is unsatisfactory because of Patrick's incontinence. Patrick has no privacy himself and his brother is subjected to unpleasant smells. Patrick also saw incontinence as his greatest problem because of the leaks which he found 'embarrassing', especially 'when I am at home'.

Patrick attended a residential special school for most of his school years. He actually entered the school at 2 years 10 months when his mother died of asthma which developed, according to his father, 'as a shock reaction to the doctor's bluntness in telling her that Patrick was handicapped. They said he would never sit up and would be mentally handicapped'. Patrick's brother was only ten months old when his mother died and his father could not cope alone with the baby and a handicapped son. Patrick returned to live at home when he was eight years old after his father had remarried. He attended a day special school until he was eleven when his father and stepmother separated, at which point he returned to his previous boarding school. His father married again when he was thirteen, but Patrick remained at boarding school throughout the secondary stage.

Although Patrick's family life has been rather unsettled, he has not been too disturbed by this and is a cheerful, independent and mature boy and a keen student. His stepmother described him as having an 'amazing character' because of his determination, willpower and resilience. Patrick is very close to his brother and they spend a great deal of time together when he is at home. Although Patrick does not have any friends of his own at home, he goes out with his brother and *his* friends.

Since leaving school Patrick has suffered a setback in health due to a bad pressure sore on his buttock. This developed during the summer when he was at home, before going to college. As a result he was unable to join in the normal curriculum and social life at college after the first two weeks, when he was confined to bed for the rest of the year. He followed most of the O level syllabus, but because he had to work on his own he felt his work had suffered greatly, and of course has not been able to make any new friends at college or to follow any other interests. Patrick said that he got very depressed and fed up at times because of this isolation. He was in hospital for a skin graft when interviewed for the second time and expected to be there for the entire summer. He said he only hoped that the graft would work and that he would be able to return to college in the following year.

## Spina bifida: a brief account

Spina bifida is a condition which results from arrested foetal development, which occurs some time in early pregnancy at a stage when the nerve cord is being formed. The causes are not known but 'genetic predisposition plays some part in aetiology as do intrauterine environmental factors' (Carter, 1969). In England it is found in about two per 1000 births and it occurs more frequently in girls than in boys.

Children suffering from this defect are born with a spine which is 'bifid' (i.e., split in two) and the tissues surrounding the nerve cord or even the cord itself are exposed on the surface of the body. Where the underlying tissues protude, a cyst or fluid-filled sac forms on the back. If this sac contains only the tissues which surround the nerve cord (the meninges) and not the nerve cord itself, then the defect does not usually cause any handicap. This less serious type of spina bifida, called meningocele, is not so common, causing handicap in less than 20 per cent of children with this condition. In myelomeningocele the spinal cord itself is abnormal and the nerves are exposed or lie close to the surface of the skin. These children have paralysis of some or all of the muscles which are controlled by the damaged portion of the spinal cord, and the muscles of the hips, legs and feet as well as those controlling bladder and bowel functions may be affected. Between a third and a half of the children with myelomeningocele are paraplegic, while most of the others have significant locomotor problems. Depending on the type of defect, the position of the defect on the spine, and the extent of the damage to the nerve cord, a child may be totally paralysed from the waist down or virtually normal in function.

In addition, the child may have associated abnormalities either present at birth or arising later as a consequence of the damage present at birth, including abnormalities of the rib cage, scoliosis (when the spine is twisted sideways), kyphosis (curvature of the spine), dislocated hips, or other 'fixed limb' deformities of the ankles and knees. These 'fixed limb' defects occur because only the muscles on one side of the limb are paralysed (an imbalance of muscle power) resulting in the limb being pulled out of shape. Orthopaedic surgery may be necessary to help correct these deformities, the aim being to improve the balance of muscles pulling on a limb. Most surgery is carried out in the early years, but in the teens some final corrective surgery may be required.

Unlike children with cerebral palsy, however, the damage is not confined to the motor nerves only, and there is usually a loss of sensation in the lower part of the body as well, which leads to additional problems of control and the constant danger of skin damage. If pressure is applied to any part of the body for a long period this will cut off the supply of oxygen to the skin, which will then become damaged producing a discharging ulcer or 'pressure sore'. People with normal sensation experience discomfort and change their position as soon as pressure builds up. Those without sensation have to take precautions throughout their lives to prevent pressure sores from arising, but accidents can easily happen, so this is a constantly recurring health problem. Similarly, it is very easy for burns to occur if an individual can't feel and therefore fails to notice the presence of even quite mild heat, such as a cool radiator.

Because of poor circulation, pressure sores or burns are slow to heal in spina bifida; hence damage caused by half an hour's carelessness may take weeks to heal.

Most of those with myelomeningocele have problems with incontinence of urine and faeces, due to paralysis and loss of sensation in the bowel and bladder. The bladder may be flaccid with little capacity for retention and so constantly dribbles urine, or it may be retentive but with little or no bladder sensation, holding urine until it is full, when it begins to overflow. The retentive type of bladder cannot empty itself fully without 'expression', that is, the application of pressure to the stomach, and even with a flaccid bladder expression may be needed to ensure that the bladder is completely emptied. For both these groups, the problem is not simply a social one. Urine that lies static in the bladder for even a short period easily becomes infected, and if the infection travels back up to the kidneys then there are very serious dangers to the child's health and life. Regular monitoring is required of the urine and the urinary system to detect infection or damage to the kidneys.

Although in a few children incontinence can be controlled through manual expression coupled with social training, most of those with myelomeningocele will have to use some sort of artificial urine-collecting device. Incontinence in boys can usually be managed by the use of a suitably designed flexible sheath (urinal) fitted over the penis and draining into a plastic bag which is strapped to the thigh (known as a 'penile bag'). For girls the problem is more difficult, the most common alternatives being either incontinence pads and protective rubber pants or a urinary diversion – an operation to by-pass the bladder. The most common form of by-pass operation is the ileostomy where the ureters are separated from the bladder and implanted into a spout made from a piece of ileum (the small intestine). The spout or 'stoma' is brought onto the surface of the abdomen, slightly above and to one side of the naval, so that a collecting device – usually a plastic bag – can be fitted over it. This operation will also be carried out for boys if there is a serious risk of kidney damage. Both types of bag are fitted with a tap so that they can be emptied without having to remove the whole system.

In recent years, some surgeons have advocated management of incontinence in girls by means of a catheter inserted into the urethra, whenever this is possible, as an alternative to the by-pass operation. The catheter may be inserted intermittently into a retentive bladder whenever it needs emptying, or it may be indwelling permanently (i.e. changed every few weeks) and attached to a bag in which to collect the urine.

Malfunction in the urinary system is frequently associated with problems in sexual functioning. In myelomeningocele loss of sensation in the genital area is common both in boys and girls. This usually will not prevent conception; however, erections may be difficult to initiate or maintain, and control of emissions may also be faulty. However, sexual functioning in males is innervated in such a complicated way that it is difficult to generalize and whether a male with spina bifida can have genital intercourse or father a child depends very much on the level and severity of the spinal lesion.

About 90 per cent of children born with myelomeningocele are also likely to have hydrocephalus, or 'water on the brain'. This means that the cerebro-spinal fluid (CSF) which normally circulates around the brain begins to accumulate. In a young baby, the bones of whose skull are still not set, the accumulating fluid will cause the head to grow rapidly; once the bones of the skull are set, however, any further build-up of fluid will cause damage to the brain from pressure or stretching of the tissues.

In some cases the hydrocephalus is not progressive, that is, the fluid does not continue to build up. These children with 'naturally arrested hydrocephalus' usually have heads of normal size once their body growth is complete, and their intelligence is relatively unimpaired. However, if the hydrocephalus does progress early surgery is required, and a 'shunt' or valve is inserted in the head, designed to drain off the excess CSF and reduce the pressure to a normal level. The shunt system consists of a catheter and valve leading from the central cavity (ventricle) of the brain, so that the fluid is drained into the blood stream where it can be re-absorbed.

This procedure will prevent severe brain damage and, if completely successful, the child will be of normal or near normal intelligence. However, the treatment can lead to complications, any of which may cause further damage to brain cells. The catheter may become disconnected from the valve, they may need lengthening as the child grows, and the shunt system may become blocked or infected. Symptoms of a malfunction are severe headaches, vomiting and drowsiness, or the sudden appearance of a squint; urgent treatment is then required.

Because of the risk of brain damage, some degree of impairment in intellectual functioning is common in spina bifida children with shunt-treated hydrocephalus. Many have deficits in visual perception and in visuo-motor or spatial skills that are very similar, though less marked, to those found in cerebral-palsied children, and many spina bifida children have difficulties with number concepts. Other problems associated with the presence of hydrocephalus are permanent squints and difficulties in hand control. Although this is never as grossly impaired as it can be in cerebral palsy, careful testing commonly reveals a degree of clumsiness and a lack of speed in manual tasks among spina bifida children that has a detrimental effect on school work.

Readers who would like more detailed information about the medical problems of cerebral palsy should consult Bleck and Nagle, *The Handicapped Child. A Medical Atlas for Teachers* (1975); and for spina bifida they should look at the various booklets published by the Association for

Spina Bifida and Hydrocephalus, or Anderson and Spain, *The Child with Spina Bifida* (1977), chapter 1.

## Section B: The sample and their disabilities

### Overview of the sample

The sample consisted of 119 young people, nearly three-quarters (eighty-nine) with cerebral palsy and one-quarter (thirty) with spina bifida. All but one of the spina bifida children also had hydrocephalus. As expected, there were more boys than girls in the cerebral-palsied group, fifty boys (56 per cent) compared to thirty-nine girls, while the reverse was true for the spina bifida group – nineteen girls (63 per cent) and eleven boys. When first interviewed the handicapped teenagers were between fifteen and nineteen years old. Although most of the non-handicapped controls were in the younger age range, the average age in both groups was about fifteen and a half. (Further details of the sample are given in Appendix A.)

### Severity of handicap

One of the key factors we wished to look at was the effect of the severity of handicap on psychological functioning and social life, and this had therefore to be assessed as objectively as possible. The assessment had to be such that a non-medical person could rate the teenager from questions put to the mother, and from records where available, about the ways in which the disability affected day-to-day functioning; it had to provide an objective method of distinguishing between those who were mildly, moderately and severely handicapped; and it also had to allow for the possibility of comparing degrees of impairment between different functional handicaps (for example, to show whether hand control was more impaired than mobility).

The system chosen was a modified form of the Pultibec system proposed by Linden (1963). This classification is based on an assessment of a range of functions including hand control, locomotor difficulties, toileting, intelligence, behaviour disorders, eyesight, and speech and hearing impairments. It has been used successfully in earlier studies (Anderson, 1973, where it is discussed more fully; and Cope and Anderson, 1977). Details of the scoring system are given in *The Disabled Schoolchild*, Appendix B (Anderson, 1973).

The overall severity of handicap in the two diagnostic groups is shown in Table 1.1. Clearly, more spina bifida teenagers were severely handicapped – about 70 per cent, compared with only about one-third of those with cerebral palsy, because a much higher proportion of the spina bifida group were incontinent and heavily reliant on wheelchairs. Within

Table 1.1 *The sample – type and severity of handicap*

| Severity | Type of handicap | | | | | |
| | Cerebral palsy | | Spina bifida | | Total | |
| | N | (%) | N | (%) | N | (%) |
|---|---|---|---|---|---|---|
| Mild | 23 | (26) | 3 | (10) | 26 | (22) |
| Moderate | 36 | (40) | 6 | (20) | 42 | (35) |
| Severe | 30 | (34) | 21 | (70) | 51 | (43) |
| Total | 89 | (100) | 30 | (100) | 119 | (100) |

each diagnostic category the ratings on severity of handicap were roughly the same for both boys and girls.

Table 1.1 does not show the multiplicity of handicaps from which many young people often suffered, and in Table 1.2 we have therefore shown, irrespective of severity, the total number of problems of the young people within each diagnostic group. Twelve different problems were included: impaired mobility, impaired hand function, abnormal bladder function, abnormal bowel function, speech defect, visual defect, hearing defect, presence of a valve, obesity, marked facial or bodily abnormality, epilepsy, and IQ below 85. Most of these problems are discussed individually and in much more detail later in this chapter, but the purpose of this table is simply to bring home to the reader the large number of handicaps suffered by these teenagers.

Only about 10 per cent of the teenagers had simply one problem to contend with. Within the cerebral-palsied group over one-third had two or three problems and one-half four or more problems, while in the spina bifida group an even higher proportion, nearly three-quarters, had four or more problems.

The rest of this section gives brief details of the handicaps present in the teenagers. It is inevitably a rather barren account and perhaps the reader would prefer to skim through this section, rather than try to read it closely at this stage, and then refer to it again from time to time, as the different handicaps are mentioned later in the text.

Table 1.2 *Multiplicity of handicaps in the different groups*

| No. of problems | Cerebral palsy | | Spina bifida | |
| | N | (%) | N | (%) |
|---|---|---|---|---|
| 1 | 8 | (9) | 3 | (10) |
| 2–3 | 33 | (37) | 5 | (16) |
| 4–6 | 41 | (46) | 20 | (67) |
| 7 or more | 7 | (8) | 2 | (7) |
| Total | 89 | (100) | 30 | (100) |

Table 1.3 *Mobility*

|  | CP (N = 86) | | SB (N = 30) | |
|  | N | (%) | N | (%) |
|---|---|---|---|---|
| No problems | 6 | (7) | 1 | (3) |
| Minor problem | 38 | (44) | 4 | (14) |
| Moderate problem | 28 | (33) | 7 | (23) |
| Severe problem | 14 | (16) | 18 | (60) |

## (i) Mobility

Mobility problems are shown in Table 1.3. Teenagers rated as having minor problems could run and walk but with less than usual dexterity and speed: those with moderate problems could manage only short to moderate distances with or without aids, and included those who tended to fall rather easily. Those rated as having severe problems had no useful walking, all this group depending heavily on wheelchairs. Comparing the two diagnostic groups, a much larger proportion of the spina bifida young people had moderate or severe mobility problems, nearly two-thirds of them being mainly dependent on wheelchairs, compared with less than 20 per cent of the cerebral-palsied group.

## (ii) Hand control

Over 60 per cent of the cerebral-palsied group had a moderate or severe degree of dysfunction in one or both upper limbs (see Table 1.4). A moderate dysfunction meant definite difficulty in using the limb, but

Table 1.4 *Upper limb dysfunction in the cerebral-palsied group*

|  | N | (%) |
|---|---|---|
| *No or minor problems* | 34 | (39) |
| Dysfunction in *either* right *or* left arm and hand: | | |
|     Moderate dysfunction (13 right, 6 left) | 19 | (22) |
|     Little or no effective use (7 right, 5 left) | 12 | (15) |
| Dysfunction in *both* upper limbs: | | |
|     Moderate dysfunction in both | 12 | (14) |
|     Moderate dysfunction in one, little use in other | 4 | (4) |
|     Little/no effective use in either | 5 | (6) |
| Total: | 86 | (100) |

nonetheless a useful degree of control, whereas severe dysfunction meant little or no effective use because of spasticity or uncontrollable involuntary movements. Only three of the spina bifida teenagers (10 per cent) had obvious hand function problems, and only one had difficulty in using both hands. However, other research suggests that about four in five children with spina bifida and hydrocephalus have problems of hand control which is revealed only by special testing, and consequently most of the spina bifida teenagers probably had some difficulties in this respect (Anderson 1975; Anderson and Plewis 1977).

### (iii) Incontinence

*(a) Bowel incontinence.*   Twenty of the thirty spina bifida young people (67 per cent) were reported by parents as having abnormalities of bowel functioning, as was one boy diagnosed as having cerebral palsy and spina bifida. When mothers were asked whether they had by now worked out a good routine for coping with this, only about one-third (seven) reported that a really infallible routine had been established. In one case accidents were very common (nearly every week) while in the remainder accidents occurred about once per term. The routines involved varied, some relying on suppositories, others on manual evacuation or on 'keeping her slightly constipated', while others had evolved some other sort of routine which, coupled with attention to diet, seemed to be satisfactory. Accidents tended to occur if the routine was broken or if there was a change of diet, or occasionally if the teenager had a sudden shock.

*(b) Bladder incontinence.*   Only three of the cerebral-palsied group had abnormalities of bladder functioning, one being a boy diagnosed as having both spina bifida and cerebral palsy. One coped with nappies, and two with frequent visits to the toilet. In contrast, over 80 per cent of the spina bifida group had bladder incontinence. One who had a problem over retention of urine managed to cope in the normal way, but the rest required urinary appliances. Sixteen (64 per cent) had urinary diversions (only two of these were boys), seven (28 per cent) had penile bags, while one girl had an indwelling catheter.

In cases of urinary diversion the mothers were asked if it had been a success. Only seven (44 per cent) thought that it had been, while four (25 per cent) thought that it was definitely not successful, and five (31 per cent) had mixed feelings. When the teenagers themselves were asked if they were glad 'on the whole' that they had had the operation, only two had strong negative feelings, but many of the others expressed some reservations and described the trouble they experienced. Most accepted it because they saw it as the only alternative to nappies. The problems most commonly complained of were either difficulties in getting the bag to stay firmly in place, or with the bag perforating or tearing, the former being the most serious. A number of complicated routines have to be followed to fit the bag over the stoma – the skin must be cleansed thoroughly and kept dry while adhesive is spread on to the skin and covered with a circular patch to which the bag can then be adhered, and finally the whole affair is held in place with a metal plate and a belt. If the skin is not thoroughly cleansed, or if the stoma leaks urine onto the skin during the process, then the bag will not adhere well and will gradually loosen so that leakage occurs. Finding the right type of adhesive, cleanser, patch, bag or belt to suit any particular child can take years of trial and error, as will the evolution of a routine which is quick but sufficiently thorough to avoid the problems of leakage. In some children, progressive deformities of the spine and the rib cage result in a stoma, well sited initially, being poorly placed to fit the bag securely; this is a most difficult problem to overcome.

In contrast, five of the seven mothers whose sons had penile bags felt that this was satisfactory, although two mentioned many problems in the past in finding bags which fitted well. Four of these mothers thought that their sons also found it satisfactory (e.g., 'I don't think it bothers him, he's had it since he was four years old'), while one didn't know because her son wouldn't discuss this at all.

Of the five spina bifida teenagers with normal bladder/bowels, four were completely dependent for toileting, and the fifth independent with adaptions. In the case of the eighty-three cerebral-palsied teenagers who were normally continent, however, seventy-two were completely independent, and a further two independent with appropriate adaptations; only nine (10 per cent) required toileting assistance. Six of the nine were athetoids who could not cope alone because of a combination of poor hand function and poor balance; the other three were confined to wheelchairs.

## (iv) Speech defects

Speech defects were reported in nearly 60 per cent of the cerebral-palsied group but in only two of the spina bifida children, both with very mild defects. Fifteen of the cerebral-palsied children had moderate and eleven had severe defects – nearly one-third of the total cerebral-palsied group altogether – while twenty-three had mild defects. A moderate defect meant that one would have considerable difficulty in understanding the teenagers, while in severe cases he or she was either intelligible only to family and close friends, or had no useful speech (four cases).

## (v) Hydrocephalus

Twenty-two teenagers in the spina bifida group (73 per cent) had shunts, while eight had hydrocephalus which arrested spontaneously. In the cerebral-palsied group there were two teenagers with hydrocephalus and valves, and one-third in whom hydrocephalus was suspected. Some teenagers had continuing difficulties with their shunts (see Section ix).

### (vi) Epilepsy

Mothers were asked whether their children had ever had a fit or convulsion or any blank spells, or if they were on anticonvulsant medication. Twenty-three teenagers (four with spina bifida, nineteen with cerebral palsy) had some definite form of epilepsy. Eighteen were on some form of medication, but fitting was still common in eleven cases and in some cases had become worse at puberty. All the teenagers who fitted monthly or more were cerebral-palsied.

### (vii) Sensory disabilities

*Hearing.*   None of the spina bifida children had any significant hearing loss, but in the cerebral-palsied group hearing loss was reported in nine cases (10 per cent). Five of these had loss sufficient to require hearing aids while the other four had only minor hearing losses.

*Eyesight.*   Nearly 40 per cent of both groups wore glasses, generally because of short-sight. Squinting was a common problem in both groups, affecting half the spina bifida group and over one-quarter of the cerebral-palsied group. In addition, one cerebral-palsied teenager was blind in one eye, and another was partially sighted.

### (viii) Obesity

The problem of obesity is frequent in teenagers who have severe mobility problems and are therefore unable to take enough exercise. In spina bifida this problem is further complicated by the fact that individuals with hydrocephalus are particularly prone to put on weight and that short stature is also common. The problem is not just a cosmetic one, important though that is especially for young people with a physical deformity. Excess weight makes it harder to walk with calipers and puts pressure on unstable joints, especially the hips, as well as making it harder for others to lift or move the handicapped person.

Mothers were asked whether anyone (e.g., a consultant, GP, member of school staff) had ever suggested that their child was overweight, and if so whether or not the teenager was on a special diet. Only nine cerebral-palsied teenagers (11 per cent) were thought to be overweight, six being on a special diet, compared to 43 per cent of the spina bifida group, nearly one-third of whom was on a diet. Many of those who had an overweight problem but were not currently on diets, had been prescribed one previously but were now simply 'eating sensibly'.

Two extreme examples show the problems overweight can cause. One spina bifida boy had, two years previously, become so grossly obese that he had one day collapsed, since when he has been on a very strict diet. A more typical problem was a wheelchair-bound cerebral-palsied teenager who also had a dislocated right hip. As she got heavier, the pain in her hip increased. Strict dieting had relieved this considerably and had also led to a great improvement in her appearance.

### (ix)  General health problems during the twelve months prior to the interview

The mothers were asked to detail any health problem their children had had over the last twelve months. We did not include as a 'health problem' chronic conditions which are an integral part of the handicap (e.g. epilepsy or soiling) but urinary infections, which are extremely frequent in spina bifida children, were included. In general, ill health was much more common in the spina bifida group. Only 6 per cent of the cerebral-palsied group had needed to go into hospital in the previous year (a similar proportion to the control group) compared with nearly a quarter of the spina bifida group.

Eight teenagers – all but two with spina bifida – were classified as having severe problems currently, either because these were acute or potentially life-threatening, because they had necessitated long periods of hospitalization or because they were long-term problems. For example, there were two cases of shunt failure which necessitated a three-week stay in hospital to have a catheter change. Another girl burnt her foot on a radiator and because of gangrene two toes had to be amputated. While in hospital she broke her leg and the prolonged stay in bed resulted in sores which required a skin graft, and she missed about nine months' schooling in consequence. A boy who was admitted to hospital for a leg-straightening operation fell and broke a leg while at home for Christmas. The fracture was not discovered immediately and in consequence he was in traction for several months, the whole period of hospitalization extending over seven months in all.

Among the less serious health problems reported were severe headaches (which in a child with hydrocephalus is very worrying), asthma, a two-week period in hospital for an orthopaedic operation on the ankle, pressure sores, kidney problems and protracted fits requiring hospitalization. Over half of the spina bifida group had suffered from one or more urinary infections in the past year.

### Section C

### School placement

This section describes the type of school (i.e. ordinary, day special, or residential special) attended by the pupils in the study and briefly.

indicates the characteristics of these schools. The pupils' experiences and feelings about them are discussed, as well as their current preference for ordinary or special education. The parents' overall satisfaction with the type of placement and with the individual schools attended by their children is also considered.

## Past and present placement

Table 1.5 shows the school placement of the young people at the time of the interview and also indicates the type of school they had attended before their current secondary placement, if this had been different.

Table 1.5 *School placement by diagnostic groupings*

| Type of school | Cerebral palsy | | Spina bifida | | Total | |
|---|---|---|---|---|---|---|
| | N | (%) | N | (%) | N | (%) |
| Ordinary schools[1] | 31 | (35) | 6 | (20) | 37 | (31) |
| Special secondary schools[2] | 7 | (8) | 1 | (3) | 8 | (6) |
| All-age special schools[3] | | | | | | |
| Child joined in junior section | 29 | (32) | 11 | (37) | 40 | (34) |
| Child joined at 11+ | 22 | (25) | 12 | (40) | 34 | (29) |
| Total | 89 | (100) | 30 | (100) | 119 | (100) |

[1] Four had transferred from special schools at 11+
[2] Four had transferred from ordinary schools at 11+
[3] Five had transferred from ordinary schools at 11+

Of the total sample, thirty-seven (just under one-third) were attending ordinary schools and eighty-two (69 per cent) were attending special schools. A higher proportion of the cerebral-palsied than of the spina bifida children were attending ordinary schools (35 per cent compared with 20 per cent). Transfers between the two types of school were relatively uncommon, particularly from special primary to ordinary secondary (only four in all) and only ten children (9 per cent of the total sample) had transferred from ordinary to special schools at 11+. One of these was untypical in having come from the Caribbean to join her family, and no less than six of the rest came from the same LEA, an authority which had recently opened its own special school. There was no evidence from this study, therefore, to support the commonly held view that it is often necessary for handicapped children attending ordinary schools at the primary stage to have to move to special schools at secondary level, because of the difficulties in layout and accessibility in large modern comprehensives. Problems of this kind occurred in one or two cases but they were in fact surprisingly rare.

Only eight of the children in special education attended schools which catered solely for the secondary age groups (six being from the same

Table 1.6 *School placement related to severity of handicap*

| Type of school | Severity of handicaps | | | | | | |
|---|---|---|---|---|---|---|---|
| | Mild | | Moderate | | Severe | | Total |
| | N | (%) | N | (%) | N | (%) | N |
| Ordinary | 18 | (72) | 15 | (35) | 4 | (8) | 37 |
| Day special | 6 | (24) | 21 | (49) | 27 | (53) | 54 |
| Residential special | 1 | (4) | 7 | (16) | 20 | (39) | 28 |
| Total | 25 | (100) | 43 | (100) | 51 | (100) | 119 |

school). All the rest were in all-age schools, usually very small, the majority with less than 100 pupils in total (see Table 1.8). In fact nearly half of the sample attending special schools had spent all or most of their whole school career in the same small establishment.

School placement was, of course, closely related to severity of handicap, as is shown in Table 1.6. Nearly three-quarters of the mildly handicapped teenagers were in ordinary schools, while over 90 per cent of those with severe handicaps were in special schools. Nevertheless, 20 per cent of the children with moderate or severe handicaps were coping within the ordinary school system (all but four of whom were cerebral-palsied).

To some extent placement was also closely related to intellectual level, although it is difficult to be precise about this, since IQ data were available for very few children in ordinary schools, and even in special schools many had never been formally assessed. Where IQs were not available, teachers were asked to classify the child as 'above average', 'average', 'somewhat below average' or 'very poor', and these data are shown in relation to type of school in Table 1.7. The table reveals very marked differences in placement according to ability, there being many more children of below average ability in the special schools as might be

Table 1.7 *Teachers' opinion of how teenagers' attainments compare to other children of a similar age*

| | Very much above average | Somewhat above average | Average | Somewhat below average | Very poor | Total |
|---|---|---|---|---|---|---|
| Controls | 1 | 10 | 12 | 8 | 1 | 32 |
| | (3) | (31) | (38) | (25) | (3) | (100) |
| Handicapped pupils in ordinary schools | 4 | 5 | 5 | 19 | 3 | 36 |
| | (11) | (14) | (14) | (53) | (8) | (100) |
| Handicapped pupils in special schools | 0 | 5 | 5 | 47 | 24 | 81 |
| | (0) | (6) | (6) | (58) | (30) | (100) |

expected. However, the PH children in ordinary schools also showed a wider spread of ability than did the controls. It is interesting to note also that, in terms of numbers, there were almost as many handicapped children of average and above average ability in the special schools as in the ordinary schools.

### Characteristics of schools

The schools attended by the children varied in size, location and organization; their main characteristics are summarized in Table 1.8. One of the most striking things about this table is the great contrast between the average size of the ordinary LEA schools and of the special schools, the largest of which had fewer pupils on roll than the smallest of the ordinary schools. Even the non-LEA ordinary schools were considerably larger on the whole than the special schools.

Table 1.8 *Characteristics of the schools*

| Type of school | No. of survey pupils | No. of schools | Average size of school | Range |
|---|---|---|---|---|
| *Ordinary* | | | | |
| Day LEA schools | 36 | 31 | 893 | 470–1650 |
| Non-LEA schools | 4 | 3 | 288 | 100–394 |
| Total | 40 | 34 | 840* | 100–1650 |
| *Special* | | | | |
| Day PH schools | 50 | 12 | 94 | 52–150 |
| Residential or mainly residential | 34 | 14 | 91 | 27–318 |
| Total | 84 | 26 | 93* | 27–318 |

* Overall average

The day special schools were all run by LEAs, as were two of the residential schools, the others were run by a variety of voluntary organizations. Nine of the residential schools were for the physically handicapped and the others included one for the maladjusted, a Rudolf Steiner school for pupils of mixed handicaps, a school for epileptic pupils, one for deaf pupils and one for deaf pupils with additional handicaps.

### The teenagers' views about type of school placement

All the young people interviewed were asked questions at several points in the interview to elicit their opinions about and their satisfaction with current school placement, and about what alternatives if any they would prefer. First, they were asked directly whether they were happy at school. The majority of both handicapped and control pupils (over three-quarters) said they were happy 'most of the time', and there were no differences relating to sex and type of handicap. Comparing the physically handicapped children in ordinary schools with the control children it was interesting to find that the percentage expressing unhappiness (20–25 per cent) was very similar, and there was no evidence therefore that the disabled children in ordinary schools were having more difficulties in coping with school life than their non-handicapped peers. Happiness at school was also looked at in relation to type of school attended, and this showed that the proportion who were not happy in school was higher for those in residential placement (about 30 per cent compared with 17 per cent in day special schools) usually because they would have preferred to live at home. Only about one-quarter of the boarders went home each weekend, about one-half made home visits once or twice a term, while the remainder went home only in the summer holidays.

The teenagers were then asked which type of placement – special or ordinary – they would prefer to be in, and the results were quite conclusive and consistent. Apart from one who was undecided, every pupil currently placed in an ordinary school preferred ordinary school placement, while nearly one-quarter of those in special schools said they would have preferred ordinary school placement, and 20 per cent were undecided. The four children who had transferred at eleven years from special to ordinary schools all preferred their current placement, while of the ten transferring from ordinary to special schools, six were content, three were undecided, and one would have preferred to have stayed in an ordinary school.

Later in the interview, the teenagers were asked: 'As far as friends are concerned, which of these kinds of schools would you prefer to be in: a special school for handicapped children only; an ordinary school in which you knew there would definitely be several other physically handicapped pupils; or an ordinary school where you might be the only handicapped pupil?' Again, all of those pupils who were already in ordinary schools (usually the only handicapped pupils there) opted to remain as they were. It is interesting to note that the most popular choice in each of the diagnostic groups (40 per cent) was for an ordinary school where there would be some other handicapped pupils. Given this option, which is now becoming more of a reality with the increasing trend towards special units attached to selected ordinary schools, only one-quarter of CP children and just over a third of the spina bifida group opted for special school placement. Thus from the point of view of friends, the majority of children in both groups would have liked ordinary school placement.

The other point to note here is the difference between the cerebral-palsied and the spina bifida group; more of the latter preferred special schools, and this is probably related primarily to the anxiety they feel (see chapter 6) about their incontinence and its management, and also to the fact that a greater proportion were severely handicapped.

*Teenagers' perception of the advantages and disadvantages of special and ordinary schools*

The teenagers were asked what they saw as the advantages and dis-advantages of special and ordinary schools. A minority had experienced both: the others spoke about what they liked and disliked about the kind of school they were actually in and what they thought they would like or dislike about the alternative. Because it is unusual to hear how handi-capped pupils themselves feel about school placement we are reporting their comments here in some detail.

As already noted, those in ordinary schools generally preferred their current situation and most were straightforwardly in favour of ordinary schools. One boy, a hemiplegic, previously in a special school and now in an Inner London mixed comprehensive said that he was very happy there: 'It's a better atmosphere. It was a strain at first . . . I got used to it over a few years. It was less sheltered.' He added: 'You get used to normal life better . . . it makes you better able to cope.' Another boy with a similar early experience said: 'Special school was too small. There was no chance really to do anything and no competition for your work.' Many of those in ordinary schools had not had an easy time, particularly in the first two or three years there, but they still preferred, overall, ordinary school placement. One boy said: 'I wasn't happy at first . . . I was the oddball . . . the target for aggression . . . to some extent I was bullied.' He had refused to go to school after continuous teasing during his first ten weeks in a comprehensive, but after his parents complained to the Head, most of the teasing stopped. Others mentioned difficulties in keeping up with the work, but they preferred the challenge nonethe-less. One heavily handicapped spina bifida girl said, 'I have my bouts of not being able to keep up, especially if I've been away in hospital or ill for a few days', but it 'helps you to cope with the outside world. Not everything will be [specially] equipped when you leave'. Most of those in ordinary schools were content with being the only handicapped pupil. However, those who had been teased, two boys in particular, were strongly in favour of an ordinary school where there would be some other PH pupils: in one boy's words 'the [PH] kids wouldn't take the mickey out of me'.

Of those who preferred special schools, most gave as their reason anxiety about the reactions of the non-handicapped children. These are some typical comments: 'Here they are all handicapped so they under-stand me . . . I think they'd take the mickey at ordinary school.' 'I wouldn't make friends easily from a wheelchair.' 'I wouldn't like to go to an ordinary school. I've been to my sister's school and they look rough – they might not be, but they looked it.' A cerebral-palsied girl who had been in an ordinary school said: 'There are too many bullies . . . they make fun of my walking . . . one girl pushed me over because I was staring at her.' In contrast, one spina bifida girl who had transferred at the secondary stage to a special school said she would have preferred to stay in an ordinary school. She liked the opportunities in her new school for riding and drama and the other 'facilities' it offered, but disliked being 'grouped together with handicapped people different from everyone else'. In an ordinary school she felt she had been 'considered as an ordinary person . . . the teachers don't treat you differently'.

A few other factors were mentioned, apart from these social ones, why special schools were preferred. One severely handicapped cerebral-palsied boy had been to look at an ordinary school but 'there were too many stairs and you had to change rooms every lesson. Special schools have no stairs, and handrails on slopes . . . you get extra help in school work when you can't do things, and the classes are smaller'. One girl said that at fourteen she had wanted to go to an ordinary school to make non-handicapped friends but 'Mum and Dad wouldn't let me go. . . . Now I would turn it down because I couldn't keep up with the work and the number of children.'

*Parents' preferences about type of schooling and satisfaction with their child's particular school*

Parents as well as teenagers were asked whether they thought the school their child was currently attending was the right kind for him or her to be in. The great majority felt their child was in the right kind of school. The exceptions were seven parents of children in special schools (five with spina bifida, two with cerebral-palsied children) who felt that they would have been better off in ordinary schools, either from the social or the educational point of view, and three parents of deaf CP children who had had particular problems. This seems to be in line with findings from other studies which suggest that parents are generally satisfied with the kind of placement actually available.

All the parents whose children were in ordinary schools thought that this was, overall, the right placement. 'We're very fortunate . . . they've a good pastoral care system . . . he likes it as it's near home and his brother is there.' Another mother: 'I've given a lot of thought to this . . . I think it's better to put her in this wicked world now.' Another mother said much the same: 'We'd never consider a special school; she's got to have a challenge.' (They made certain, however, by discussion with the school, that the challenge was not too much for her.)

Parents sometimes mentioned aspects of special schools that they would have liked, although they preferred ordinary school placement: 'We like to think he's with ordinary kids . . .', although, in the local special school, 'he'd be better off in terms of the time spent [by teachers] with individuals'. Another parent said: 'She's better off with ordinary children . . . but I've had my doubts . . . it's getting harder and harder . . . she's doing all right, but finds it hard to keep up, and worries quite a bit.' She had also discovered that in the local special school 'they take them away for the holidays which would give the mothers a rest'. In fact, all the things mentioned by the parents and the teenagers as being the advantages of special schools were facilities which need not have been denied to the child because the parents had opted for an ordinary school, if the gap between special school and ordinary school provision was not so discrete and distinct as is currently the case. Where the special school was preferred, the reasons also included the special facilities there: 'The staff are good . . . they have everything there, physio' and speech therapy', but more often the feeling expressed was that the child just couldn't have coped in an ordinary school: 'She wouldn't be able to stand it . . . it would be too rough. And she needs extra education.' 'There wasn't a secondary school in the area that would take him because of the steps.'

However, even parents who thought special school placement on the whole preferable often referred to aspects of special provision they were unhappy about. 'They don't make enough effort to spend time on his academic difficulties.' 'She lacks the rubbing-off effects from other [i.e., ordinary] children.' 'He might have coped more with life if he'd gone to an ordinary school from the beginning. He did go for one day a week [at secondary level] but couldn't cope with the standard of work. He seemed to be happy with the children, but the work bothered him.'

As well as being asked about their placement preference in general, the parents were also asked whether there was anything they felt dissatisfied with about the particular school their child attended. The results suggest only slight differences between the feelings of the control group parents and the parents with children in ordinary schools, over three-quarters of whom were content, while parents of children in special schools tended to be rather more dissatisfied (over 40 per cent). Any dissatisfaction expressed by parents of children in ordinary schools was usually mild, for example: 'I don't think he's had as much direction in remedial work as he might have benefited from . . . but on the whole the school has been very helpful indeed. He's had the same class teacher for three years, an excellent person and the Year Head is very sympathetic and has helped him a lot.' Only two parents were very dissatisfied. In one case the father complained about his daughter's bad behaviour, and attributed this to the school; he also complained that she was always getting into trouble and being bullied. In the other case the mother felt the staff were always 'picking on her son' and making him 'a social outcast'. The boy was only mildly handicapped and the staff did not seem to have made much effort to help him.

In contrast, many more parents of children in special schools were critical, and this was often strongly voiced. One mother, herself a headmistress said, '[the school] is a silly, stupid place, inadequate and not educationally based'. Others made similar comments: 'They should push them more: they don't learn enough'; 'Sometimes I feel they should push them a bit more academically.'

The consistency of the complaints about the lack of drive on the education front within the special schools suggests that many of these schools do need to consider how to provide more stimulation for their pupils than they do at present, especially in view of the findings from the GLC survey of spina bifida children, which suggests that in a sample matched for IQ the attainments of the more able children in special schools were considerably lower than for those in ordinary schools. (Janet Carr, personal communication, 1980.)

Children who are both cerebral-palsied and have serious hearing losses are relatively rare, but great problems are posed in finding a school which can cater for all aspects of this handicap. There were five such teenagers in the study (6 per cent of the CP group); three parents reported major problems over finding a suitable school, and even in the other two cases the situation was not entirely satisfactory.

*Summary*

These findings show that a very high proportion of the handicapped young people studied were moderately or severely handicapped (as assessed on the Pultibec scale) – over 70 per cent of the cerebral-palsied group being assessed as such, compared with 90 per cent of the spina bifida group. They also reveal that a high proportion were multiply handicapped; only about 10 per cent had a single problem, while one-half of the cerebral-palsied group and nearly three-quarters of the spina bifida group had four or more problems.

Looking at the proportion with particular kinds of handicap, the pattern differed quite markedly between the two groups. Among the spina bifida group over 80 per cent had moderate or severe locomotor difficulties, usually accompanied by bladder incontinence, and over two-thirds had bowel incontinence also. Of those who were not incontinent, all but one needed help with toileting because of severe locomotor difficulties. Those with bladder incontinence had usually been fitted with an appliance of some kind but this was not always successful, especially where a urinary diversion had been carried out. Less than half of the mothers of teenagers with urinary diversions were fully satisfied with this as a method of social control. Obesity was another common problem among the spina bifida group, over 40 per cent of mothers reporting this.

Among the cerebral-palsied group, about half also had moderate or severe locomotor problems while over 60 per cent had moderate or severe problems with one or both upper limbs. (None of those with spina bifida had upper limb problems of this degree.) Speech defects, virtually absent among the spina bifida group, affected 60 per cent of those with cerebral palsy, and about one-third had moderate or severe difficulties. Very few cerebral-palsied young people suffered from incontinence, although about 10 per cent needed help with toileting because of locomotor difficulties or poor hand control. Epilepsy, while affecting a few spina bifida teenagers, was more common among the cerebral-palsied, about 20 per cent of whom suffered from this. Deafness was a problem for about 10 per cent of the cerebral-palsied, but wasn't found at all among the spina bifida teenagers.

Visual defects of a less severe kind were common in both groups, about 40 per cent wore glasses, and squinting was found in one-quarter of the cerebral-palsied group and half of the spina bifida teenagers. Two of the cerebral-palsied teenagers had more severe visual defects.

In terms of general health the spina bifida teenagers were more likely to have moderate or severe problems than the cerebral-palsied teenagers (17 per cent compared with 3 per cent), the difference mainly being due to the fact that the spina bifida teenagers were liable to renal or shunt complications, and that more needed orthopaedic surgery. Hospitalization was also more common among the spina bifida group, nearly one-quarter of whom had been admitted to hospital in the previous year, compared with only 6 per cent of the cerebral-palsied teenagers.

In spite of the high percentage of teenagers with severe difficulties, about one-third of the sample were attending ordinary schools. Although the proportion with mild handicaps was higher in ordinary than in special schools, over half of those in ordinary school were assessed as having moderate or severe difficulties. Because of the differences in severity of handicap, a higher proportion of cerebral-palsied teenagers were attending ordinary schools compared with those with spina bifida.

School placement was also related to intellectual ability. Only about 12 per cent of those in special schools were judged to be of average or above average ability compared with nearly 40 per cent of those in ordinary schools, while 30 per cent were judged to be of very poor ability compared with only 8 per cent of those in ordinary schools.

Most of the children in special schools were in all-age schools and those tended to be very small, between 90–100 pupils on average, compared with an average of nearly 900 in the LEA and nearly 300 in the non-LEA day schools. About half of those in special schools had spent all or nearly all of their entire school careers in the same small establishment. The majority of pupils said they were happy at school regardless of placement and there was little difference in this between the control and PH children, though those in residential PH schools were more likely to express unhappiness (30 per cent compared with 17 per cent of those in day PH schools).

None of the PH children in ordinary schools would definitely have preferred to be in a special school, but one-quarter of those in special schools said they'd have preferred an ordinary school, while 20 per cent were undecided. The proportion of those in a special school who would have preferred an ordinary placement was even higher when asked to consider placement 'as far as friends are concerned', and many liked the idea of an ordinary school where there were some other handicapped pupils.

The teenagers gave very interesting and sensible replies when asked why they preferred the different kinds of placement. Those preferring ordinary school mainly saw the advantage of this in terms of it being more 'normal', although some openly admitted having problems with their peers initially, and difficulty in keeping up with homework. They also saw special schools as too small and lacking in competition. Those who preferred special schools usually expressed anxiety about ordinary school because of the reaction they feared they'd get from the able-bodied. They saw the special school as offering them more help from teachers and peers and also having the advantage of being fully accessible.

Parents mainly expressed satisfaction with whatever type of placement the child was in. Those with children in special schools commonly mentioned the advantage of accessibility and the special facilities there, such as physiotherapy. However, there was a high level of discontent with the academic standards within special schools and a feeling that the children were not adequately stimulated there.

# 2

# The attainment of independence and responsibility

Most writers on adolescence see the central developmental task at this stage in life as being the gradual attainment of personal independence. Erikson (1968), whose work has been particularly influential, describes this as 'identity formation', and views the adolescent as engaged in a gradual emotional separation and detachment from his parents. He believes (although there is little systematic evidence for this) that the young person may, because of his uncertainty about his new role, experience an 'identity crisis' which can lead to apparently maladaptive behaviour patterns. Blos (1962; 1967) whose viewpoint is somewhat similar, sees adolescence as a process of 'individuation', in which the young person takes increasing responsibility for what he does, rather than placing this on the shoulders of others, in particular on the family. The role of the parents in this context has been discussed by Framrose (1977) who considers that their 'capacity for readjustment and change . . . has an important influence on adolescent development'.

A number of writers view adolescence in terms of 'role theory'. Elder (1968) for example argues that for at least two-thirds of one's life one is building up a repertoire of roles. The adolescent years are critical in this respect, since role transitions are precipitated by the individual's growing independence from authority figures, by involvement with his peer group, and because of new sensitivities to the evaluation of others, as well as the acquisition of new roles. Sometimes the role itself does not change but the expectations of others do, for example, parents of a handicapped teenager may expect more of him as he grows older in regard to physical independence. The acquisition of new roles is often a painful and difficult process, and the question of self-image is likely to arise, that is what kind of person the youngster sees himself as now, or as becoming.

Many clinicians and researchers have implied or stated explicitly that success in carrying out these developmental tasks and the acquisition of new roles results in parent-teenager conflict or even alienation. Little evidence is produced to support this conclusion, and the most recent studies suggest that such conflict is not widespread (Rutter *et al.*, 1976). Others who have found relatively little conflict include in England Coleman (1974) and in the USA Donvan and her colleagues (e.g. Donvan and Adelson, 1966). Donvan found that where conflict did occur it reached a peak at 15–17 years and was more common among boys. This study was, of course, for non-handicapped adolescents. Handicapped young people are generally less mature and one might expect the peak of conflict to come, in most cases, from one to three years later. Coleman (1974) found that relationships between parents and adolescents were generally good, but that where conflict did occur it revolved around different issues in boys and in girls. For boys, independence of action and freedom of movement are the most common sources of conflict, whereas girls do not appear to see this as an issue but are 'much more concerned with inner autonomy . . . they want to be themselves . . . they feel threatened by the influence and forcefulness of their parents'.

These issues apply equally to able-bodied and disabled adolescents. In the case of the latter, however, the question is greatly complicated by the physical dependence of the young people on their parents. In this chapter, therefore, we have focused on three main areas out of the very large number which would have been valuable to explore. The first of these was the development of physical independence, a matter of great importance to disabled young people, while the second was that of the taking on of responsibilities and the exercise of choice. Lastly we looked briefly at vocational aspirations.

## The development of physical independence

Three aspects were investigated. First, we looked at what the teenagers actually were able to do in terms of daily living activities in the home, as well as their mobility outside the home. Next we explored their attitudes, as perceived by their parents, towards physical independence, and the parents' attitudes both as they described themselves and as they were perceived by the young people. We also looked at arguments arising when teenagers felt they were given too much help. Thirdly, the teenagers were questioned about what they knew both about the disability itself and about the benefits and allowances to which they were, or might be, entitled. Such knowledge is important in giving an individual a greater feeling of 'control' over his disability and is also of help to him in the management of interactions with others, especially social and peer interactions.

### (i) Self-help skills in the home

The parents and teenagers were asked detailed questions about the independence of the young people in a range of daily living activities in the home, such as dressing, washing, making a snack and being left alone in the house. Toileting and incontinence were considered separately.

The cerebral-palsied group were generally better at activities which required good standing skills while the spina bifida group were better if good hand function was needed. For example, one-third of the cerebral-palsied teenagers needed help with dressing and undressing, compared with less than 20 per cent of those with spina bifida. In washing, taking a shower and hair washing a higher proportion of the cerebral-palsied group coped alone, although this difference was reduced if the spina bifida young people had a basin which was accessible, or a bathroom with the necessary adaptations. In contrast nearly one-quarter of those with spina bifida but only 9 per cent of those with cerebral palsy needed help in getting in and out of bed. The majority in both groups (90 per cent of those with spina bifida and 73 per cent of those with cerebral palsy) never made a meal at home; however, two-thirds of those with cerebral palsy could make a snack (although a much lower proportion had actually done so in the last week) while this was true for only 5 per cent of those with spina bifida. For both groups about 60 per cent of mothers felt that they could leave the teenager alone in the home for at least four hours in the daytime, but over 40 per cent of parents with cerebral-palsied and nearly 60 per cent of those with spina bifida children said that they never left them in the evenings.

When self-help skills were considered in relation to severity of handicap there was little difference between the mildly and the moderately handicapped group except in activities involving hand function, such as dressing, hair washing, and making a meal. However, even on simple activities such as washing, there were very marked differences in self-help skills between those with moderate and those with severe handicaps.

The findings indicate that a very substantial proportion of the young people still relied heavily on their parents for help with many activities of daily living. In the cerebral-palsied group poor hand control was the main factor responsible, while among those with spina bifida locomotor handicap was the main problem. But in both groups, especially in those with spina bifida, a much larger number of young people could, we considered, have been more independent if they had been living in homes which had been adapted for the disabled (in particular kitchens, but also bathrooms), and if more had been done by parents *and* by their schools or other bodies to foster independence in the home. The Association of Spina Bifida and Hydrocephalus has now recognized this need, and runs an increasing number of Independence Training Weeks for young people. These can only touch the tip of the iceberg, however, and a major problem has been the lack of follow up in the home. Some, though not all, special schools (see chapter 10) have tried hard to foster independence, but many still do very little, and even those which do make great efforts in this direction often fail to liaise with parents so that the teenager does not put into practice at home what he or she has learned at school. Much more needs to be done to discover the extent to which the very severely disabled could achieve greater independence.

*(ii) Management of incontinence*

Mothers with incontinent children were asked whether their children could empty or change their bags unassisted. All were able to empty their bags competently, but only seven of the sixteen teenagers with urinary diversions and four of the seven boys with penile bags were completely independent in coping with their appliances. Some of the others thought that their children were being taught to change their appliances at school, but as one said: 'I'd rather do it myself since then I know she's clean.' Another said: 'It's quicker if I do it.'

We asked how co-operative the teenagers were about emptying their appliances regularly. A third of those with diversions and three of the seven with penile bags were very responsible about this, but the rest were said to be 'lazy' and needed frequent reminders, especially if it interrupted something interesting. As one mother pointed out, this sort of laziness was probably the same kind one would meet in non-handicapped teenagers over other aspects of personal hygiene or tidiness. In a few cases, all from families under stress of some kind, quite severe problems were reported, with the teenager being exceptionally awkward or difficult about incontinence management. One mother said it was a 'battle' every time to get her daughter to empty her bag or look after the appliance properly. For example, if it leaked she'd 'patch it up with a piece of plaster rather than starting again'. Another said that her daughter would never empty the bag till it was overfull, and refused to wash when necessary.

For those who are incontinent, the care of their appliance is probably the most crucial area of all for independence. While anyone can help a handicapped youngster to wash or dress, only those with knowledge of and practice in appliance fitting can undertake the task of changing the bag. Outside the family it is, of course, very rare for anyone to have this knowledge except for a few professionals. Unless independence is achieved, therefore, the teenager and his parents (often the mother alone) are tied together in a very restricting way. They will not easily be able to spend a night or even a whole day apart, especially in those cases where the appliance is unreliable and readily becomes detached. It is most disturbing, therefore, to find such a high proportion of teenagers over fifteen years still unable to care for themselves in this respect.

*(iii) Mobility outside the home*

A high proportion of teenagers in both groups (83 per cent with spina bifida and 49 per cent with cerebral palsy) had moderate or severe mobility problems and a series of questions were asked about the young people's means of transport. Asked about their *usual* means of transport just over one-third (36 per cent) of cerebral-palsied teenagers said that they used public transport most commonly for getting about, compared with only 7 per cent of those with spina bifida. About half the teenagers in both groups relied mainly on their parents' cars, and in the spina bifida group as many as 14 per cent had to rely on taxis because their parents had no cars. Heavy reliance on parents or taxis for transport will of course reduce the young person's opportunity to be independent.

As well as being asked about their *usual* means of transport, the teenagers were also asked specifically whether they *ever* used public transport, and if so whether they had done so over the past two weeks. Only 13 per cent of the cerebral-palsied group never used any form of public transport, compared with 40 per cent of those with spina bifida, again reflecting the much greater incidence of severe locomotor problems in the latter group. Those who had used public transport were asked whether they did so alone or, if not, who usually accompanied them, and the findings are summarized in Table 2.1. About one-third in each group never used public transport unless accompanied by an adult. In the cerebral-palsied group, however, nearly half had used public transport alone at least five times in their life, compared with less than 20 per cent of the spina bifida group.

Table 2.1 *Use of public transport by disabled teenagers*

|  | Cerebral palsy | | Spina bifida | |
|---|---|---|---|---|
|  | N | (%) | N | (%) |
| Never uses it | 11 | (13) | 12 | (40) |
| Uses alone sometimes: |  |  |  |  |
| More than five times ever | 42 | (49) | 5 | (17) |
| Less than five times ever | 5 | (6) | 0 | (0) |
| Never alone, usually peer accompanies | 2 | (2) | 3 | (10) |
| Never alone, adult usually accompanies* | 26 | (30) | 10 | (33) |
| Total | 86 | (100) | 18 | (100) |

* Many of these used public transport very rarely indeed.

Teenagers aged sixteen or over were asked if they could drive or were learning. Two cerebral-palsied teenagers, both attending ordinary schools, had their own cars, one of whom was quite severely handicapped by athetosis. Three teenagers, two with cerebral palsy and one with spina bifida (two mildly and one moderately handicapped), were learning to drive, and a fourth was about to start lessons. The others were asked whether they had discussed definite plans for learning to drive with their parents. The difference between the groups was very marked. A much larger proportion of spina bifida young people said that they were planning to learn than of those with cerebral palsy (37 per cent compared with 17 per cent). Also, about twice as many of the spina bifida group had at least raised the question of learning. This reflects the differences in types of handicap among the cerebral-palsied, including poor hand function, epilepsy, and visuo-perceptual problems. This also explains why an almost identical proportion of mildly, moderately and severely handicapped youngsters (between 45–50 per cent) had not discussed the question, since the mildly and moderately handicapped groups were made up mainly of those with cerebral palsy.

Table 2.2 *Whether parent thinks teenager will be able to drive*

|  | Cerebral palsy | | Spina bifida | |
|---|---|---|---|---|
|  | N | (%) | N | (%) |
| Teenager already has full or provisional licence | 4 | (5) | 1 | (3) |
| Definite plans for learning | 9 | (11) | 9 | (30) |
| Thinks will do so, no plans as yet | 26 | (30) | 12 | (40) |
| Thinks won't be able to | 25 | (29) | 3 | (10) |
| Don't know | 22 | (26) | 5 | (17) |
| Total | 86 | (100) | 30 | (100) |

The parents were asked whether they thought their teenager would be able to drive and the results are shown in Table 2.2. A slightly smaller proportion of parents than of teenagers said they had discussed definite plans with their children, and many parents of cerebral-palsied teenagers thought that their children were over-optimstic about this possibility, although they had not yet discussed the question. Also striking was the substantial number of parents who simply didn't know whether their child might be able to drive, or whose estimate was based solely on guess-work. No professional had ever raised or discussed the question with them and most did not know where to obtain advice. Advice given to parents and/or teenagers by special schools seemed minimal, and parents who had heard about schemes for teaching disabled people to drive had often done so accidentally – for example, through chatting to neighbours or relatives. In general, discussion about use of public transport or sources of voluntary transport did not seem to be part of the school curriculum.

## Attitudes to physical independence

*(i) Mothers' perception of the teenagers' attitude.* Although the attainment of physical independence is partly limited by the nature and severity of the disability, a great deal depends on the attitudes of the teenagers, their parents, and other members of society. The parents of all but some very severely or very mildly handicapped teenagers were asked

whether their child was the sort of person who wanted to do as much as possible for himself.

Overall, nearly two-thirds of the teenagers were perceived by their parents as wishing to be as independent as possible, and less than one-quarter as liking more help then they actually needed. There was no difference between the cerebral-palsied and the spina bifida groups in this respect. In terms of severity of handicap almost identical proportions of mildly, moderately and severely handicapped young people were judged as wishing to be as independent as possible.

The mothers of teenagers described as preferring to be as independent as possible were usually in no doubt about this: 'She doesn't really want people to help . . . she'll say "I can do it".' 'She'll go off if it's something new and try it till she's mastered it.' 'He'll try anything . . . for instance a bike . . . skateboard.'

The minority who thought the teenager preferred more help than was needed frequently used the word 'lazy' to describe their children. 'She's a bit lazy . . . prefers to be helped . . . and lacks confidence' (of a mildly handicapped cerebral-palsied girl). 'He's rather lazy . . . he's definitely not keen to be independent . . . relies on me. He does a lot more at school' (of a severely handicapped cerebral-palsied boy). 'He's quite happy to be helped . . . I may have done too much for him, but there's a lot he can't do' (of a mildly handicapped cerebral-palsied boy). 'She's lazy in my presence . . . but if I'm not there she'll do everything' (of a moderately handicapped spina bifida girl).

*(ii) Mothers' perception of their own and their husbands' attitudes to independence.* The term 'over-protection' has often, we believe, been applied unfairly to parents of handicapped children. The concept is one which has been discussed in detail by Oliver (1976). He argues that attachment and dependency have not been satisfactorily measured even in families without handicapped children, and that it is far more difficult in the case of handicap to judge what aspects of maternal behaviour are unnecessary. In our own study it was not possible to make any systematic measures of maternal over-protection, although in a very few cases where the teenager was mildly handicapped it did seem self-evident. Instead we relied on asking the mothers whether they themselves considered they gave too much help.

Overall half the mothers said that they usually encouraged independence and one-quarter agreed that they tended to give the teenager more help than he or she actually needed. A small number said that they were inconsistent, and 15 per cent that they were satisfied with the independence already achieved.

It was the mothers of the more handicapped children who were most self-critical. The proportion of mothers who thought they gave more help than was needed was 18 per cent for the mildly handicapped group,

21 per cent for those who were moderately handicapped, and 32 per cent for those with severely handicapped teenagers. The mothers who felt sure that they encouraged the teenager to be as independent as possible often mentioned that this had been their policy since the child was very young. 'We both try hard to make her independent . . . we've encouraged her ever since she was a baby' (mother of severely handicapped athetoid girl). 'I've always made her do things herself . . . she's never had any choice' (mother of wheelchair-bound spina bifida girl). A few mothers said that their attitudes had changed: 'I did give him [too much] help for many years but then he went away to boarding school . . . he could do more afterwards and it showed me what he could do' (mother of severely handicapped cerebral-palsied boy).

Most mothers who described themselves as giving too much help were aware that it was the wrong thing to do, but frequently mentioned the time factor: 'I do give more help than she needs . . . I do it for quickness.' 'It's a question of time in the morning.' 'I help too much because it's quicker, especially if I'm in a hurry.' (These were all mothers of severely handicapped teenagers.) Two mentioned that they helped for the sake of peace: 'I've given up now' [i.e., encouraging independence], 'I feel I can't stand any more scenes with her . . . I've tried everything . . . so has my husband . . . I think it's her way of getting back at us . . . other people can get her to do more than we can.'

Some mentioned that they knew they helped too much without giving reasons: 'I spoil her . . . I do everything for her . . . I'm very dependent on her and she on me . . . I did everything for her before she went away [to boarding school] . . . even fed her' (mother of severely handicapped spina bifida girl). 'I'm aware of giving him more help than he needs.' 'I think I do too much for her and spoil her.' A few mothers mentioned their child's opposition to over-protection: 'I think I tend to give him too much help to get things done quickly but he's very determined.' 'When she's home she says "Leave me alone" . . . she says she has to do it at [boarding] school . . . she gets cross.'

The mothers (or the fathers themselves if present) were also asked whether they thought their husbands encouraged the teenagers to be independent. Two trends were noted. First, the fathers were more inclined to encourage their sons than their daughters to be independent, and secondly, where the child attended ordinary school, the fathers were much more likely to encourage independence than if he or she attended a special school. (This difference was not found among mothers so it was not related to degree of handicap alone.) This suggests either that the child's placement influences the way he is perceived by his father, or perhaps that the father's attitude is very influential overall in determining placement. In several instances mothers who described themselves as too protective recognized that their husband's approach was more helpful. 'He encourages her more than me.' 'He often doesn't give him any help at all . . . quite the opposite of me.' In other cases fathers were seen as too soft, especially, although not always, for the girls. 'He's inclined to shelter her too much and to spoil her a bit.' He's softer with N than I am . . . for instance he says "you know she can't do that" if I'm trying to get her to do something.'

The mother was also asked whether the question of the teenager's independence caused much friction between her and her husband; 6 per cent reported marked friction and 19 per cent some friction. There was rather more friction over boys than girls and all the cases of marked friction involved boys. Friction arose more frequently in the case of moderately than of severely handicapped teenagers, probably because it is often less clear in the former case what the teenager can reasonably be expected to do. Friction was generally because the father considered the mother over-protective rather than vice versa. One mother said 'We argue about A most weekends . . . my husband thinks he should be able to dress himself, do his teeth and so on'. Another said 'We sometimes argue . . . he says I do too much'. (In fact during part of the interview this mildly handicapped teenager was present, and when she was addressed the father had several times to ask the mother to let his daughter 'speak for herself'.) A minority of others felt they were unjustly taken to task by their husbands. 'I know what B can do. J [her husband] doesn't . . . he criticizes me, and says "let her try".'

*(iii) Teenagers' perceptions of their parents' attitude to independence.* The teenagers were asked: 'Do you ever feel your parents want to do things for you when you can manage yourself?' About two-thirds felt this was not the case, while 20 per cent thought that their parents sometimes gave too much help, and only 14 per cent that they definitely gave too much help. No differences in the proportions were found between cerebral-palsied and spina bifida teenagers, but more than twice as many girls as boys thought they were definitely helped too much (19 per cent compared with 9 per cent). Where severity of handicap was concerned there was no difference between those who were mildly and moderately handicapped but a much higher proportion (over half) of those with severe handicaps thought that their parents did more for them than was necessary. This suggests that the aspirations of girls and of the severely handicapped for independence is often not appreciated by parents. Those who felt their parents did too much for them said that there were frequent arguments about this.

The young people were asked for specific examples of occasions when their parents did more for them than was necessary and their comments are quite revealing. 'Mum tries to treat me like a baby . . . she'll hold my coat up when I put it on . . . I'll say "I don't want you to do that, I can manage".' '[She helps too much] for instance when I'm dressing . . . or if I'm slow . . . we have arguments because I'm a bit slow . . . I get annoyed.' '. . . for example helping me in and out of cars . . . it gets on my nerves . . . Mum means well . . . but she panics if we come home late.'

Girls were more likely than boys to feel irritated or to argue with their parents when they thought they were being given too much help. Here are a few examples: 'Sometimes [they help too much] with the bag. I really want to get used to doing it on my own. I start shouting at them.' 'Yes. . . they run my bath . . . they're nervous about letting me make a cup of tea in case I burn myself.' 'The main thing is washing my clothes . . . Mum wants it done and finished with . . . as I'm very slow, she won't let me do it.' 'I have arguments with Mum all the time . . . she even holds my hand when I'm walking. I feel frustrated . . . I tell her I can do it on my own. The last argument was when I was getting off a chair and she put her hand out to help me . . . and she tries to help me out of the bath' (severely handicapped athetoid girl who attends a boarding school where there is considerable emphasis on independence training).

The majority who were allowed to do things for themselves appreciated this and made comments such as 'They let me get on with it'; 'They know what I can do and let me'; 'I've been encouraged not to ask unless I really need help.'

*(iv) Teenagers' perceptions of other adults and peers as giving too much help.*  The teenagers were also asked whether they thought there were any adults at their schools who tried to give them more help than they really wanted. A similar proportion (about 20 per cent) of those both in ordinary and special schools felt this regardless of type of handicap. The young people were also asked if their peers helped them more than they wanted, and again the proportion answering Yes was very small indeed – about 10 per cent. There was no evidence that handicapped teenagers attending ordinary schools were any more likely to receive too much help from adults and peers than those attending special schools, although this is an argument commonly used against placement in ordinary schools.

## Knowledge of disability, and of statutory benefits and allowances

An important aspect of the development of autonomy and responsibility is that young disabled people should be informed about their own disabilities and about the benefits to which they may be entitled. The young people were therefore asked a series of questions about their knowledge of their own handicaps, where they had obtained their information, and whether they would like to know more. They were also asked what they knew about benefits and allowances.

*(i) Naming and describing the condition.*  The question of the teenager's knowledge of his or her disability was put in this way: 'One thing

we're very interested in is how much boys and girls actually know about their physical handicaps and also how much more information they want. Let's imagine that I've never met anyone with your kind of handicap. I want you first of all to tell me what it's called and then explain to me what it *is*.' After the teenagers had given the name and a description of the condition, the interviewer then probed areas which had been omitted or only very vaguely referred to, saying, for instance, 'And what about your legs/arms/speech etc. . . . Can you tell me a bit more about why you can't/have difficulty in walking/using your hands/speaking etc.?' Probes were also made about the shunt and about urinary incontinence and diversions where appropriate.

While all but two spina bifida teenagers knew the name of their condition, nearly 60 per cent of those with cerebral palsy either did not know (many said they'd 'no idea') or gave an incorrect name such as polio, while three described themselves as 'spastic'. Those who were severely handicapped were more likely to know that they had cerebral palsy (50 per cent compared with only 30 per cent of those with moderate or mild handicaps) and consequently a higher proportion of those in special schools than in ordinary schools (57 per cent compared with 40 per cent) were able to name their condition. It was disturbing to find that only fifteen of the thirty-seven disabled teenagers in ordinary schools could give their peers the correct name of their disability.

Table 2.3 *Rating of teenagers' knowledge of disability*

|  | Cerebral palsy | | Spina bifida | |
|  | N | (%) | N | (%) |
| --- | --- | --- | --- | --- |
| Poor: No/very little information or inaccurate information) | 52 | (60) | 12 | (40) |
| Mixture accurate/inaccurate | 3 | (4) | 8 | (27) |
| Fair or good | 31 | (37) | 10 | (33) |
| Total | 86 | (100) | 30 | (100) |

It was difficult to evaluate the description of the condition given by the teenager, but an attempt at a threefold rating was made and the findings are shown in Table 2.3. Again, a rather higher proportion of those with spina bifida were able to give some kind of information about their handicaps, but even so 40 per cent could produce little (compared with 60 per cent of those with cerebral palsy). No relationship was found between level of knowledge and degree of handicap, but while half the sample could give little information regardless of type of placement, a slightly higher proportion of those in ordinary schools were able to give a fair or good description of their handicaps (43 per cent compared to 32 per cent). Examples follow which show the great variability among the young people as to how well they were informed about their handicaps.

Here are some descriptions from cerebral-palsied teenagers who knew very little about their condition or whose ideas were muddled and inaccurate. 'I don't know how to describe it as I don't even know myself why I'm in this school. I may have a slight limp but that may be because of my shoes rubbing . . . I don't know' (mildly handicapped boy attending day special school who definitely wanted to know more). 'All I know is I stammer. Sometimes it affects me and sometimes it doesn't' (moderately handicapped boy). 'My talking and my walking are not right' (severely handicapped girl). One mildly handicapped boy who attended an ordinary school said correctly he was a hemiplegic, but continued: 'I know it's only temporary. The right side is not developed properly. I've got the right hand and leg of a five year old. I could reverse the situation if I stopped using the left side but the left side wouldn't stay as it was. I still wouldn't be right handed.' A mildly handicapped girl attending an ordinary school said she limped because 'I think I've got a bone broken inside'.

Some young people's explanations were rated as fair, although often rather limited, for example: 'When I came out of Mum the blood missed a bit in my head. Basically one side of me tenses up more than the other. The muscles in my neck – when I'm nervous my head is affected.' Only a minority were able to give a clear description of their condition, such as one mildly handicapped girl who said, 'I have brain damage through lack of oxygen given to the brain, as I was born three months early. And I have a damaged motor nerve which carries a message from the brain to the right-hand side and if I want to move it it doesn't work. It affects all my right side.'

Spina bifida with accompanying hydrocephalus is a much more complex condition to explain, and again the young people's knowledge was extremely varied. In many cases their information was either very limited or confused: 'It's trouble with the spine which involves the bottom half of you, it gets bent or something like that' (moderately handicapped boy who couldn't explain his mobility problem or why he needed a penile bag). 'I'm paralysed in the legs . . . I can't feel anywhere from the waist down . . . it's something to do with the spine . . . exactly what I don't know' (severely handicapped girl). 'Spina bifida . . . it's something to do with the back and legs' (mildly handicapped girl). 'I've got a valve in my head, I don't know what for' (severely handicapped girl). '

A boy whose knowledge was accurate as far as it went, although rather limited, said: 'I have spina bifida with a myelomeningocele and hydrocephalus. When I was born I had a lump on my back. I had a valve put in for my hydrocephalus, I think, and they closed my back which was open . . . that's all I really know about it.' When prompted about his legs and penile bag he said: 'It must have been that my muscles were so weak that I can't walk . . . I can't feel from below there [points] so that's why I have the bag . . . it's probably caused by not feeling.' When asked about the valve he said it 'goes from my brain into my heart . . . a long tube that runs down the side of my neck', but couldn't explain what its function was. Some could give quite a clear picture, however. One moderately handicapped but not incontinent boy said, 'There is a gap in the back and this forms a lump which must be covered up when you're a baby. The nerves are damaged and that is why you can't move your legs.' Asked about his hydrocephalus he said 'Some of the spinal fluid goes up to the head and puts pressure on the brain and it has to be pumped out by a valve.'

Since urinary incontinence is so great a cause of anxiety we thought it particularly important that teenagers should be clear about the nature of the problem, especially those who had had urinary diversions. Of the seven boys with penile bags, three could give no information and all that one of the others could say was: 'I have a bag because of kidney infections.' The other three explained it thus: 'I can't control myself because I'm paralysed.' 'I can't feel from below there so I can't tell. That's why I have to have a bag. It's probably caused by not feeling.' The third said 'My muscles are too weak to control my bladder because of my back problem.' Sixteen young people had had diversions. One said he 'had no idea' why the diversion was done, and several could offer only very simple explanations such as: 'It's so I can go to the toilet, otherwise I'd be wet.' 'To stop me being in nappies . . . as I can't feel myself'; 'Because I find it easier to cope with; my Mum thought it would save changing nappies'; 'Because I'm not able to feel I'm going, it was all caused by my back'.

Only three girls with diversions offered explanations which were anything like adequate. One said: 'To stop you wetting you have an ileal loop operation; a sort of artificial bladder outside the body.' While another said, 'I'm paralysed from the waist and have no bladder control. I had the urinary diversion because I had nappies till then and it was inconvenient when I went out. Part of the intestine is brought out through the stomach through a stoma'.

These questions revealed a level of ignorance among the teenagers about their own handicaps which is quite astounding. Many of the young people were below average ability but not so severely limited in intelligence that they were quite unable to understand a simple explanation. The main reason for their lack of information, as we shall show, was that no systematic attempts appeared to have been made to ensure that they did understand or that they had a vocabulary to explain their handicaps to others.

*(ii) From whom had the teenagers obtained their information?* The teenagers were next asked which people had given them information on their condition and whom they had learnt most from. Two very mildly handicapped cerebral-palsied young people in ordinary schools said that

no one had ever said anything to them about their condition. More commonly, teenagers reported that they couldn't remember how they had learnt about it: 'I was very young when it all started . . . the doctor, I think.' 'I can't remember . . . I couldn't walk and that was it. You pick up information at school and from doctors.' 'Nobody told me . . . I just learned through the years.' One boy said, 'My mother used to talk to people and I used to overhear . . . it was in the street when I heard I was injured at birth, . . . I couldn't really ask what happened . . . I feel I might embarrass or upset her . . . or both of us.'

A great many simply said that 'Mum told me': some added a precise time, although there was no way of checking how reliable this was. 'Mum told me straight away . . . I asked her, two years before my operation' (at seven years). 'Mum told me I was spina bifida when I was young, about four or five. Now I realize what it is from my own experience at hospital and school and so on.' 'I learnt mostly from my Mum but also from Link [the ASBAH magazine] . . . at the hospital they wouldn't tell you anything I suppose.'

Although parents were mentioned much more often than anyone else, some teenagers said they had learnt about their condition from doctors or consultants. This was more likely to be true for those with spina bifida than those with cerebral palsy. A few made revealing remarks about how they had 'picked up' information. One boy said, 'I've overheard what doctors say to student doctors all huddled around me . . . I felt like hamsters . . . like I was in a zoo . . . but it didn't bother me to the point of protesting . . . Mum gave me the exact name after I'd already known.'

It was rare for teenagers to say that they had taken any initiatives themselves in learning about their handicaps, but a few had done so. A cerebral-palsied girl said that she had 'Asked the doctors . . . I guessed it was brain damage because the brain makes the whole body work', and a boy said that he had 'looked up a lot myself when I was doing my CSE project' (about mentally handicapped children).

When asked who had given them *most* information from a list of possible people read out by the interviewer, the person mentioned most frequently (in well over half the sample) was a parent, usually the mother, followed by a hospital consultant (in about 20 per cent of cases). Five young people said that their physiotherapist had given them most information. Others mentioned (in each case by one or two teenagers only) included the school doctor, the school nurse, the GP, a speech therapist, a biology teacher, a TV programme, and a helper at a club. A larger proportion of mildly handicapped teenagers gave parents as their main source of information than of moderately or severely handicapped young people.

The teenagers were also asked specifically whether they '*ever* talked to a person with medical knowledge . . . a school doctor or nurse or anyone like that . . . about your handicap'. Nearly 40 per cent of those with cerebral palsy and over 50 per cent of those with spina bifida said that they had had such a discussion, usually with a hospital consultant, but the majority said that they had never talked to a person with medical knowledge about their handicaps. This finding was unrelated either to the severity of their handicap or to the type of school attended.

*(iii) Did the teenagers want to know more about their handicaps?* The question which was of particular intererst was: 'Do you feel you would like to know more about your handicap?' The findings suggest that about two-thirds of the teenagers felt the need for more explanation especially those with cerebral palsy (who were more likely to be ill-informed). A much larger proportion of those in special than in ordinary schools wanted to know more about their handicaps (71 per cent compared with 46 per cent) this being related to severity of handicap, but it was still noteworthy that about half of those in ordinary schools (nearly all cerebral-palsied pupils) would have liked to have known more.

Most of the teenagers who didn't want to know more were mildly handicapped young people who either were not interested or felt that to know more would be irrelevent. They made comments such as: 'I'm not bothered.' 'I don't really need to . . . I'm not bad . . . I can walk.' 'I haven't any problems.' Some teenagers considered that they were already sufficiently well-informed about their condition. 'I know enough' (mildly handicapped cerebral-palsied girl who was in fact very confused about her condition). 'I know the basics and that's sufficient.' A very few teenagers didn't like the idea of finding out more: 'Because if I did I would find out more that was worse – wrong with me' (mildly handicapped cerebral-palsied girl). '. . . it would be very complicated' (severely handicapped spina bifida boy).

Many of the young people, however, were enthusiastic about the idea of obtaining more information and, in a few cases, indignant that they had not been better informed. While most were severely handicapped they included some who were mildly handicapped. A number of themes emerged from what they said. Some were anxious to know what caused the condition as well as understand what it really was. 'I would like to know what caused it . . . but I've got my own version . . . I was born at home and there was a doctor who wasn't very good . . . the midwife said every baby where this doctor was had a handicap.' 'If I could find something on it, I'd like to read it. I'd like to know why it happens to some people . . . on the scientific side.'

Some teenagers mentioned specific aspects of their condition: 'I'd like to know why my arm and leg are like this . . . why I suffer from epilepsy. For instance I can't drive now.' 'I don't want to take drugs. Is it all right to come off them?' 'I'd like to know why I can't use my arm.' 'What exactly are they going to do in the operation on my ankle?' 'There are certain things I've never asked, like will I be able to have a child and will they be all right? – all I want is a son who can do everything.' 'And what happens to your bag when you're pregnant?'

Several young people wanted to know more in the hope that they would be able to 'improve' physically. 'I want to know what's really wrong with me . . . and what I could do to make things better.' 'I'd like to know the things that could be done to improve it.' '[If I knew more] I could perhaps be told how I could help myself and walk by myself one day.'

Teenagers sometimes mentioned that if they knew more about their handicaps they would be in a better position to explain to other people, particularly their peers. 'I'd like to know the full story . . . because then I can tell people . . . when I was in hospital I heard a doctor say part of my brain was damaged.' (Interviewer: 'Did you ask him about this?' Teenager: 'I should have done, but I didn't.') 'I don't understand all my handicap . . . if someone comes up and asks about my handicap I wouldn't be able to tell them.' 'I just feel I should know more . . . If someone asks you, you feel really silly not being able to answer.'

Finally, a telling comment from a severely handicapped girl with spina bifida who attended a residential special school where there were many other young people with spina bifida: she wanted to know more because, as she put it, 'It is *me*, and although I haven't been told, I shouldn't have to ask. They should tell you what's happened and what is going to happen'.


## Knowledge of benefits and allowances

A good deal of research has now been done on the take-up of benefits by disabled people showing that many do not know all the benefits to which they are entitled. The teenagers in our study, all of them fifteen years or older, were quite capable of being taught exactly what they were entitled to, or which benefits their parents were already receiving on their behalf. Giving disabled teenagers information of this kind is an important aspect of their social education and one of the ways in which they can be helped to acquire a greater sense of autonomy and responsibility for their own lives, again irrespective of the severity of their handicaps. The young people were therefore asked a number of questions about allowances and benefits.

*(i) Mobility allowance.*   This benefit is payable to parents until the child is sixteen, and from that age to the young people themselves. The teenagers were asked whether they had heard of the mobility allowance, and if so, what it was. Just over half of the spina bifida teenagers had fairly accurate information about this, compared with only 35 per cent of those with cerebral palsy, probably because knowledge about this

allowance was closely related to severity of handicap. About half of those with moderate or severe handicaps had fairly accurate information, compared with only 13 per cent of the mildly handicapped group. When asked whether they got the mobility allowance and if they knew how to claim it, approximately 10 per cent didn't know whether or not they got it. Of those who said they received it, just under half of those with cerebral palsy but less than one-quarter of those with spina bifida, knew how to claim it. Some teenagers knew how to claim, although not being very sure what it was: 'A form for anyone who's not mobile' (no idea how to claim). 'It's £5 a week to make sure a child gets what he needs . . . I went to the doctor about it but didn't get it.' 'It's money towards parts of a car and petrol' (not sure whether he got it). 'It's money which Mum gets and puts in the bank for me . . . I've no idea what it's for. You fill in a form in the Post Office. I just sign it.'

*(ii) Knowledge of other benefits and allowances.* We next asked whether, apart from the mobility allowance, they had heard of *any* 'allowances or benefits or help which disabled children or adults are entitled to', and obtained a description from them. We then asked if they could suggest where a disabled person could go to find out what benefits he or she might be entitled to. Finally, the interviewer asked specifically whether the young person had heard of the Attendance Allowance, the Non-contributory Invalidity Pension (NCIP) and the Chronically Sick and Disabled Persons Act, and if so what these are.

On the basis of the information obtained, the young people were given a fourfold rating (see Table 2.4) which took into account both their actual knowledge and whether they mentioned an appropriate way of obtaining more information, other than from their parents. Since virtually none of the teenagers had heard either of the NCIP or the Chronically Sick and Disabled Persons Act, the ratings principally reflect their knowledge of the Attendance Allowance. Responses considered as appropriate answers to the question of where to go for information included a social security office, a social worker, the Post Office, a doctor, nurse or member of the school staff, a named voluntary organization, or the Citizens Advice Bureau. What we were really interested in was not so much the actual choice of place at which to enquire, but whether the teenager had any idea at all of how to set about obtaining information for him- or herself, rather than depending on parents. Many young people were not able to make any suggestions but said things like: 'I leave it to my parents' or 'haven't a clue'. Over 45 per cent did not know where to find out more, and less than one-third of the teenagers were really well informed. Those who knew least were the mildly handicapped teenagers, but many of those with moderate or severe handicaps were also poorly informed.

The social education programme in schools is discussed in more

Table 2.4 *Teenagers' knowledge of benefits and how to obtain them*

|  | N | (%) |
|---|---|---|
| No/vague  –  Doesn't know how to find out | 37 | (32) |
| No/vague  –  Does know how to find out | 25 | (22) |
| Knows one or more  –  Doesn't know how to find out more | 16 | (14) |
| Knows one or more  –  Does know how to find out more | 37 | (32) |

detail in chapter 10, but these findings clearly show that there is still great scope for more to be done about teaching young people which benefits they are entitled to and where they can obtain further information.

## The exercise of responsibility and choice

Wall (1968), in his book on adolescence, points out that 'self-knowledge, independence, and a sense of responsibility paradoxically can only come as a result of responsible action and choice, and both depend upon a genuine autonomy'. In this section we look at some of the ways in which the disabled young people can and do take on responsibilities and exercise choice, and compare them with the teenagers in the control group. Areas investigated included responsibilities in the home, outside the home (i.e., part-time jobs), the exercise of choice in such matters as clothes and hair styles, and freedom of movement outside the home. The amount of conflict which the exercise of such choices gave rise to was also looked at, as were parental attempts to encourage responsibility.

### (i) Responsibilities in the home

The teenagers were asked various questions about the chores and jobs, both unpaid and paid, for which they were responsible. First they were asked in detail about helping at home. Chores were categorized as 'minor' or 'major' using the definitions derived from the Manchester Scales of Social Adaptation (Lunzer, 1966). Examples of minor chores included making the bed, laying the table, and giving assistance with the washing up. Major chores included helping to prepare or preparing the main meal, cleaning one's own room, washing, ironing, housework lasting at least 35 minutes, responsible errands, gardening, child-minding, decorating and household repairs. The chore had to be done regularly and as a matter of course, where appropriate at not less than weekly intervals (or in the holidays in the case of boarders).

According to their replies, the teenagers were placed in one of three categories: (i) those who did no chores or only one minor or major chore; (ii) those who did two or more minor chores; (iii) those who did two or more major chores. The results are given in Table 2.5.

Table 2.5 *Responsibilities for chores according to teenager*

| | Controls (N = 26) | | PH* (N = 116) | |
| --- | --- | --- | --- | --- |
| | N | (%) | N | (%) |
| No/only one minor or major chore | 8 | (31) | 79 | (68) |
| Two or more minor chores | 11 | (42) | 20 | (17) |
| Two or more major chores | 7 | (27) | 17 | (15) |

* *PH* = physically handicapped.

There was little difference on this measure between those attending ordinary or special schools. In general, a much higher proportion of the control group had responsibilities at home. Among both the handicapped and non-handicapped, fewer boys than girls did chores. Responsibility for chores was not closely related to severity of handicap, and in fact moderately handicapped teenagers reported doing slightly more chores than those who were mildly handicapped, although the severely handicapped did few chores.

The mildly and moderately handicapped girls who helped at home mentioned a wide range of activities including making the beds for all the family, washing up, cooking or preparing meals, doing the weekend shopping, helping with the housework, cleaning the family car and going to the launderette. From what they said they were expected to help in very much the same ways as were non-handicapped girls. Few severely handicapped girls did many chores but there were notable exceptions, such as a severely handicapped spina bifida girl whose mother, a single parent, had been ill for two weeks and who had been responsible for running the home apart from cooking. (She had shopped with a neighbour.) In some cases girls said that they would have liked to help but 'Mum won't let me', or in one instance that it wasn't possible to help as 'Mum is very tall – everything is built to her height' (from a spina bifida girl in a wheelchair), a cerebral-palsied girl who was also wheelchair-bound but loved domestic tasks: 'I can't do any [chores] really – our flat is too small. I can't get in the kitchen, it's only for one person. But I love cooking. I can make coffee and so on at school, but at home it's too high. I like to be independent and do everything for myself.'

The boys, in contrast to the girls, reported doing comparatively little. Those who had major responsibilities included a moderately handicapped boy with a single parent who said that in the holidays he gave a lot of help with housework as his mother was out at work all day, several who did the washing up on a regular basis, and a severely handicapped boy who said that in the holidays his jobs were to wash up after breakfast, do the hoovering, help in the garden and wash the car. In most cases, however, the boys' chores were confined to making their own beds and tidying their rooms, or occasionally washing up.

The mothers as well as the teenagers were asked whether the young people helped at home, and although they were not questioned in such detail their replies confirmed what the young people themselves had told us. They were also asked whether they thought the teenager did his or her 'fair share of chores', taking into account the nature and severity of the disability, or whether they did not expect as much from the young people as they were capable of.

Over half the mothers thought that their children were not helping at home as much as they could have done, this being particularly true of the boys, and the mildly and moderately handicapped. Some revealing comments were made about the disabled boys, many mothers blaming themselves for not asking their sons to do as much as they were capable of: 'His Dad thinks he's lazy . . . I've always done too much for him.' 'He loves to help . . . but he's no regular job . . . I probably don't ask him as much as I should, but I've got a seventeen year old daughter.' In contrast there were a number of mothers who were very proud of the help which their sons (some of whom were severely handicapped) gave at home: 'He makes his own bed, cleans his room, lays the table, does baking and housework and often volunteers to clean . . . he likes to do things to be helpful' (mother of severely handicapped cerebral-palsied boy). 'He does a lot, cleans his bedroom, washes up every night for pocket money . . . more than most boys do' (mother of moderately handicapped cerebral-palsied boy).

In the case of the girls there was also a group of mothers who simply did not ask much of their daughters, particularly those whose children were only at home in the holidays. 'No [she doesn't do much] I feel as she's only at home in the holidays she should enjoy herself with her friends.' 'No . . . she's on holiday when she's at home. It would be different if she was here all the time.' A number made the point that the fact that their daughter didn't do much was not related to her disability: 'No, none of the others do either . . . I just let them do what they feel like doing.'

As in the case of the boys, there were mothers who were proud of their daughters, several of whom were severely handicapped: 'She does everything when she's at home . . . she's an especially good cook, and very tidy . . . she does more than her fair share.' 'She's very good in the house . . . very domesticated. She enjoys it . . . she cleans her own room and takes a pride in it . . . washes up, and so on . . . she's very helpful' (severely handicapped cerebral-palsied boarder). 'She loves to help . . . keeps her bedroom and the bathroom tidy, tidies the living room, hoovers the floor on her knees' (severely handicapped athetoid girl).

## (ii) Responsibility outside the home: spare-time jobs

Many teenagers approaching school leaving age try to find spare-time jobs to do during the week, at weekends, or in the holidays. In the case of handicapped young people, having such a job is both an indicator of a certain level of responsibility and independence, and a great help in developing feelings of responsibility. The teenagers were therefore asked (and a check was also made with their parents) whether or not they had a spare-time job in the term time; when they did this job; how many hours per week were involved; and how much they were paid. It was found that 43 per cent of the controls had spare-time jobs (the main ones being paper rounds and working in shops) compared to 27 per cent of the physically handicapped (PH) pupils in ordinary schools and only two (3 per cent) of those in special schools.

The jobs done by the handicapped pupils, most of whom were mildly disabled, included babysitting, cooking at a nursery, walking dogs for neighbours, taking parcels to the post office for a political organization, a paper round, an evening cleaning job, working in a shop, working in a relative's firm, working in the father's pub, helping mechanics at a local garage, and doing sub-contract work at home. A few other teenagers mentioned spontaneously that they gave unpaid help, two for example in their parents' shops, and one gave regular voluntary help at a club for mentally handicapped adults. Two girls with spina bifida had had week-end jobs but had been unable to hold on to these. One 'got the sack because she was too slow', the other, who had had a Saturday job, 'was hopeless . . . [she] left after three weeks because of [her] inability to give change'.

Nearly half of the controls had had a holiday job, compared with only about one-fifth of PH pupils in ordinary schools and only 5 per cent of those in special schools. The handicapped teenagers who did have jobs usually kept on their term-time job in the holidays, but three had found different holiday jobs. One typed envelopes after her mother had replied to an advertisement in the local paper, one helped her parents who were stallholders, and one had a job in a chemist. Several teenagers in both groups said that they would very much like holiday jobs and that it 'wasn't for want of trying' that they hadn't been able to find one.

*(iii) Exercising choice as an aspect of growing up: clothes and pocket money*

For a number of reasons it is very difficult to compare disabled and non-disabled young people when it comes to the exercise of choice, since the latter are often so restricted by their handicaps. In matters like the choice of clothes, however, such comparisons can be made, and the teenagers were asked whether or not they chose their own clothes.

Nearly three-quarters of the controls chose most of their own clothes compared with about 60 per cent of the physically handicapped attending ordinary schools, and only 46 per cent of the special school group. Some of the latter were of course so severely handicapped that it was difficult for them to get out to choose clothes. However, on the whole we found that even the most handicapped teenagers were fashion conscious, with definite views about the clothes they liked, and we believe this was one area in which, with more thought, the difference between the groups need not have been as marked.

The teenagers were also asked whether their parents gave them pocket money, whether they saved any regularly, and the sort of things they spent their money on. Because so many of the control group had jobs, a much larger proportion of this group (39 per cent) said that they did not get pocket money, compared with the PH pupils in ordinary schools (19 per cent) and those in special schools (15 per cent). Among those who did get pocket money, the group who tended to save most were those in special schools – 86 per cent of whom saved some of their money regularly each week, compared with 66 per cent of the PH pupils in ordinary schools, and only 37 per cent of the controls. This finding probably means that the PH teenagers, especially those in residential schools, went out less and so had less opportunity to spend.

## (iv)  Choice regarding freedom of movement

The young people were asked if they went out in the daytime with friends of their own age and if so whether their parents always wanted to know where they were going. The pattern between controls and handicapped in ordinary schools was very similar, almost half the parents in each case being very strict about this. A similar figure was given by those in special schools, but the comparison was hardly fair, since over half never went out without their parents or another adult. In the evening, 78 per cent of those in special schools compared with only 14 per cent of the controls never went out without an adult.

## (v)  Parent-teenager conflicts in areas involving choice

In order to investigate the extent of parent-teenager disagreements, the teenagers were asked a number of specific questions about their parents' responses to choice of clothes and of hair style as well as what their parents thought of their friends. They were also asked more general questions about the frequency of disagreements with parents, and about how strict they perceived their parents to be in comparison to parents of other teenagers.

Disagreements over clothes and hair style were only minor sources of friction, as has been found in other studies (e.g., Rutter et al., 1976). Over one-quarter of the controls reported some friction over clothes, compared with about 14 per cent of the PH pupils in ordinary or special schools. When teenagers were asked whether their choice of hair style was a cause of friction, again the proportion reporting conflict was small, and no marked differences appeared between the groups. Also, only thirteen handicapped teenagers (11 per cent) reported any friction over choice of friends (in four cases the parent had stopped them from seeing friends considered undesirable). A higher proportion of control group teenagers (about one-quarter) reported some parental disapproval of friends, but only one parent had stopped their child from seeing a friend.

The teenagers were also questioned about the frequency of disagreements with their parents about matters such as where they went, what time they came home in the evening, and the time they went to bed, this latter being a potential source of argument even for severely handicapped young people. The number of those who had frequent disagreements (i.e., weekly or more) was very small in all groups, but the proportion having between one to three disagreements over the last month did differ, over one-third of the controls having disagreements this frequently compared with one-fifth of handicapped pupils in ordinary schools, and only 11 per cent of those in special schools. A much higher proportion of handicapped pupils than of controls said that they *never* disagreed with their parents – over 60 per cent compared with only 36 per cent of the controls. This may reflect not only the fact that there were fewer potential sources of disagreement (for example, going out in the evening), but also the fact that many handicapped teenagers were quiet and lacking in confidence, and many were also probably at an earlier stage of adolescent development than were the controls.

In the handicapped group, much the most common source of argument was about going to bed, and in particular about staying up late on weekdays to watch television. Generally, the parents 'won' the argument. A few of the more mildly handicapped boys had arguments about the time they came in from playing (usually on the estate) in the evenings.

Overall, however, serious parent-teenager disagreements or altercations were the exception rather than the rule, and this was confirmed by the teenagers' responses to the question of whether they considered their parents to be more or less strict than parents of other teenagers, or 'about the same'. Overall, comparing our findings with those from the Isle of Wight Study (of fourteen and fifteen year olds), as well as with our own small control group, a much higher proportion of handicapped young people perceived their parents as less strict than average. However, handicapped teenagers attending ordinary schools were more likely to perceive their parents as strict compared with those in special schools (22 per cent compared with 6 per cent), several being mildly handicapped young people whose parents were indeed markedly protective towards them. Typical comments were 'They don't just let me go round anywhere . . . they keep a strict eye on me'. 'More strict in some ways, especially when I was younger . . . everyone else went cycling . . . it's for my own good . . . but they don't shelter me.' 'They get worried about me going out.' One of the saddest comments, however, was from a very personable, moderately handicapped teenager attending a special school and totally reliant upon his parents for social life, who simply said: 'I don't know many other teenagers or what their families are like.'

## (vi) Parental encouragement of the development of responsibility

The parents were specifically asked whether there were any other ways in which they were 'trying to build up X's sense of responsibility' apart from those already discussed. The results suggest that, the more severe the handicap, the more the parents tried to make definite efforts to build up the teenager's sense of responsibility – only 15 per cent of those with mildly handicapped teenagers made definite efforts in this, compared with 30 per cent of those with severe handicaps. In some cases, those with mildly handicapped teenagers may have been right in thinking there was nothing special they needed to do, but in many others their youngsters clearly needed help of this kind as much as did those who were severely handicapped. Among those who were not doing anything were some parents with very severely handicapped teenagers. One mother said, 'No, because he can only go so far . . . he must always be helped', and another 'No . . . there's not much we *can* do to make her independent'. In a very few the attitude was *laissez-faire*: 'I haven't pushed him . . . I'm leaving it to him to mature and cope with life.' Or an admission of over-protection: 'I know I've kept her young because of her problems.'

Those whose answers indicated that they were making rather vague efforts included a few who said they encouraged responsibility by not treating their handicapped teenagers as 'different' from his or her sibs. 'I just don't fuss . . . he does everything himself . . . just like the others.'

Others were making efforts in a particular area: 'Personal hygiene . . . she's beginning to take a pride in her hair.' 'I'm trying to get her to write thank you letters.' 'I've tried to make her go on a bus with a sister waiting at the other end.' Others had more general aims, for instance: 'I'm trying to teach him the value of money', or 'by talking to her . . . I'm trying to get her to start thinking ahead about the future'. One mother of a teenager whose hand control was poor mentioned letting him drive despite her anxieties (he did in fact eventually pass his test) and letting him use a power-drill. Some parents concentrated on encouraging their young people to go out on their own; one took her wheelchair-bound spina bifida daughter to the shopping precinct and encouraged her to use the supermarket on her own. Another, whose daughter also depended on a wheelchair, had eventually helped her to make the journey to school on her own, and she also went to the town centre (a new town with underpasses and comparatively few curbs) in her wheelchair with her sister. A mother of a wheelchair-bound boy gave him the house key and sometimes made sure that she arrived home after he did so that he had to let himself in after being dropped by the school bus. Parents sometimes mentioned encouraging the teenager to join a club or to go out to the local pub. In some cases the emphasis was on encouraging financial responsibility: 'I've made her buy her own clothes, make-up, records and so on from the attendance allowance.' 'We've got him to open an account at a building society.' 'We leave her to handle her own post office savings account.' Another way of encouraging responsibility was to involve the teenager in any family discussions.

Although many parents were making very determined efforts to encourage responsibility, it was also clear that they often wanted to do so but felt at a loss to know exactly what they could or should do. As one parent of a mildly handicapped cerebral-palsied boy put it: 'It's because I'm not sure what to do.' This whole area is one in which discussions between parents or school staff starting in the early teens would be of immense value.

## Vocational aspirations

From about fourteen years onwards most teenagers begin to think seriously about what they will do when they leave school. A number of questions were put to the teenagers and their parents to find out how much thought they had given to school leaving, whether they were looking forward to it, and what their hopes and expectations were. Only fifteen (13 per cent) of the disabled teenagers had made definite arrangements for post-school placement at the time of the first interview, mostly in further education or training, and only three of the controls (8 per cent) had made definite arrangements, all being for open employment.

The teenagers who did not have anything definite arranged for when they left school were asked, as were their parents, what they thought it was most likely that they would do when they left. The results are shown in Table 2.6. The parents' expectations closely resembled those of the teenagers, except that a smaller proportion of those with disabled teenagers thought they would get a job on leaving school.

The expectations of the controls and the handicapped pupils in ordinary schools were very similar, with the highest proportion (about 40 per cent) in each group mentioning a job. Only six teenagers in special schools (8 per cent) expected this; the majority (67 per cent) thought they would go on to further education or training, usually in a special college. There was, however, a marked difference between the spina bifida and cerebral-palsied teenagers, almost all (89 per cent) of the former expecting to go on to further education or training, compared with only 46 per cent of the latter.

The teenagers who did expect to get a job were asked what sort of job they wanted to do and what their chances were of obtaining this. Most

Table 2.6 *Teenagers' expectations about their most likely placement on leaving school*

| | | Job | Higher education | Further education or college | Other type of training | Day centre | Don't know | Total |
|---|---|---|---|---|---|---|---|---|
| Controls | N | 12 | 3 | 8 | 4 | 0 | 3 | 30 |
| | (%) | (40) | (10) | (27) | (13) | (0) | (10) | (100) |
| Handicapped teenagers in ordinary schools | N | 12 | 4 | 5 | 6 | 0 | 5 | 32 |
| | (%) | (38)[1] | (13) | (16) | (19) | (0) | (16) | (100) |
| Special schools | N | 6 | 0 | 27 | 21 | 3 | 15 | 72 |
| | (%) | (8)[2] | (0) | (38) | (29) | (4) | (21) | (100) |

[1] Proportion of parents expecting this was 24 per cent
[2] Only two parents expected this (3 per cent)

of the controls and the handicapped teenagers in ordinary schools thought that their chances of getting their preferred job were very good or fairly good (about 68 per cent), but four of the six teenagers in special schools mentioning jobs said they did not know what their chances were.

On the whole, the young people's expectations were more realistic than is often supposed, at least in predicting their short-term future after leaving school (see Table 7.4, p. 181). However, the percentage expecting to go to a Day Centre was far below the reality, nor was it clear if those who expected to go on to further education or training realized that this would not necessarily result in a job. Most serious of all, however, is that about twice as many of the handicapped compared with the control group had no idea what they would do on leaving school, and there was little difference between those in ordinary and special schools in this respect.

### (iii) Attitudes to work or post-school occupation

The teenagers were asked a series of questions to discover what they considered important about work or a job. They had to rate eight statements about work as 'not important', 'quite important', or 'very important'. Although the replies of handicapped and non-handicapped young people showed a broadly similar pattern, there were some interesting differences. One of these differences related to the social aspects of work. While all the teenagers thought it very important to have friendly people to work with, nearly twice as many handicapped teenagers in special schools (44 per cent, compared with 24 per cent of those in ordinary schools) thought that it was very important to have a job where they worked closely with other people. A higher proportion of the teenagers in special schools (43 per cent compared to 27 per cent) also thought that it was very important that their work gave them the opportunity of helping others.

When it came to the nature of the job, about three-quarters of teenagers in special schools expressed a preference for jobs which involved using their hands, compared to only half the disabled teenagers in ordinary schools and just over half the controls. A smaller proportion of the handicapped than of the control group preferred jobs which would involve 'using your head and which needs concentration'. A somewhat higher proportion of handicapped than of control group pupils (52 per cent compared with 39 per cent) considered it very important that their job was well paid.

The main difference between the groups concerned the location of the job. A substantial proportion (40 per cent) in special schools said that it was very important that their work was near home, compared with only 16 per cent of the handicapped in ordinary schools and of the controls. This difference probably reflects both their greater physical dependence on their parents and their lack of self-confidence.

*Summary*

The majority of teenagers, regardless of their degree of handicap, were perceived by their parents as striving for independence. The differences in self-help skills noted were based partly on the type of disability – the cerebral-palsied group could manage more activities which required reasonable standing skills, while the spina bifida group did more of those activities requiring reasonable hand function. However, there was overall a high degree of dependency in many of the basic skills, and in many cases it was apparent that the teenager could (and wanted to) be more independent than his or her parents allowed, though in some cases lack of independence was directly related to the physical conditions of the home. There is no doubt that more could be done to help the young people achieve independence if parents were helped to realize what their children were capable of from an early age, and if suitable adaptations were provided within the home. Incontinence management in particular was an area where parents needed help in allowing their teenagers to become more independent, and where unnecessary restrictions were placed on both parent and child as a result of his or her lack of skills in this respect. The severely handicapped teenagers, in particular, felt that their parents did too much for them, but parents would certainly need guidance in helping these teenagers to do more, because they would obviously be concerned in case the teenager came to any harm and therefore quite naturally would be inclined to be very protective.

One of the most striking facts revealed by this investigation was the very poor level of knowledge the teenagers had about their handicaps, especially among the cerebral-palsied group, 60 per cent of whom did not even know the *name* of their condition and had very little or inaccurate information about it. When asked about their sources of information, over half gave their parents as the main source and between 40–50 per cent had never spoken to a medically trained person about their condition. The majority wanted to know more and it is, of course, their basic right to have this knowledge. The findings suggest that not nearly enough is done by schools and hospitals to ensure that the young people are given appropriate information about the nature and cause of their handicaps.

Information on benefits and allowances was also rather scanty, with the exception of the mobility and attendance allowances which were known to about 40 per cent of those with cerebral palsy and 60 per cent of those with spina bifida. Furthermore, only about half the group had any idea how to find out more information about what they were entitled to. Again this kind of knowledge is crucial if handicapped people are to feel any degree of autonomy or independence.

In terms of helping in the home, and the exercise of choice over such things as clothes, there was great variability among the handicapped youngsters, but on the whole they were more accepting of their parents' standards than were the non-handicapped teenagers. What gives cause for optimism is the fact that quite severely handicapped young people did manage to do a lot for themselves and contribute to the running of the household when they were allowed to do so. One had the impression of much undeveloped potential in this area, and again it was apparent that parents badly needed advice. They were very unsure about what they should expect of their teenagers, and although a substantial proportion were fully aware of the importance to the young person of feeling that he was a contributing member of the household, many were quite oblivious to the young people's needs in this respect, or that to allow them to do more would increase their self-confidence and self-respect.

# 3

## Social life: friendships and the use of leisure

This chapter will look at friendships and the use of leisure among the young people in our study to discover to what extent the pattern of friendships and leisure activities is affected by the fact of handicap. Since most of the disabled young people in this study were too severely handicapped to be able to get a job in open employment, as we shall show in chapter 7, it is most important to consider how well prepared they appeared to be for an adult life where most of their satisfactions would have to come from things other than work, or at best from unpaid activities.

There is little theoretical work on the sociology of leisure which, as Parker (1975) points out, has been a very neglected field. He makes a number of points, however, which are very relevant to the consideration of leisure activities among the handicapped. First, he suggests that the main reason why leisure has not been considered as a suitable area for study is that it has tended to be regarded

> as part of the superstructure rather than the base of society [since] cultural norms . . . socialize us into the belief that work is good and idleness reprehensible. So the long-term unemployed . . . who ought to be able to adjust to a life of total leisure, in fact mostly find this extremely difficult. They cannot envisage leisure as an autonomous sphere of activity which can be enjoyed for its own sake. Instead they – and most others – see leisure as a marginal period of recreational time, which can be legitimately enjoyed only in conjunction with the experience of work.

Since so many of the handicapped will be permanently unemployed in the sense of never having a paid job in the open market, it is likely that given this cultural norm they will find their situation difficult to accept. Without considerable help in reorientating their value-judgements, they are likely to view themselves as failures because they are not working, and will find it difficult to achieve a constructive use of their time which will at least give them some personal satisfaction and, if possible, a sense of dignity and personal worth. In fact, as Parker points out, 'There is plenty of evidence that large sections of the population are only instrumentally committed to their work roles and that it is in their leisure lives that they feel they are expressing their real personalities.' Furthermore, leisure activities for many people compensate for what is lacking at work, even for those whose jobs give some satisfaction (see Mott, 1973).

In addition many people spend much of their unpaid time in activities such as politics, or community or voluntary work, which others do for a living, and they may gain at least as much satisfaction from these pursuits as they do from their paid work. For this reason it is inappropriate to class some activities as entirely work or entirely leisure (Young and Wilmott, 1973). Consequently, the distinction between 'work' and 'leisure' activities is not entirely clear-cut in our society, and many people face problems similar to those of the handicapped in that they have to gain their sense of dignity and personal worth mainly, if not wholly, from unpaid activities usually described as leisure activities. Those with jobs are more advantaged, of course, than the permanently unemployed, in that they are at least fulfilling the cultural stereotype of what constitutes basic dignity by earning their own living, even if in a way which is not wholly satisfying, emotionally or intellectually. Even the retired have the advantage of feeling that the pension they receive has been 'earned', by years of work and contributions paid into a pension fund. However, it is apparent that the realization that unpaid activities can be just as personally satisfying and as constructive (in the sense of making a contribution to the community) as paid activities can make all the difference to whether an individual can face the prospect of permanent unemployment, through age or disability, without feelings of inferiority.

Another theme which will frequently occur throughout this chapter is the social isolation experienced by many of the handicapped young people. Although it is about a completely different age group, Townsend's *The Social Minority* (1973) makes some very useful points about social isolation among the elderly which apply equally to the handicapped of any age. He points out that the concept of 'social isolation' can be applied in many senses, to individuals who cannot properly communicate their feelings; to members of a group which is not integrated into the community as a whole (even if the members have a great deal of mutual contact); or to individuals who have few relationships and activities compared with others in society, in particular their peers. Handicapped young people may experience isolation in any or all of these senses.

Townsend points out that while we can measure objectively the 'extent to which an individual interacts with society . . . how he feels is another matter', though it is just as important to assess this since some people are distressed by relatively mild degrees of isolation while others appear genuinely to enjoy a great deal of solitude. Townsend uses 'social isolation' in the objective sense (that is, the frequency of social contacts) and defines 'loneliness' subjectively as 'an unwelcome feeling of lack or loss of companionship which is not necessarily coincident with social isolation'. Indeed he found that 'over two-fifths of isolated persons living alone . . . maintained they were never lonely', while 'of those who were often lonely . . . one-fifth were living with spouses and one-third with children'. Loneliness, therefore, 'cannot be regarded as the single direct result of social circumstances, but is rather an individual response to an external situation to which other . . . people may react quite differently'.

Townsend also makes the distinction between familial and extra-familial participation in social life. For the elderly it is the former which appears to be most important, but for the young people in our study it is more likely to be the amount of extra-familial social contact which will determine whether or not the young person experiences loneliness (except in those cases where family relationships are very strained, which is itself likely to result in increased feelings of loneliness).

Looking at the correlates of social isolation in the elderly, Townsend found that one of the main variables was infirmity. 'With increasing incapacity far fewer people reported going out for a walk, shopping or meeting friends', although more frequent visits from others did compensate to some extent. He noted that 'even watching TV decreased among the incapacitated'. Feelings of loneliness were also likely to be increased by infirmity even if objectively the number of social contacts was relatively high. 'People with moderate or severe handicap were more likely to say that they were often alone than those with little or no incapacity', regardless of objective ratings of social isolation.

For the old people, what seemed to be more important than the actual number of contacts was the difference both in ability to get about and in the number of social contacts relative to an individual's earlier experience. Those who were recently widowed, for example, often felt far more isolated, even if they were living with a daughter, than did old people living quite alone but who had done so all their lives. Social isolation in comparison with their peer group did not appear to be so important for this age group therefore, but with younger people the difference between themselves and their peers is likely to be of overwhelming importance.

Of course, many handicapped young people have little or no experience of the real facts of the social life led by the non-handicapped because they have so little contact with able-bodied peers. For many this may be a protection against feelings of extreme loneliness, but in some respects, for example in relation to anxieties about feeling unattractive to members of the opposite sex, the young people's ignorance of the fact that many of their fears are similar to those of non-handicapped teenagers serves only to enhance their feelings of isolation and difference.

## Studies of non-handicapped teenagers

Several surveys exist which can be used to establish how non-handicapped young people spend their leisure time, how frequent are their peer contacts, and how common their experience of feeling lonely. Two which involve large representative samples are the National Child Development Survey (NCDS) of sixteen year olds and the Isle of Wight Study of fourteen year olds (Rutter, 1979). Both confirm that in the mid-teens the amount of peer contact outside school hours is very high, both in terms of the number of times peers are seen and in the number of different friends seen in one week. In the Isle of Wight Study less than 10 per cent of teenagers were said by their parents to have had no peer contact within the previous week, while over half had had three or more contacts. Over 40 per cent had seen four or more friends during the week according to the teenagers' own report. Membership of a gang was not very common (less than 30 per cent claimed to be definitely a member) although almost half were members of a club and a quarter had been to a club at least twice in the previous week. Over 70 per cent claimed to have a special friend (usually one of the same sex) and three-quarters were on regular visiting terms with these friends. At this age few teenagers went out regularly with their parents; over one-third never went out with them at all, and only 10 per cent as often as once a week.

In terms of use of leisure time, the National Child Development Survey found that watching television was very common (confirming Parker's (1975) suggestion that this is 'the leisure pursuit which occupies more time of more people than any other') but so was reading, since nearly 30 per cent said that they read 'often' and less than one-quarter read only 'rarely'. In the Isle of Wight Study nearly half the teenagers had read at least two books during the previous month. Going to the cinema was another common activity, nearly half having been at least once in the previous month, and a quarter had been two or more times. Playing outdoor games was also popular, nearly 40 per cent of the teenagers in the NCDS playing 'often' and over one-third playing 'sometimes'. As one might expect, with this great flurry of activity, very few young people said that they felt lonely 'often' (about 6 per cent, a very similar figure being given also by the parents), while nearly 60 per cent said that they never felt lonely.

## Studies of handicapped young people

There are relatively few studies of how handicapped young people spend their time. Stephen Dorner's papers (1976, 1977) on teenagers with spina bifida, and Brian Rowe's (1973) study of young people (aged 18–35) with cerebral palsy being two which should be mentioned. Both show a very high level of social isolation among the handicapped. In Rowe's study nearly 20 per cent had never been outside the house at all, except to go to their work centre, during the preceding two weeks, while less than 40 per cent had been out five or more times. Over 60 per cent said that they'd like to go out more often, and cited difficulties with transport and lack of accessibility of places of entertainment as being reasons why outings were so infrequent. Those who could drive were very emphatic about the difference this had made to them. Being self-conscious about their disability did not appear to be a problem to the majority of those questioned, only 12 per cent saying that they felt people stared at them and that this bothered them. However, over one-third said that this used to bother them, especially during their early teens, until they gained the confidence to ignore other people's reactions. Watching television and listening to the radio or to records were the most common leisure activities named. Reading was not so popular, nearly one-quarter saying that they actually found reading difficult. However, nearly half did something as a 'hobby' (though this included listening to records, a very passive activity).

In Dorner's study, while nearly all the young people had friends at school or college, friendships outside school were very limited indeed, especially for those who were in special schools or colleges, over half of whom saw no friends at all in the evenings or weekends or out of term-time. Social isolation in his study related closely to locomotor disability, and virtually all those with definite mobility problems were judged to be socially isolated. Loneliness as such was not asked about, but feelings of misery and depression were found to be closely related – at least in girls – to social isolation.

The teenagers in our survey were asked about a wide range of activities to discover how they spent their leisure time, and how much contact they had with their friends, as well as questions to them and their parents about their feelings of loneliness or how they thought their social life compared with that of other young people.

**Interests, hobbies, leisure-time activities**

*(i) Home activities*

As one might expect from the studies previously mentioned, watching television was a very common pastime for most of the young people in the study. However, whereas less than half the control teenagers watched four or more nights a week, far more of the handicapped young people watched it frequently (see Table 3.1), indeed nearly 60 per cent of those in special schools watched six or seven evenings each week. The handicapped teenagers, particularly those who were severely handicapped, thought that they watched television more than other members of their family.

Listening to music was also a very common activity – over 90 per cent of all teenagers said that they enjoyed doing this often, but the handicapped teenagers were more likely to have their own radio or record player than were the controls (81 per cent compared with 70 per cent for

Table 3.1 *Home activities (%)*

|  | | Handicapped | |
|  | Controls | In ordinary school | In special school |
|---|---|---|---|
| Watches television four or more evenings per week | (48) | (67) | (74) |
| Reads papers daily | (70) | (62) | (30) |
| Read at least one book in last month | (77) | (65) | (57) |
| Plays indoor games at home | (88) | (89) | (80) |
| Watches sport on television (boys only) | (40) | (39) | (39) |
| Total (N) | 33 | 37 | 80 |

radios, and 50 per cent compared with 39 per cent for record players), which perhaps indicates that they listened to music more often. Playing indoor games at home (mainly board games and cards) was also a frequent leisure-time pursuit for all the teenagers.

However, reading was much less common among the handicapped, only 57 per cent of those in special schools having read at least one book in the last month, compared with 77 per cent of the control group (see Table 3.1). The difference between the groups was even greater when considering reading newspapers – 70 per cent of the control teenagers said they read papers regularly compared with only 30 per cent of those in special schools. No doubt this is due in part to differences in reading skills, since many of the cerebral-palsied young people, in particular, would have perceptional difficulties, and generally there were more young people of below average ability among the handicapped group whose reading might not have been fluent. However, there are now many books of a suitable interest level for teenagers but requiring relatively slight reading skills which the young people did not appear to know about, while reading newspapers is at least partly dependent upon how much one is encouraged to do this by family and school, since the reading skills required for most of the 'dailies' are of a fairly low level.

Reading papers and keeping abreast with what is going on in society at any one time, even if this is mainly at the gossip level of news, is important so that one can participate in conversation with others and contribute to general discussions. Having few topics of conversation will greatly inhibit the ability to make casual social contact, and will make the handicapped person seem less interesting to talk to.

Watching sport is also an important activity for facilitating social intercourse, particularly for boys, since knowledge of sport is the common coinage of much casual conversation. The proportion of handicapped boys who watched sport in some form was very similar to that of the controls. However, far fewer of the handicapped boys, especially those with severe disabilities, watched live sport, although most sports stadia do have limited facilities for wheelchairs. Among girls the number watching sport in all groups was very low.

### (ii) Playing an instrument

Despite the fact that most teenagers said they were interested in music and enjoyed listening to it, relatively few played a musical instrument, particularly the controls (less than 10 per cent compared with nearly one-third of the handicapped teenagers). However, none of the teenagers said that they played or sang in a group, so it did not appear that this skill was being used to make contact with others with a like interest, or to facilitate communication with the able-bodied.

### (iii) Indoor and outdoor sports

*Swimming.* The majority of control teenagers and those in special schools were learning to swim or could already swim, but nearly 40 per cent of the handicapped in ordinary schools could not swim at all. In special schools, of course, the children are encouraged to swim because this is seen as a therapeutic exercise and there are specialist teachers available. It seems unfortunate that the handicapped in ordinary schools do not benefit as readily from this activity. In fact, this was one of the few activities which more of the severely handicapped were taking part in, compared with those with mild handicaps. The handicapped in ordinary schools went swimming from school far less often than those in special schools (over 70 per cent never went, compared with less than 40 per cent). It is interesting to note in relation to swimming outside school, however, that over 40 per cent of the handicapped never went, compared with only 10 per cent of the controls. (Over three-quarters of the spina bifida young people never swam outside school.) No doubt this is largely a reflection of the lack of special swimming clubs for the disabled, and the difficulties for the disabled in using unadapted facilities, especially for those who are incontinent. But unless the habit of going swimming from home is established in the pre-teen years, before the young people become too embarrassed by their exposed bodies, they are unlikely to continue with this form of exercise once they have left school and this does seem a great pity, since not only is this good exercise, but being a member of a swimming club also provides an opportunity for social intercourse.

*Playing outdoor games and sport.*  A very similar pattern exists in relation to outdoor sports. While about three-quarters of the young people in special schools and of the controls played outdoor sport in school, only about half of the handicapped in ordinary schools did so. Presumably, many of the mildly handicapped do not wish to participate because they are unable to compete on equal terms, while no facilities are available for the more handicapped to do so. However, very few of the handicapped from special schools (only about one-quarter) played outdoor games outside school compared with nearly 70 per cent of the controls. Again, this is a reflection of the poor sports facilities available for the handicapped, but it does suggest that, once they have left school, very few of the handicapped are likely to continue with outdoor sports or use this interest as a means of making friends.

*Indoor games and sports.* Special schools seem to offer a better programme of indoor sports to their students than do ordinary schools, and over 80 per cent of the handicapped in special schools participated in these, compared with only 46 per cent of the handicapped in ordinary schools and 55 per cent of the controls. Once again, very few of the handicapped teenagers appeared to pursue these as an interest outside school.

## (iv) Other interests and hobbies

About one-quarter of the controls and 20 per cent of the handicapped teenagers mentioned another interest, apart from those already discussed, which occupied at least one evening a week, while a further 20 per cent in both groups did something less frequently than once a week. These included making mobiles, fishing, riding and tinkering with a bike, crochet, etc. Again, very few of the handicapped were using their interest directly as a way of making friends, although the fact that they had a hobby would mean they had something more to talk about.

## (v) Going to cinema, discos, parties

When the teenagers were asked if they ever went to the cinema or theatre, a much higher proportion of the handicapped than of the controls never did so with friends, though some went with their parents. Of course their mobility problems and difficulties of access would make it harder for them to do this without an adult companion. Twice as many of the control teenagers had been to dances or discos in the last month as had the handicapped teenagers (33 per cent compared with 16 per cent). Going to parties was also a much more common activity for the controls, over two-thirds of whom had been to a party in the last year compared with less than half of the handicapped young people. Most of the parties attended by the handicapped teenagers were mainly for adults or were supervised teenage parties, and less than one-quarter were unsupervised

Table 3.2 *Teenagers' report of friends at school*

| | Total N | No friends N | (%) | One friend N | (%) | Two or more friends N | (%) |
|---|---|---|---|---|---|---|---|
| Controls | 33 | 0 | – | 1 | (3) | 32 | (97) |
| Handicapped in ordinary schools | 37 | 0 | – | 1 | (3) | 36 | (97) |
| Handicapped in special schools | 79 | 5 | (6) | 10 | (13) | 64 | (81) |

teenage parties, in contrast with the controls, over two-thirds of whom usually attended unsupervised teenage parties.

### Friendships

*(i) Number of friends*

When asked to name their friends at school all but five handicapped teenagers were able to name at least one (see Table 3.2). This is a similar result to Dorner's, who also found that very few of the spina bifida teenagers he interviewed had no friends at school. However, rather more of the teenagers in ordinary schools, compared with those in special schools, named two or more friends. This must be due in part to the fact that special schools are very small, and cover a wide range of handicaps and spread of ability within each age group, and that in consequence the choice available of suitable friends is somewhat restricted. However, opportunities to develop close friendships are more limited for the handicapped than the able-bodied, and this must also be an important factor.

Of the five handicapped teenagers without friends at school, three had severe speech defects, which was thought to be the main reason for the lack of friends, and the speech difficulties of two of these were compounded by language problems, one being from an Urdu-speaking and the other from a Spanish-speaking home. The fourth was a severely handicapped boy of quite low ability who had spent most of the previous year in hospital. He attended a very small special school (there were only four children in his class) and his mother felt that there were no suitable companions at school within his age range. The fifth was a moderately handicapped boy with many emotional problems, who had difficulties in his relationship with his parents and his rather odd manner at school made him a butt for teasing. He found it difficult to talk to other boys and his mother said, 'I've never met a boy his age who wants to make contact with him'.

When the teenagers were asked if they had any friends who were not at

Table 3.3 *Whether teenager has handicapped friends*

| | None are PH | | Most not PH | | Mixture | | Most are PH | | Total |
|---|---|---|---|---|---|---|---|---|---|
| | N | (%) | N | (%) | N | (%) | N | (%) | |
| Controls | 24 | (75) | 8 | (25) | 0 | – | 0 | – | 32 |
| Handicapped in ordinary schools | 33 | (92) | 3 | (8) | 0 | – | 0 | – | 36 |
| Handicapped in special schools | 4 | (5) | 3 | (4) | 25 | (33) | 44 | (58) | 76 |

their school, a substantial proportion said that they did not, the figures from all three groups being quite similar (30 per cent of controls, 41 per cent of the handicapped in ordinary schools, and 40 per cent of the handicapped in special schools). The pattern of friendship in relation to the opposite sex was very similar, although more of the controls reported having an opposite sex friend (18 per cent, compared with 8 per cent of handicapped pupils in ordinary schools and 6 per cent of those in special schools).

## (ii) Whether teenager has handicapped friends

The teenagers were asked whether or not their friends were handicapped, and their replies are shown in Table 3.3. More of the controls than of the handicapped teenagers in ordinary schools said that they had a handicapped friend, which is probably the result of the way in which the controls were selected, since they all come from the same class or tutor group as the physically handicapped teenagers (and sometimes the friend of a handicapped pupil was chosen by the school to be the control). Perhaps more significant is the fact that nearly sixty of those in special schools had mainly handicapped friends, and only 5 per cent said that none was handicapped, compared with over 90 per cent for the handicapped in ordinary schools. Having all or mostly handicapped friends can obviously have advantages in terms of feeling that they can understand and share in personal experiences, especially since about half of these friends had the same handicap as the survey child. However, it also has serious disadvantages in that it makes seeing friends outside school hours more difficult, and restricts the teenager's range of activities and opportunities for mixing with the able-bodied.

## (iii) Teachers' perception of peer relationships in school

As part of the Rutter questionnaire, teachers were asked whether the survey children were 'not much liked by other children', or if they tended to be solitary. The results in Table 3.4 show that while there were very few children in any group who were said to be definitely disliked, a higher percentage of handicapped than of control children were thought to be 'somewhat disliked'; over one-third of the handicapped children in ordinary schools fell into this category compared with only 6 per cent of the controls, while the equivalent figure for the children in special schools was 18 per cent. Many handicapped children were said to be solitary to some extent; this applied to nearly three-quarters of the handicapped children in ordinary schools, compared with less than one-quarter of controls, and almost half of those in special schools (see Table 3.4).

Table 3.4 *Teachers' ratings of popularity and solitariness*

|  | Controls | | Handicapped in ordinary schools | | Handicapped in special schools | |
|---|---|---|---|---|---|---|
|  | N | (%) | N | (%) | N | (%) |
| Not much liked by others: | | | | | | |
| somewhat applies | 2 | (6) | 13 | (35) | 15 | (18) |
| definitely applies | 1 | (3) | 1 | (3) | 4 | (5) |
| Tends to be solitary: | | | | | | |
| somewhat applies | 5 | (15) | 19 | (51) | 31 | (38) |
| definitely applies | 2 | (6) | 8 | (22) | 7 | (9) |
| Total | 33 | (100) | 37 | (100) | 82 | (100) |

It must be remembered, of course, that there is some difficulty in making a direct comparison of the teachers' judgements for children in ordinary and special schools since they were likely to be using different standards of comparison resulting from the differences between the two types of school. Nevertheless, the results indicate that many more of the handicapped children were seen by the teachers as having difficulties in peer relationships. The fact that more of the handicapped in ordinary schools were perceived to have problems compared with those in special schools, however, is at least as likely to be attributable to differences in the standard of comparison used as to real differences between the two populations.

*(iv) Teasing*

Teenagers were asked about teasing in school since this might also reflect popularity or difficulties in peer relationships. The most striking fact was the very similar proportions who reported teasing from each group (about 40 per cent). However, while among the controls and those in special schools the majority of those teased thought that this was 'no more than for other children', the handicapped children in ordinary schools were much more likely to see themselves as being teased more frequently than their peers (30 per cent compared with 12 per cent of controls and handicapped in special schools). Since the overall proportions reporting teasing are so similar, this may indicate a difference in the perceptions of those children rather than any real difference in the amount of teasing aimed at them. Also, while teasing did cause distress, as the following quotations show, it should be remembered that in spite of the teasing these children still preferred to be in ordinary schools.

In the ordinary schools the teasing given to the handicapped pupils was frequently to do with an awkward gait, and more commonly came from children in other classes, particularly those new to the school. One boy said, 'It's about my gait, . . . they imitate me. Sometimes I just ignore it and sometimes I make sarcastic remarks, depending on my mood.' Another said, 'I'm teased about the way I walk, . . . by the first and second years. I take no notice . . . I'm more annoyed if it's the big kids than the little ones, as they should know better.' One boy with a mild hemiplegia, who was reluctant to admit to being handicapped, eventually admitted to being teased 'because I'm lazy . . . in a sense of walking. I'm sometimes called "bionic dread" by my friends.'

What is often not realized is that a good deal of bullying and teasing also goes on in special schools. One cerebral-palsied girl reported having been beaten up by a 'gang' in her day PH school. Another who was unhappy at school said, 'I get tormented more than anything.' She described how the other pupils, who were always 'having a go at me because I'm too slow', took her radio and put it on a shelf out of her reach (she is wheelchair-bound). A hemiplegic boy in a day PH school said that he was 'always getting bullied around and kicked . . . if I say something to them they don't like . . . they're jealous I think, probably because I can walk and they can't'. In fact this boy seemed to provoke the other children, perhaps because his reaction was to fly into a rage. One teenager who was very unhappy at his residential school said that another boy 'knows he can beat me up and get me to do what he wants'. This happened three or four times a term, and he didn't dare tell the staff. 'He pulls my bed to bits . . . takes my things, for instance my radio, and keeps it locked in his case.'

Overall, there was no strong evidence that handicapped teenagers in special or in ordinary schools attracted a great deal more teasing than did non-handicapped children. The difference was that for the disabled teenagers in ordinary schools the focus of the teasing was likely to be the handicap itself, although, as with the control children, for special school pupils it was probably the child's own personality which attracted the teasing most often rather than any physical oddity. There is also a suggestion in this data that the handicapped children in ordinary schools were more sensitive to teasing and more likely to see it as being caused by their handicap.

*(iv) Parents' perception of peer relationships*

When parents were asked how well their child got on with their peers, about 40 per cent of the handicapped teenagers were said to have difficulties, compared with only 9 per cent of the controls, although the majority of problems were said to be mild or moderate rather than severe (see Table 3.5). There was very little difference between those in ordinary and special schools in the proportion said to have difficulties, and neither severity of handicap nor incontinence appeared to be important.

Table 3.5 *Parents' report of how well teenager gets on with peers*

|  |  | No problem | Mild/ moderate problem | Severe problem | Total N |
|---|---|---|---|---|---|
| Controls | N | 29 | 3 | 0 | 32 |
|  | (%) | (91) | (9) | (0) |  |
| Handicapped in ordinary schools | N | 22 | 12 | 1 | 35 |
|  | (%) | (63) | (34) | (3) |  |
| Handicapped in special schools | N | 44 | 30 | 4 | 78 |
|  | (%) | (56) | (39) | (5) |  |

In general the problems described by the parents were remarkably similar. Only a few mentioned anti-social conduct and by far the majority described their child as withdrawn, shy or self-conscious, making comments such as 'he doesn't mix with other boys', 'She's always been solitary', 'Quite a loner', or 'She always sits in the background, doesn't push herself forward', 'She's shy because of being handicapped, especially with new people and boys outside school', 'She thinks she doesn't have things to say'. When asked if their child preferred solitude to company, only 6 per cent of controls, compared with 17 per cent of the handicapped in ordinary schools and 14 per cent of those in special schools, were said to prefer solitude. Although more of the handicapped than of the controls appeared to their parents to enjoy solitude, the majority actually would have preferred company and wanted to have friendships.

Of the five teenagers who had severe difficulties, three had problems of various kinds with family relationships, while another was in a school for the maladjusted because she had many emotional difficulties. The fifth was a girl in an ordinary school, described by her mother as being very withdrawn and lacking in self-confidence.

The parents' judgements confirm those of the teachers, therefore, and taken together they imply that many handicapped teenagers were too introverted and withdrawn to be able to relate easily to other people, and that their shyness and lack of self-assertion made them appear to adults to be both isolated and not very attractive to other young people as friends.

## (vi) Seeing friends outside school hours

To get a measure of social isolation, questions were asked of both parents and teenagers about how many friends were seen outside school hours and how frequently this happened. Table 3.6 shows the number of friends the teenagers had who were seen outside school hours. Figures from the Isle of Wight Study of fourteen year olds are also given for comparison (Rutter, 1979).

Table 3.6 *Friends teenager sees – parents' report*

| | Total N | Sees no friends (%) | Sees one friend only (%) | Sees 2–3 friends (%) | Sees 3 or more friends (%) |
|---|---|---|---|---|---|
| Handicapped in special schools | 81 | (61) | (17) | (14) | (9) |
| Handicapped in ordinary schools | 35 | (31) | (20) | (37) | (11) |
| Controls | 32 | (3) | (19) | (28) | (50) |
| IOW sample | 180 | (10) | (18) | (16) | (56) |

These results show a very striking difference between the controls and the handicapped teenagers, in that less than 10 per cent of the former were said to see no friends outside school compared with nearly one-third of the handicapped in ordinary schools and over 60 per cent of those in special schools. By contrast, nearly 80 per cent of the control group saw two or more friends outside school, whereas this was true for less than one-quarter of the handicapped in special schools and only half of those in ordinary schools. Taking these figures in the context of the earlier findings, that less than 20 per cent of handicapped teenagers were thought by parents to be solitary from choice, these results indicate a very serious problem of social isolation for the handicapped, especially those in special schools.

The teenagers themselves were asked if they had seen any of their school friends within the last week (for at least 5 or 10 minutes) and how often they had met. The results are shown in Table 3.7, and indicate that despite the fact that nearly all the young people had at least one school friend, over 80 per cent of those in special schools had not seen their friends outside school hours during the previous week, compared with only one-quarter of the controls. The handicapped in ordinary schools were in a much better position than were those in special schools, but were still very isolated in comparison with the control group. In range of contacts also, substantial differences appeared between the groups. Over one-third of the controls had seen two or three different friends in the last week, compared with only 14 per cent of the handicapped in ordinary schools and a mere 2 per cent of those in special schools.

Table 3.7 *Number of times the teenager has seen a school friend in the last week*

| | None | | Once | | 2–3 times | | 4 or more times | | Total |
|---|---|---|---|---|---|---|---|---|---|
| | N | (%) | N | (%) | N | (%) | N | (%) | N |
| Controls | 8 | (24) | 1 | (3) | 7 | (21) | 17 | (52) | 33 |
| Handicapped in ordinary schools | 14 | (40) | 7 | (20) | 7 | (20) | 7 | (20) | 35 |
| Handicapped in special schools* | 45 | (83) | 7 | (13) | 2 | (4) | 0 | (0) | 54 |

* Twenty-eight residential placements excluded.

Parents were asked how often their son or daughter had been out with friends of their own age in the last week (or a typical week in the holidays for those in residential school). Their reports confirm the picture which the young people painted: nearly three-quarters of those in special schools had not been out at all during the week, compared with 43 per cent of the handicapped in ordinary schools, and less than 20 per cent of the controls, most of whom went out with friends several times each week.

Since virtually all the teenagers claimed to have friends within school it is surprising that such a high proportion never saw them outside school hours. A major determining factor was the mobility of the teenagers themselves, as Table 3.8 shows, since two-thirds of those with severe problems saw no friends outside school compared with just over half of those with moderate difficulties and 40 per cent of those with a mild locomotor handicap. By the same token most of the teenagers in special schools had friends who themselves had mobility problems. These results confirm Dorner's (1975) finding that mobility is an important factor in social isolation.

However, an additional factor must have been that many more of the friends of special school pupils lived far away. Nearly three-quarters of the controls and about half of the handicapped in ordinary schools had friends who lived within walking distance, but this was true for only one-quarter of those in special schools. None of the teenagers attending ordinary

Table 3.8 *Parents' report of friends seen by mobility*

| Mobility problems | No friends seen | | Sees one friend only | | Sees two or more friends | | Total |
|---|---|---|---|---|---|---|---|
| | N | (%) | N | (%) | N | (%) | N |
| Mild | 16 | (38) | 10 | (24) | 15 | (38) | 42 |
| Moderate | 19 | (54) | 5 | (14) | 12 | (36) | 35 |
| Severe | 21 | (66) | 5 | (16) | 6 | (19) | 32 |

schools had friends living more than an hour's distance, whereas over one-quarter of those in special schools did, especially those who were attending residential schools. This lack of opportunity to see friends regularly without adult supervision must reduce the likelihood of close friendships developing, and contribute to the isolation and general immaturity of the young people.

### (v) Visiting friends

For the same kinds of reasons, visits between friends' homes were far less common among the handicapped. While only one control visited his friends' homes 'never or rarely', this was true for nearly one-quarter of the handicapped in ordinary schools and over half of those in special schools. Mobility was a major factor, since over 40 per cent of those with a mild or moderate handicap had made a visit in the last month, compared with only 13 per cent of those with a severe locomotor handicap. However, this is not the whole story, since nearly one-third of those with a mild locomotor handicap never paid any visits and a further one-third had not done so in the last month. Similar results were obtained for visits to the teenagers by their friends. Distance and ability to use public transport must be important variables which act to the advantage of the non-disabled and those in ordinary schools. But once again, problems of handicap and distance do not account for all the differences observed, since all the handicapped in ordinary schools had friends who were not themselves handicapped, and there is no reason why they could not have been visited as commonly as were the controls.

### (vi) Peer contact in the holidays

Since the handicapped teenagers, especially those in special schools, see their friends outside school quite infrequently, the implication is that during the holidays there will be quite serious social isolation, so we asked the teenagers how often they usually met their friends, apart from attendance at clubs, during the school holidays. The results are shown in Table 3.9. This gives further confirmation of the previous findings on

Table 3.9 *Meeting friends in the school holidays*

| | Less than once a week | | 1–3 times a week | | More than three times a week | | Total |
| | N | (%) | N | (%) | N | (%) | N |
|---|---|---|---|---|---|---|---|
| Controls | 1 | (3) | 6 | (18) | 26 | (79) | 33 |
| Handicapped in ordinary schools | 9 | (24) | 14 | (38) | 14 | (38) | 37 |
| Handicapped in special schools | 49 | (62) | 14 | (14) | 19 | (24) | 79 |

Table 3.10 *How often teenager is at home in summer holidays (%)*

|  | 3 or more days at home | 1–2 days at home | Goes out each day | Total N |
|---|---|---|---|---|
| Controls | (3) | (28) | (69) | 32 |
| Handicapped in ordinary schools | (34) | (26) | (40) | 35 |
| Handicapped in special schools | (32) | (33) | (35) | 81 |

social isolation. While only one control met friends less often than once a week, over 60 per cent of the handicapped in special schools, and nearly one-quarter of those in ordinary schools rarely saw friends during the holidays. Once again, overall, severity of handicap and degree of loco-motor handicap were important correlates of visits, but this does not fully account for the findings, since those with a mild locomotor handi-cap were still visiting far less often than were the controls. Handicap in itself cannot account for why nearly one-quarter of those in ordinary schools saw friends so infrequently, although they all had school friends who were not themselves handicapped. In fact, many of the handi-capped from ordinary or special schools appeared to spend most of the school holidays sitting indoors. Only just over one-third went out daily (compared with nearly 70 per cent of the controls), and about one-third were at home three or more days a week (see Table 3.10), and 10 per cent of those in special schools appeared never to go out at all, or at most only once a week.

*Special friend.* Closeness of relationships is more important in many ways than having a large number of more shallow contacts. Especially during the school holidays, what may be important is not the number of times friends are seen but the depth of any friendship and the fact that the teenager has a close confidant of his or her own age. Teenagers were asked if they had any special friend – someone that they especially enjoyed going out with or whom they confided in. These results are shown in Table 3.11 and indicate that twice as many handicapped

Table 3.11 *Whether teenager has a special friend – teenager's report*

|  | No special friend N | (%) | Special friend, same sex N | (%) | Special friend, opposite sex N | (%) | Total N |
|---|---|---|---|---|---|---|---|
| Controls | 7 | (21) | 24 | (73) | 2 | (6) | 33 |
| Handicapped in ordinary schools | 16 | (43) | 20 | (54) | 1 | (3) | 37 |
| Handicapped in special schools | 38 | (48) | 36 | (46) | 5 | (6) | 79 |

youngsters as controls, whether in ordinary or special schools, had no close friends. This is something that cannot be explained in terms of handicap *per se*, although all the findings quoted so far suggest that many of the handicapped were withdrawn, self-conscious and non-assertive, and for these reasons perhaps found it more difficult to make close relationships than their non-handicapped peers. Also, the fact of infrequent contact with friends no doubt tended to keep relationships at a rather superficial level, compared with the control teenagers who had the opportunity to see their friends often and so develop a deeper understanding of each other. This is particularly true for those in special schools, over three-quarters of whom had a close friend who was also handicapped, which greatly affected how often they could meet. Half never saw their friend at all in the holidays, and only 14 per cent saw them as often as four times a week, in contrast to the controls and the handicapped teenagers in ordinary schools, about half of whom saw their close friends at least four times a week. These findings suggest that the significance of a 'special friend' was quite different for the teenagers in special schools who just did not have the opportunity to develop those close ties and loyalties which give one the confidence to trust and confide in another.

Teenagers were also asked if they went out with a group of friends, since this is quite a common pattern for some young people and may be a substitute for having a special friend. Among the control group, nearly one-third reported that they went out regularly in a group, whereas this was true for only 8 per cent of the handicapped in ordinary schools and for 5 per cent of those in special schools. There is no evidence here therefore that the handicapped teenagers went out in groups more commonly as an alternative to having a special friend.

*Clubs.*   Information gathered about membership of clubs suggested that the handicapped were making more use of these as a source of social interaction than were the able-bodied youngsters. As can be seen from Table 3.12, the pattern of club membership was very similar for the controls and the handicapped pupils in ordinary schools, nearly half of whom belonged to at least one club. In contrast, nearly three-quarters of

Table 3.12 *Club membership by type of school (%)*

|  | None | One club | Two clubs | More than two clubs | Total N |
|---|---|---|---|---|---|
| Controls | (55) | (31) | (12) | (3) | 33 |
| Handicapped in ordinary schools | (54) | (32) | (11) | (3) | 37 |
| Handicapped in special schools | (26) | (54) | (13) | (7) |  |

those in special schools belonged to clubs, and a rather higher proportion were in more than one club than with the other two groups.

However, it appeared that many more of those in special schools attended clubs attached to their schools than did those in ordinary schools, and a much smaller proportion belonged to clubs close to home, where they would be likely to meet with and make friends with neighbouring teenagers. In clubs attached to school, the majority of members would be schoolmates so that the club would not be a source of new friends. Furthermore, over one-quarter of the special school pupils attended clubs which only operated during the term, and would do nothing to help the young person through the long school holidays.

Because their clubs were so near home, the majority of those in ordinary schools were able to get there by walking or public transport, whereas over half of the handicapped went by special transport and over a quarter in their parents' car or the car of a friend. Most of the clubs attended by those in special schools were specifically for the handicapped (45 per cent), while one-third attended mixed clubs (for able-bodied and handicapped), and less than one-quarter were in ordinary clubs (i.e., ones which did not cater for the handicapped in any special way). In contrast, three-quarters of the handicapped in ordinary schools attended ordinary clubs.

Considering how the young people heard about their clubs, we found that the majority of the young people in ordinary schools, whether handicapped or not, heard about their clubs from a friend or a member of their family, whereas most of those in special school heard about their clubs from school, or from a professional or a handicapped organization of some kind. Membership was initiated by adults in the majority of cases rather than by peers. The whole pattern of club attendance for the handicapped in special schools therefore appeared to be rather different from that of their counterparts in ordinary schools. Membership and attendance was much more adult-controlled and organized, and their clubs were far less likely to provide a location where they could meet with the able-bodied and make friends with neighbouring children. Many provided companionship during the term-time only.

*Going out with parents.* As we mentioned earlier, studies of non-handicapped teenagers suggest that going out with parents is much less common for young people of this age than is going out with peers, and indeed our control group's parents reported that their teenagers usually went out with peers, while only 3 per cent commonly went out with their parents. For the handicapped in ordinary schools this figure rose to nearly one-quarter, but for those in special schools nearly 70 per cent usually went out with their parents. There was a close relationship between severity of handicap and how common it was to go out with parents, but even the mildly handicapped were quite different in this respect from the controls, 27 per cent commonly going out with parents and only 40 per cent with a peer.

When teenagers did go out with their peers during the day, although the parents of the handicapped teenagers did not insist on knowing where they were going more frequently than did the parents of the controls, the handicapped youngsters (those in special schools particularly) were much more likely to volunteer the information. Very few of the handicapped young people went out in the evening with their peers, although this was normal behaviour for the controls.

In general, the handicapped teenagers in special schools, and to a lesser extent those in ordinary schools, had a pattern of outings much more similar to that of younger children in that they far more frequently went out with parents rather than with peers, rarely went out in the evenings without an adult, and felt the need to report their comings and goings to their parents more often if they ever did go out with peers. To some extent this is both inevitable and proper, of course, but it is one more indication of the lack of autonomy that handicapped teenagers experience in comparison with their able-bodied peers, and a further indication of lack of self-confidence and maturity.

*Overall social life ratings.* In this chapter so far we have discussed a number of ways in which the handicapped teenagers were disadvantaged compared with their peers in their experience of friendship and use of leisure time. However, this does not give us the overall picture, since while a handicapped person may lack a special friend and rarely go out with peers, he might be a member of several clubs and go out with a sib quite regularly. Another might have few social outlets outside the family, but have one very close friend whom he saw at least weekly. In this way deficiencies in one area of social contact might have been compensated for to some extent by others, so that the young person was contented, even though not having as full or exciting a social life as most of his able-bodied peers.

In order to see how many had restricted social lives overall, therefore, we considered all the information available to us from the teenager himself and from his parents, and rated each person on a three-point scale: those considered to have a 'satisfactory' social life, those whose social lives appeared to be 'limited' and those whose social life was 'very restricted'. For example, a young person attending one club regularly and having one friend whom he saw from time to time, but who otherwise only went out with his family, would be classed as having a 'limited' social life. 'Very restricted' implied a severe degree of social isolation, applying in the main to teenagers who were almost totally reliant on their parents for social stimulation.

Table 3.13 shows the social life ratings for the controls and the handicapped. Over 90 per cent of the controls were rated as having a 'satisfactory'

Table 3.13 *Quality of social life related to overall severity of handicap (%)*

| Quality of social life | Controls | Handicapped teenagers | | | Total |
|---|---|---|---|---|---|
| | | Mild | Moderate | Severe | |
| Satisfactory | (94) | (30) | (26) | (12) | (21) |
| Limited | (3) | (58) | (40) | (27) | (38) |
| Very restricted | (3) | (15) | (33) | (61) | (41) |
| Total (N) | 33 | 26 | 42 | 51 | 119 |

social life, compared with only 21 per cent of the handicapped. At the other extreme, while over 40 per cent of the handicapped were thought to have a 'very restricted' social life, only 3 per cent of the controls (one individual) was so rated. In other words, there were many teenagers in whom all the individual measures of social isolation were combined, and who were relying almost entirely upon their parents for their social life. For many, their only other social outlet was one school-based club which didn't operate during the holidays; they never saw school friends outside school, they had no other friends close to home, were too timid to go out on their own even to the local shops, and because of their locomotor handicap longer journeys could only be made by car, which meant relying again upon their parents. Our findings confirm those of other studies. Very similar results were found by Dorner (1975) who, using rather different criteria, estimated that about half of the spina bifida young people in his study suffered from social isolation. Parallel results were also found for spina bifida teenagers in Sheffield (Lorber and Schloss, 1973) and in Australia (McAndrew, 1977). The majority of subjects in Rowe's study (1973) of cerebral-palsied young people also showed a high degree of social isolation.

Considering quality of social life in relation to severity of handicap and mobility ratings it was obvious that both factors were of great importance. Only 15 per cent of those with a mild handicap were thought to have a very restricted social life, compared with over one-third of those with a moderate handicap and over 60 per cent of those with a severe handicap (see Table 3.13). Similarly, poor mobility appeared to be a major cause of social isolation in that nearly twice as many of those with a severe locomotor handicap were thought to have a restricted social life compared with those who only had a mild locomotor handicap (see Table 3.14). However, the fact that only one-quarter of those with a mild locomotor problem were thought to have a satisfactory social life suggests that although mobility is important it is not the only factor which influences the making of friendships and mixing with others outside the family. Further evidence for this is the fact that a small number of those with very severe handicaps nevertheless led quite full

Table 3.14 *Quality of social life related to locomotor handicap (%)*

| Social life | Overall mobility rating | | |
| --- | --- | --- | --- |
| | Mild | Moderate | Severe |
| Satisfactory | (26) | (29) | (9) |
| Limited | (40) | (37) | (23) |
| Very restricted | (33) | (40) | (63) |
| Total | 42 | 35 | 32 |

and active social lives. Looking at handicaps other than mobility, severe speech defects appeared to be a significant factor in determining quality of social life, but incontinence was not. Little difference was found between the cerebral-palsied and spina bifida teenagers which could not be attributed to differences in severity of handicap.

Looking at quality of social life in relation to type of school (see Table 3.15), we can see that although compared with the control group, the handicapped teenagers in ordinary schools were less likely to have a satisfactory social life, nevertheless a greater percentage of them were leading active social lives compared with those attending special schools (43 per cent compared with 11 per cent). Those in residential schools appeared to be in the worst position – nearly 80 per cent being rated as having 'very restricted' social lives when at home, compared with 37 per cent of those in day PH schools and 19 per cent of those in ordinary schools. The difference between those in ordinary and those in special schools can be accounted for partly in terms of degree of handicap, but there were no great differences in handicap between those in day special and those in residential schools (see Table 1.10). This difference is probably due largely to the fact that because the teenager is away from home for much of the year he is unable to make or retain social contacts there, while his school friends live too far away to make visits. It may also be due in part to the fact that many of those at residential school also had

Table 3.15 *Social life rating by type of school*

| Type of school | Quality of social life | | | | | |
| --- | --- | --- | --- | --- | --- | --- |
| | Satisfactory | | Limited | | Very restricted | |
| | N | (%) | N | (%) | N | (%) |
| Controls | 31 | (94) | 1 | (3) | 1 | (3) |
| PH in ordinary schools | 16 | (43) | 14 | (38) | 7 | (19) |
| Day special schools | 6 | (11) | 28 | (52) | 20 | (37) |
| Residential schools | 3 | (11) | 3 | (11) | 22 | (78) |

poor relationships with their families, and therefore could not make contacts through their parents and sibs as readily as other teenagers.

What we have been considering here so far are our own ratings of social isolation, based on objectively measured variables such as whether or not the teenager has a special friend or how many times a week he goes out. As we pointed out in the introduction, however, social isolation and the experience of loneliness are not necessarily coincident, and what we need to consider separately is what the parents and the teenagers themselves felt about their social life, whether social isolation made the young people feel unhappy, and how they accounted themselves for the lack of social contact.

### Attitudes and feelings about social isolation

#### (i) Parents' feelings about teenagers' leisure time and how many friends they have

The parents of the handicapped were asked whether they felt that their teenager had as good a social life as others of the same age and whether they had as many friends as non-handicapped teenagers. Their views were strongly related to the degree of handicap in the teenager, as one would expect given the facts quoted previously. Of those with mildly handicapped children about half (54 per cent) thought that they had fewer friends than the able-bodied, compared with two-thirds of those with a moderate handicap (67 per cent) and 84 per cent for those whose handicap was severe.

Severe speech difficulties appeared to the parents to be an important factor, as indeed they are, and all those with severe difficulties were rated as having fewer friends, compared with two-thirds of those with moderate speech difficulties and about half of those with mild problems. Other handicaps such as epilepsy and incontinence were not related to the parents' judgements about how many friends their children had. The parents' judgements seemed to be based more on the frequency of visiting and the closeness of the relationships between their teenager and his friends, rather than on friendships at school, and in general, their assessments agree quite well with our objective findings.

When asked how the teenager's leisure activities compared with other young people of the same age, however, the majority of parents thought that although their activities were limited, the young people were generally content. Only a third of those with children in special schools and about 20 per cent of those whose children attended ordinary schools thought that their son or daughter had an unsatisfactory social life. For those in ordinary schools the parents' estimate agrees well with our estimate of the number with a 'very restricted' social life, but where the child was in a special school, the parents' estimate of the numbers with an unsatisfactory social life was considerably lower than our rating.

## (ii) Teenagers' own opinion of leisure time

The teenagers were asked whether they themselves thought that they went out as much as other teenagers. By far the majority of the controls (62 per cent) thought they went out as much as others, whereas nearly three-quarters of the handicapped felt that they went out less, there being little difference between those in ordinary and those in special schools in this, although objectively there were quite substantial differences in the amount of activity between the two groups. This suggests that while those in ordinary schools do usually lead more active lives than those in special schools, their expectations are probably higher, and the level of discontent is correspondingly higher, especially since they are more aware than those in special schools just how much their lives differ from those of the able-bodied.

## (iii) Teenagers' feelings about loneliness in the holidays

The young people were specifically asked about loneliness in the holidays because it seemed that the special schools were offering many young people some social outlets during term-time, but that the holidays were relatively bleak. The contrast between term-time and the holidays seemed likely to be particularly great for those in residential schools. The teenagers were asked if they found themselves spending more time alone in the holidays than they really wanted, or if they saw enough friends of their own age. The majority of controls (nearly 80 per cent) thought that they saw enough of friends, but the position was reversed for the handicapped in special schools, two-thirds of whom said they were too much alone in the holidays. The handicapped in ordinary schools did not feel this so commonly (and indeed objectively they did spend more time out of the house and with friends in the holidays), but over 40 per cent still felt themselves to be too much alone. In relation to severity of handicap, less than 40 per cent of those with a mild handicap felt themselves to be too much alone, compared with two-thirds of those who were severely handicapped, and again this agrees well with earlier findings on the frequency of contact with friends.

The teenagers who thought they spent too much time alone were asked if there were any problems that made it difficult for them to spend more time with friends in the holidays. Of the six controls who thought they spent too much time alone, two said that their friends did not live very near, one that she had to look after her younger brothers and sisters, but the others were rather vague about the reasons. The handicapped teenagers were much more specific about problems. Over one-quarter

Table 3.16 *Social life rating related to feelings of loneliness*

|  | Satisfactory social life | | Limited social life | | Very restricted social life | | Total |
|  | N | (%) | N | (%) | N | (%) | N |
|---|---|---|---|---|---|---|---|
| Never lonely | 26 | (84) | 22 | (51) | 14 | (31) | 62 |
| Sometimes lonely | 5 | (16) | 13 | (30) | 12 | (27) | 30 |
| Often lonely | 0 | – | 8 | (19) | 19 | (42) | 27 |
| Total | 31 | (100) | 43 | (100) | 45 | (100) | 119 |

felt that restricted mobility was the main difficulty, and over 40 per cent said the problem was that their friends lived too far away. Interestingly, almost as high a proportion of day special school pupils gave this as a reason as did those who were boarders – about one-third in both cases. Only 17 per cent said that they had very few or no friends.

### (iv) Experience of loneliness and quality of social life

The teenagers' responses as to whether they felt lonely during the school holidays were related to our rating of overall quality of social life, and the results are shown in Table 3.16. They bear out Townsend's thesis that social isolation, objectively measured, and the experience of loneliness do not correlate precisely. However, over 80 per cent of those rated as having a satisfactory social life said that they were never lonely, while none said that they were often lonely; conversely all those who claimed to be often lonely were given a social life rating of 'limited' or 'very restricted' (in fact over 70 per cent of teenagers 'often lonely' were rated as having very restricted social lives).

The discrepancies arose mainly in that there were twenty-two young people who were rated as having a 'limited' social life but who claimed never to be lonely; clearly many of these teenagers were quite accepting of their situation, particularly those who were more severely handicapped. Also there were fourteen young people who had a 'very restricted' social life who claimed that they never felt lonely during the school holidays, although many of these were boarders who had in fact complained of boredom in the holidays. Most of this group were girls, who possibly did not expect to be able to go out as much as boys, and several were very timid and lacking in self-confidence and claimed to be quite happy staying at home in the warmth and security of the family. Some perhaps did feel lonely but were inclined to deny this when asked directly.

What the results indicate is that having a satisfactory social life does in general protect the young people from feeling lonely, as one might expect, and that young people who frequently experience loneliness are usually the ones who go out very rarely. However, having a restricted social life does not necessarily lead to feelings of loneliness, since this depends more on the young person's expectations about what he should have, and possibly his knowledge about the social life of the able-bodied, and how content he is to stay at home with his family. It was notable that among the young people with a very restricted social life and who frequently felt lonely, many came from families where relationships were quite strained.

## Summary

Although on the whole they were quite a mobile group, the handicapped teenagers in ordinary schools were found to have a limited social life in comparison with their able-bodied peers. For example, one-third rarely saw their school friends outside school, compared with less than 10 per cent of able-bodied teenagers, and they were also much more likely to go out with a sib or their parents than were the controls. However, as a general rule, the handicapped teenagers in ordinary schools did have far more outings than did those in special schools, and far more contact with peers and with the able-bodied. However, in a few respects the two groups were very similar; for example, the frequency with which they went out in the holidays (one-third in both groups were at home three or more days a week compared with only 3 per cent of the controls) and only about 60 per cent of both handicapped groups had a special friend, compared with nearly 80 per cent of the controls.

In respect to active sports carried out in school hours, the handicapped in ordinary schools were at a disadvantage compared with those in special schools. Fewer went swimming from school or played outdoor or indoor games at school. However, those from special schools rarely took part in active exercise outside school including swimming, and in terms of using active sports as a means of making friends or widening the social contacts, there seemed to be little difference between the two handicapped groups.

Many of the handicapped in special schools suffered from a high degree of social isolation. Over 60 per cent never saw their school friends outside school; over half had never visited their friends' homes, and only one-quarter had made such a visit in the last month. (Comparable figures for the controls are 3 per cent and one-half.) In the holidays especially they were very isolated, and only one-third left their home for an outing every day, compared with 70 per cent of the controls. Half of those who had special friends never saw them during the holidays, compared with less than 10 per cent for the controls and of the handicapped in ordinary schools. When these teenagers did go out, nearly three-quarters usually did so with a member of the family, in contrast with the controls who almost invariably went out with peers.

However, many more of the handicapped in special schools belonged to clubs – over three-quarters were members of at least one compared with less than half of the controls and the handicapped in ordinary schools. It appeared that many of those in special schools joined clubs as a way of compensating for the lack of informal peer contact, but to what extent it was successful is doubtful, since most were in clubs solely or primarily for the handicapped, and over one-third were school-based clubs, most of which did not run during the school holidays. Nevertheless, club membership was most important to these teenagers for whom it was their only regular social outlet, and on other nights they spent most of their time watching television. In general, those in special schools spent far more time watching television and rather less time reading books or newspapers than the controls and the handicapped in ordinary schools, and had few well-established hobbies with which to occupy themselves constructively.

Overall degree of handicap, and especially the degree of locomotor handicap, was very closely related to the amount of social contact that the teenagers had. Considering such things as seeing friends outside school, visiting friends in their homes, peer contact in the school holidays and the overall rating of social life, the more severely handicapped were consistently at a disadvantage, while the more mildly handicapped consistently led the most active lives.

For those who were in special schools their greater degree of physical handicap was compounded by two other factors. First, the majority of these teenagers had friends who were themselves handicapped and therefore on both sides of the relationship there were physical difficulties in making regular contact. Secondly, while most of those attending ordinary school, whether handicapped or not, had friends who lived close by, less than one-quarter of those in special schools had a friend living within walking (or wheeling) distance. However, physical factors such as poor mobility and distance from friends do not account for all the differences observed between the handicapped and the controls in the amount of social contact. We still have to account for why fewer of the handicapped in ordinary schools than of the controls had a special friend; why nearly 40 per cent of the mildly handicapped, most of whom could either walk or use public transport, never saw their friends outside school; and why it was, since most of their friends were not themselves handicapped, 40 per cent of the handicapped in ordinary schools had not been visited at home by a friend within the previous month.

Apart from mobility, no particular handicap appeared to influence peer relationships, except that those with moderate or severe speech difficulties were much more likely to be solitary and to have fewer peer contacts. Incontinence did not appear to interfere with the making of friends.

Probably because contacts with friends were less frequent and because there were far fewer opportunities for them to have unsupervised contacts with friends, the handicapped teenagers were less likely to develop close relationships with their school friends, according to their own reports. This lack of closeness is reflected in the finding that only a very small proportion of the handicapped teenagers ever spoke to their friends about their handicap and its problems, even though most of those in special schools had friends who were themselves handicapped, and indeed a high proportion had a similar diagnosis.

The parents' and teachers' perceptions of the difficulties with peer relationships give some indication, perhaps, of what was happening. While there was no evidence that the handicapped in ordinary schools were really rejected by their peers (for example they complained of teasing no more frequently than did the controls, and very few of them were said to be 'definitely not much liked' by their peers), both the parents and the teachers more often thought that the handicapped teenagers had difficulties with peer relationships compared with the controls. The teachers more often described the handicapped teenagers as solitary, and although the parents thought that most of the young people on the whole preferred company to being alone, a higher proportion of those with handicapped children, whether in ordinary or special schools, said that their child preferred to be alone.

When parents were asked to describe the kind of difficulties in personal relationships that their children had, they usually talked about shyness, lack of self-confidence and self-consciousness. These are all problems that many young people have at this age, when there is so much awareness of appearance and physical characteristics, but someone with a physical deformity of any kind will be particularly prone to shyness and timidity in peer relationships. We shall see later (in Chapter 5) that timidity and lack of self-confidence are characteristics of many of the handicapped teenagers in the survey.

# 4

# Fears and aspirations about marriage and relations with the opposite sex

In the first section of this chapter we discuss whether the handicapped teenagers had been out with members of the opposite sex, whether they wished to do so, how much knowledge they had about intercourse and contraception, and what kind of worries they had about mixing with the opposite sex. The second half is concerned with issues relating to marriage and having children.

## (i) Experience of dating

We started by asking whether the teenager had *ever* actually 'been out with' a boy or girl, leaving the interpretation of this question to the teenager, and followed this up by asking whether, if they had not done so, they would like to. The teenagers' responses are shown in Table 4.1.

Table 4.1 *Whether teenager has been out with member of the opposite sex, and if not, whether would like to*

|  | Handicapped | | Controls | |
|  | N | (%) | N | (%) |
|---|---|---|---|---|
| Has been out | 29 | (25) | 25 | (76) |
| Hasn't been out: | | | | |
|    would like to | 61 | (53) | 5 | (15) |
|    wouldn't like to | 20* | (17) | 3 | (9) |
|    doesn't know if wants to | 3 | (3) | 0 | (0) |
|    hasn't been out and not asked if wants | 2 | (2) | 0 | (0) |
| Total | 115 | (100) | 33 | (100) |

* Fourteen boys and six girls.

Over three-quarters of the control group compared with only one-quarter of disabled teenagers had ever been out with boy or girl, but the great majority of those who had not said that they would like to. Neither type of handicap nor, more surprisingly, severity of handicap appeared to be a factor in influencing experience of going out with a member of the

Table 4.2 *Pupils in ordinary schools who say they have gone out with a boy or girl*

| Experience of dating | Handicapped | | | | | | Controls | | | | | |
|---|---|---|---|---|---|---|---|---|---|---|---|---|
| | Boys | | Girls | | Total | | Boys | | Girls | | Total | |
| | N | (%) | N | (%) | N | (%) | N | (%) | N | (%) | N | (%) |
| None | 12 | (63) | 18 | (100) | 30 | (81) | 4 | (27) | 4 | (22) | 8 | (24) |
| Some | 7 | (37) | 0 | (0) | 7 | (19) | 11 | (73) | 14 | (78) | 25 | (76) |
| Total | 19 | (100) | 18 | (100) | 37 | (100) | 15 | (100) | 18 | (100) | 33 | (100) |

opposite sex. However, one of the problems in interpreting these results is that the teenagers used their own judgement about what was meant by 'going out', and it was our impression that those in special schools interpreted this question rather idiosyncratically. We therefore looked only at those in ordinary schools in more detail to compare with the controls; the results are shown in Table 4.2.

This table shows a great contrast between the handicapped pupils in ordinary schools and the control group, and also a clear difference between the handicapped boys and girls, although of course the numbers are very small. None of the latter had ever been out with a boy, compared with less than one-quarter of the control girls. The situation for the handicapped boys was somewhat better; just over one-third had dated a girl, compared with nearly three-quarters of the able-bodied group. (For the handicapped pupils in special schools the difference between the boys and girls was less marked and slightly in the opposite direction.)

Those who had been out with a boy or girl were questioned in a little more detail about their experience, including the age at which they had their first date, and the number of boys or girls they had dated. The only aspect of sexual experience they were asked about was the age at which they had first kissed a boy or girl. The findings suggested that the experience of the comparatively small group of handicapped teenagers who had dated had been rather different from that of the controls. They had tended to date at a later age and been out with a smaller number of partners, and while all the controls had experience of kissing this was true for only one-quarter of the handicapped pupils who had dated.

Table 4.1 shows that while the majority of the controls and of the handicapped teenagers who had no experience of dating wished that they had, about twice as many handicapped as control teenagers either didn't want to or weren't sure if they wanted to go out with a member of the opposite sex. This is no doubt largely a reflection of the fact that many handicapped teenagers were immature compared with the controls, and did not yet think of themselves as adult or as having adult needs, but it may also in part reflect the fears that many handicapped young people have about what such a relationship might involve. The lack of opportunity for those in day PH schools, compared with those in residential schools, to pursue a friendship with a member of the opposite sex may also be important, however, since nearly three-quarters of those in boarding schools declared that they were interested in such relationships (a similar proportion to the controls) compared with less than 40 per cent of those in day special schools.

### Teenagers with boy- or girlfriends

The differences between handicapped and non-handicapped, in whether they had now or had ever had a steady boy- or girlfriend, were striking. Nearly half the control group currently had or had once had a steady boy- or girlfriend, while over one-quarter went out with one sometimes. In contrast, the great majority of the handicapped pupils (80 per cent) reported that they had little or no experience of dating.

Overall, the number of teenagers who currently had steady boy- or girlfriends comprised nine controls (27 per cent), one handicapped pupil in an ordinary school (3 per cent), six pupils in day special schools (12 per cent), and five in boarding special schools (18 per cent). All the teenagers attending ordinary schools had able-bodied boy- or girlfriends, as did five of the six pupils in day special schools. The reverse was true for the five boarders, four of whom had boy- or girlfriends who were also physically handicapped.

One of the boys who attended an ordinary school had a girlfriend, as did five of the six pupils in day special schools, while four of the five boarders had boy- or girlfriends who were also physically handicapped. The teenagers were asked if they felt they had enough opportunities to be alone with their boy- or girlfriends and also how often they were able to meet. Most of the handicapped teenagers met their boy- or girlfriends less than once a week, two about twice a week, and four more than twice a week. Only one teenager with a current boyfriend (a handicapped girl attending a day special school) said that her mother disapproved of her able-bodied boyfriend. However, 'Mum just keeps out of the way when he comes'.

### (ii) Sexual knowledge

All the parents of the control teenagers, all but one of the parents of handicapped teenagers in ordinary schools and all but five of those in special schools thought that their son or daughter knew about sexual intercourse. Most thought that their teenagers had first found out either from a parent (39 per cent of the disabled teenagers and 31 per cent of the controls) or from lessons at school (40 per cent and 50 per cent respectively). Only a small number of parents of both groups (9 per cent and 16 per cent) thought they had gained this knowledge from peers.

When the teenagers themselves were asked, most said that they knew

Table 4.3 *Teenagers' accounts of how they first learned the facts of life*

|  |  | Mother | Father | Teacher | Friends | Books | Other | Total |
|---|---|---|---|---|---|---|---|---|
| Controls |  |  |  |  |  |  |  |  |
| Boys | N | 1 | 1 | 7 | 10 | 1 | 1 | 17 |
|  | % | (6) | (6) | (41) | (59) | (6) | (6) | (100) |
| Girls | N | 14 | 1 | 7 | 5 | 2 | 0 | 19 |
|  | % | (74) | (5) | (37) | (26) | (11) | (0) | (100) |
| Handicapped |  |  |  |  |  |  |  |  |
| Boys | N | 11 | 4 | 31 | 30 | 2 | 7 | 60 |
|  | % | (18) | (7) | (52) | (33) | (3) | (12) | (100) |
| Girls | N | 27 | 5 | 18 | 7 | 5 | 8 | 54 |
|  | % | (50) | (9) | (33) | (13) | (9) | (15) | (100) |

the facts of life. Only one control, one handicapped teenager in an ordinary school, and eight (10 per cent) handicapped teenagers in special schools said they did not know; but this did not appear to be related to the severity of the handicap. However, the account the teenagers gave about who first told them about the facts of life differed considerably from that of their parents (see Table 4.3), a much higher proportion naming a peer, as has been found in other studies of handicapped teenagers. More handicapped than control boys quoted their mothers as a source of information and both boys and girls frequently quoted some 'other' source, such as a sib or a doctor or television. The majority of girls in both groups quoted their mothers as their source of information and teachers were frequently mentioned by both boys and girls.

When asked about contraception, most of the parents of controls (84 per cent) and the handicapped teenagers in ordinary schools (66 per cent) thought that their teenager knew about this compared with under half (43 per cent) of the parents of teenagers in special schools. Many parents of the handicapped teenagers (28 per cent in ordinary schools and 36 per cent in special schools) said they had no idea if their teenager knew about this. The majority thought that their child had first found out about contraception at school or from them, and only a small proportion mentioned peers. There was little difference between the parents of controls and the handicapped.

From the teenager's own account of whether he/she knew about contraception the parents' impression was corroborated, in that those in special schools were much more likely to have no information or inaccurate information than the teenagers in ordinary schools. One-third of pupils in special schools said that they did not know what contraceptive precautions a couple could take compared with about 10 per cent of controls or handicapped pupils in ordinary schools. The more severe the handicap, the less likely it was that the teenager possessed accurate information about contraception, less than 20 per cent of the severely handicapped having accurate information, compared with one-quarter of the moderately handicapped, and nearly 60 per cent of the mildly handicapped.

In chapter 10 we shall discuss the sex education programmes of the ordinary and special schools taking part in the study: while special schools are today making a much greater effort over sex education than was recently the case, the findings above suggest that it is still inadequate.

### (iii) Worries about boy- or girlfriends

Little systematic research, other than that of Dorner (1977), has been reported in the UK about the extent to which physically handicapped teenagers have worries about boy- and girlfriends. For this reason we report in some detail the teenagers' answers to the question, 'Most boys and girls your age worry quite a lot about boy (or girl) friends. Do you worry about this sometimes?' Having asked this general question, we then asked about a number of specific worries which often elicited more information than did the general question.

The proportion of handicapped boys and girls who said they worried was very similar to that of the control group, except that the spina bifida girls worried much more than any of the other groups. No significant differences related to severity of handicap were found, nor were the major differences related to the type of school attended. The great majority of those in the handicapped group said quite explicitly that they worried about the reaction of a boy or girl to their handicaps. Here are examples of the kinds of comments made. The first is from a good looking, intelligent, mildly handicapped hemiplegic boy attending an ordinary school. 'They [girls] make you feel you're not normal . . . they call you names . . . for instance, "you f......g spastic, f.... off" . . . it still surprises me when it happens. People who do that are ignorant anyway.' Another boy, diplegic, again personable and intelligent and attending an ordinary school, began by saying that he hadn't talked to his parents or any other adult about this, but he definitely felt a girl might be 'put off'. When once he'd talked to a close friend, the friend had 'laughed it off' and said his handicap 'didn't matter', but the boy thought that 'really it must . . . particularly the first impression'. Another boy, rather more severely handicapped but also in an ordinary school, said 'Mum tells me girls won't think of me having something wrong with me . . . [but] . . . a girl may think of me as spastic . . . she may go out with me only when she can't get a normal boy. My mum tells me it's personality, but I can't see that really. I see a girl with glasses and I think "ugh . . . she's ugly".' A few of the boys mentioned specific aspects of their disability, for instance a mobility problem or 'bag' problem (only one boy raised this spontaneously).

The disabled girls tended to worry more than the boys, although this difference was equally true of the control group. Again, the most frequently voiced worry was about the reaction of a boy to the disability itself. One girl, in a wheelchair and incontinent but attending an ordinary girls' school, was, according to her own account and her mother's, almost obsessed by the problem. She said she discussed it frequently with her mother and another adult, and her mother described her as 'boy mad'. As her remarks showed problems typical of the feelings of many disabled young people, we have quoted verbatim:

You feel left out when you go out with others and they've got [boy] friends. I've got spots . . . I'm not good-looking . . . I just lose hope . . . I don't think I'll ever have one. Boys don't want handicapped girlfriends. You don't hear of many. You hear of spina bifidas marrying each other but not of boys who're not handicapped marrying a girl who is . . . I like the able-bodied boys better . . . I'm funny like that . . . I've never met a good-looking handicapped boy around. I'm particularly worried about telling them about the bag . . . Even if you did [have a boyfriend] I suppose he'd soon walk out if he found I had an ileal loop . . . Mum says I'm too conscious of my handicap . . . [She went on to mention the scars on her body, and what a boy would think of that] But you've got to tell him sometime . . . If a boy says nice things to me I don't think he really means it . . . he's either being kind or doing it because he has to from a sense of duty. I just think they're joking when boys say you look nice.

Here is another girl speaking, an attractive, talented girl with diplegia, who depends heavily on a wheelchair: 'I'd like to go out with a boy . . . but it's very difficult if you're handicapped as people make a lot of judgements on first appearances. If people see you're handicapped they avoid you or adopt a special attitude unconsciously. They feel you're not capable of going out with people and having a special relationship . . . that's if they've never encountered handicapped people before . . . Usually [boys] are wary . . . they don't try to get involved.' She gave examples of boys whom she might have become interested in who were, she felt, put off because she was handicapped.

Another question asked was whether the teenager worried about not being found attractive to members of the opposite sex. This was a major worry for all teenagers, but especially for the handicapped (see Table 4.4).

When talking about this, the handicapped teenagers frequently referred to their disability, for example: 'I wonder if my arm will turn them off', 'I worry about being in a wheelchair', or 'I worry that he wouldn't want to know me because of my handicap'.

Another specific question put to both the control and handicapped

Table 4.4 *Worries about not being found attractive*

| | Handicapped pupils | | | | Controls | |
| | Special schools | | Ordinary schools | | | |
| | N | (%) | N | (%) | N | (%) |
|---|---|---|---|---|---|---|
| No worries | 41 | (54) | 17 | (46) | 23 | (70) |
| Mild/moderate worries | 22 | (29) | 11 | (30) | 7 | (21) |
| Definite worries | 13 | (17) | 9 | (24) | 3 | (9) |
| Total | 76 | (100) | 37 | (100) | 33 | (100) |

groups was about whether they had worries connected with sex. Only three (8 per cent) handicapped pupils in ordinary schools (all boys) said they were worried about this, compared to seven (21 per cent) of the controls (five girls and two boys). The difference is likely to be due to the fact that many more of the controls, especially the girls, had had a boy-or girlfriend so this was more likely to be a real problem for them. However handicapped teenagers in special schools were three times more likely than those in ordinary schools to have worries connected with sex (24 per cent – a similar proportion to the control group). Those with spina bifida were more likely to worry than those with cerebral palsy; nearly 40 per cent of the former were worried about some aspect of a sexual relationship, no doubt because of their incontinence.

A number of the questions asked in this part of the interview were relevant to the handicapped teenagers only. One question was whether the teenager worried about mixing with able-bodied teenagers of the opposite sex. Of those who were in ordinary schools, only two (6 per cent) said they worried about this compared to nearly one-quarter (24 per cent) of those in special schools. As might be expected this worry was strongly related to severity of handicap, 19 per cent of the moderately handicapped group and 26 per cent of the severely handicapped group said they worried about this compared to none of those with mild handicaps. The next question was whether their mobility problem was a worry when it came to having boy- or girlfriends. Of the twenty-four teenagers in ordinary schools with mobility problems over one-quarter were worried, compared with nearly half of those with locomotor problems in special schools, the latter of course being more severely handicapped.

Another question put to the handicapped group only was whether they worried about explaining the visible aspects of their handicaps (these were enumerated by the interviewer) to a boy- or girlfriend. Of the 107 who were asked, over one-third (36 per cent) said that they were worried. There was, as might be expected, marked differences relating to severity of handicap. Mildly handicapped teenagers were least worried (less than 10 per cent, compared with over 40 per cent of those with moderate or severe handicaps). However, it did appear that, regardless of degree of handicap, those in special schools were much more worried about this than those in ordinary schools.

The final question put to the teenagers was what their *main* worry was. Again, the most frequently cited worry was that they would never find a boy- or girlfriend because their handicaps would make them unattractive to others. This worry was common in both girls and boys, and did not depend on the severity of handicap. Two girls who had boyfriends worried about what their boyfriend really thought of them: one very pleasant, severely handicapped girl felt very vulnerable: 'I worry because he's normal . . . in case he's leading me on a string . . . two-timing me . . . I think it's just because I have a disablement that I worry.' One of the most justifiably bitter responses to this was made by a very severely handicapped boy, who had been rather silent up to this point: 'What's the difference between you and me . . . I can't use my bloody hands properly. I can't walk. I can't talk and that's it . . . what did you think?' The second most frequently voiced worry related specifically to some aspect of having a urinary bag, either of explaining it to a boy- or girlfriend, or of practical problems, in particular the worry about the bag leaking.

Eight of the handicapped teenagers mentioned some sort of sexual problem or anxiety as their major worry. Such worries were very varied, and included a spina bifida boy who was worried he 'wouldn't be able to give a girl a baby when I'm older because of the problem'; a cerebral-palsied boy in an ordinary school who worried because he felt he was the only boy without any sexual experience; a boy with many sexual anxieties which he felt he would find very difficult to explain; and several girls who were all afraid of how they would cope with the sexual side of a relationship.

The main difference between the controls and the handicapped boys was that the latter worried mainly about ever finding, or being thought attractive by, a girl, whereas the controls tended to worry about the relationship itself. However, the fears expressed by the handicapped and control girls were very similar. Half of the non-handicapped girls worried about boyfriends, for example about not having a boyfriend, and what their boyfriend was up to when not with them. It would certainly have helped some of the handicapped girls to know that very similar worries were often expressed by their non-handicapped peers.

## Hopes and anxieties concerning marriage and children

In this section the responses of the teenagers and their parents to a number of questions relating to marriage and children are discussed. It was possible to make a direct comparison in a number of cases between the views of the young people and their parents.

*(i) Marriage*

After the questions about boy- and girlfriends, the young people were told that the next series of questions was about the future. They were first asked, 'Do you feel you'd like to get married later on?' The great majority either definitely wanted to marry (76 per cent of the controls, 61 per cent of the handicapped) or thought they would probably want to (6 per cent and 16 per cent respectively). This was true of both sexes, although the girls were more certain than the boys. There was very little difference between the aspirations of PH pupils in ordinary and in special schools in this respect.

No controls and only nine handicapped teenagers said that they did not want to marry (8 per cent of the whole group). All were severely handicapped except for two who were moderately handicapped. One girl said that she 'just didn't want to', but added that 'somebody . . . I can't remember who, said it would be better to be single', while one boy said that he definitely wanted to live on his own and couldn't imagine himself getting married.

This question was followed by the question: 'Do you think you will *probably* get married eventually?' The results are shown in Table 4.5. None of the control group and only a very small proportion of the handicapped group thought that they wouldn't marry. However about one-third of the handicapped group, compared with only 12 per cent of the controls were uncertain as to whether they would. (All these teenagers wanted to marry.) Those who were severely handicapped were the most likely to be uncertain about whether or not they would marry (44 per cent said they 'didn't know', compared with between one-fifth and one-quarter of the others).

Table 4.5 *Whether teenager thinks that he/she will probably marry*

|  | Handicapped | | Controls | |
|  | N | (%) | N | (%) |
|---|---|---|---|---|
| Probably won't | 7 | (6) | 0 | (0) |
| Probably will | 71 | (62) | 29 | (88) |
| Don't know | 37 | (32) | 4 | (12) |
| Total | 115 | (100) | 33 | (100) |

The parents of the handicapped teenagers were also asked whether they thought their child was likely to marry, and overall the responses of the parents were remarkably similar to those of the teenagers – less than 10 per cent saying no, and one-third being uncertain. Again, as in the case of the teenagers' responses, the proportion of parents who replied that they 'didn't know' was much higher for those who were severely handicapped. Several mothers referred to the severity of their child's handicaps: 'It's unlikely because he's so handicapped. But he's always talking about it and would like to'; 'I shouldn't think it likely . . . no boy would want her'; 'I always try to emphasize other aspects of life, such as a career . . . as I can't help feeling she won't get married'. 'I think it's unlikely that a girl might want to . . . because of his speech, and dribbling and the way he is at the table . . . it would just put people off' (this mother had told the interviewer that she herself found it difficult to accept these things).

Of the parents who were uncertain, some said it was too far ahead to think of: 'I haven't thought too much ahead . . . and it's out of my hands.' Others clearly had thought about it, but were unable to reach any conclusion: 'I don't know . . . but she wants to so much.' 'I'd like to think he would.' 'I don't know.' 'It's terribly important to him to have a home, but not necessarily marriage.' Others thought it would depend on the opportunities which arose: 'I think it would have to be a very special man.' 'It all depends on who she meets. If she's at a mixed training hostel she might.' Occasionally, when parents said that they thought their child would marry, it appeared to be wishful thinking. One mother of a deaf cerebral-palsied boy said: 'Yes . . . why not?' but immediately after that began to cry, saying that her family thought the boy would be with his mother all his life: she didn't mind that, but was desperately worried about what would happen when she died.

Quite a number of parents mentioned the likelihood of their son or daughter marrying another disabled person: 'I just have a feeling he will . . . I'd like him to get involved in a youth club where he could meet girls in the same boat.' One couple with an able, but very severely handicapped athetoid son said they'd talked quite a lot about this to each other. The husband thought he might meet someone with a different disability 'who would be able to look after him'. Another said, 'I don't see why not, but I think it'll probably be to a disabled person . . . if he wasn't disabled he'd have to be a very special person'. One mother of a severely handicapped cerebral-palsied boy explained that as part of her job she visited a couple handicapped by spina bifida, and knew from experience that severely handicapped people can and do get married. She'd told her son about this. 'He says he's definitely getting married.' Although most parents spoke of their son or daughter marrying if they could find a person who could cope with their disabilities, a few mothers stressed the other side, that is what their son or daughter had to offer: 'I hope so . . . she's very loving . . . not the sort to get left on the shelf.' 'I think she may, as she's so well liked.'

Most of the disabled young people wanted to marry and this was appreciated by their parents. Most parents very much wanted this for their son or daughter's sake, and expressed as much optimism about this as did their teenagers, although this was clearly an area that caused the parents as well as the young people great anxiety. There was little evidence either that parents wanted their children to cling to them, or that the idea of a severely disabled person getting married was distasteful to them.

### (ii) Parenthood

The young people who said they wanted to marry were then asked if they would like to have children. No differences at all were found between disabled and able-bodied teenagers. The great majority – well over 80 per cent – did want this, while only seven disabled teenagers and one control definitely did not want children. The parents again appeared to appreciate the teenagers' aspirations about parenthood, although one-third said they didn't know what their child thought about this, especially if their child was severely handicapped.

Among parents who thought that their teenager would not want children, or were not sure about this, only a very small number put this down to the teenager's not liking children. Others who weren't sure said spontaneously that this was because their son or daughter was afraid of having a handicapped child: 'She talks on the basis that if she had any children they'd be like her [though] I've told her it's just a rare chance and not hereditary.' (Mother of severely handicapped athetoid girl.) 'I don't know . . . I think he must be wondering about the baby.' (Mother of spina bifida boy who never communicated his feelings to his parents.)

Only rarely did mothers appear to project their own negative feelings on to their children. This mother of a mildly handicapped, hemiplegic boy, who herself found it difficult to accept his being handicapped, said that she didn't know if he would want to have children. 'My greatest worry is children, if he does get married. I suppose I'd feel sorry for the children . . . of course my husband would help him financially . . . he's [her son] never mentioned it . . . [but] I've told him it might be a great burden to his wife.' 'I don't know . . . many couples don't have children now. She'd be mad if she does, there's no future for them.' (Mother of mildly handicapped girl whose daughter did want to have children.)

Many parents were well aware that their teenagers did very much want children: 'Yes, she loves children at school and helps a lot in the nursery there.' 'Yes . . . she likes looking after small babies.' Parents of boys were as likely as parents of girls to say how much their teenagers liked and wanted children: 'He really likes young children . . . enjoys watching them play . . . home life means so much to him.' 'He notices young children . . . why they're upset . . . he's very intuitive and very good with them.' 'He loves his sister's children and he's very good with them.'

Both the handicapped teenagers and their parents who thought marriage a possibility were also asked a number of questions about areas that might cause problems in relation to parenthood. In reply to an open-ended question: 'Do you have any worries in connection with having children?' not surprisingly a much higher proportion of girls than boys (52 per cent compared with 32 per cent) had such worries, especially the spina bifida girls. Among both the boys and girls the most common reason for worry was that the child might be disabled. This was as much a worry to cerebral-palsied as spina bifida young people: 'If I do [have children] they might end up with the same problem as myself' (spina bifida boy). 'I worry in case they'd be disabled' (cerebral-palsied boy). 'I wouldn't like them to turn out like me' (cerebral-palsied boy). 'If the child will have spina bifida, if they'll be handicapped . . . that's the main one . . . I might give birth to a spina bifida baby' (spina bifida girl). Two boys, both moderately handicapped by cerebral palsy, mentioned they didn't know if they would be able to have children. Several girls worried about whether they would be able to have children: 'I'll need to get advice about whether I can have them' (spina bifida girl). 'I don't know if I can have them . . . I haven't asked anyone' (spina bifida girl). 'Yes, I feel I might not be able to have any' (cerebral-palsied girl). One boy, who was only mildly handicapped, worried about what the child 'would feel like having a disabled father', and another about the cost of having a child. One girl mentioned her urinary bag: 'I worry about my bag . . . what will happen if I have children.' Several mentioned worries about looking after the children, and several voiced fears about the pain of childbirth.

After this open-ended question, the teenagers were asked specifically (unless they had already referred to this) whether they worried in case they might not be able to have children. Their responses are shown in Table 4.6.

Table 4.6 *Teenagers who worry in case they might not be able to have children*

|  | Cerebral palsy | | | | Spina bifida | | | |
|  | Boys | | Girls | | Boys | | Girls | |
|  | N | (%) | N | (%) | N | (%) | N | (%) |
|---|---|---|---|---|---|---|---|---|
| No worry | 33 | (83) | 25 | (74) | 5 | (50) | 9 | (47) |
| Vague worry | 2 | (5) | 5 | (15) | 2 | (20) | 2 | (11) |
| Definite worry | 5 | (13) | 4 | (12) | 3 | (30) | 7 | (37) |
| Total | 40 | (100) | 34 | (100) | 10 | (100) | 19 | (100) |

Of the thirty young people who had worries, only twelve had ever discussed the question with anyone – four with parents, five with doctors, and three with house-parents. Parents also worried that their son or daughter might not be able to have children. Only twelve parents of cerebral-palsied children (15 per cent), all moderately or severely handicapped, were doubtful about this. A few went into details, for example: 'She is a true spastic . . . she gets very tight and [finds it] very hard to relax.' A much higher proportion of mothers of spina bifida children – in particular boys – were quite correctly worried about whether their son or daughter would be able to have a child. Three were definite that their sons would not be able to: 'It's not possible as far as I know.' Another mother found it very difficult to imagine her son in a sexual relationship, and said that anyway she had gathered that it would be 'physically impossible' for him to have children. Of the three mothers with spina bifida girls who thought it would not be possible, one had been told this by her doctor, another had no definite information but thought she remembered the doctor telling her this, while the third had been informed by the hospital that her daughter's kidneys were 'not strong enough'.

We then asked: 'Do you worry that you might not be able to look after children properly yourself?' Many teenagers were realistic about this, especially the girls. The responses of cerebral-palsied and spina bifida teenagers were very similar – about 40 per cent in each group – twenty-nine of those with cerebral palsy were worried, but again few had discussed this with anyone. Several who said they were not worried about looking after children added that this was because they had not yet thought about it: 'I've never thought that far . . . I think I'll need help of some sort during the day . . . especially as my husband would be out at work.' 'I think I mightn't be able to cope . . . but I've never thought about this before and I'm not worrying about it.' Among those who were worried, holding or carrying a baby was most frequently mentioned by those with cerebral palsy: 'It's difficult with a baby to hold him, it's better when children are older and more robust.' 'I've got balance problems . . . but I might be able to learn to do it a different way.' 'The lifting and carrying side . . . I might accidentally fall and drop them.'

The question which revealed the greatest amount of anxiety was whether the teenager ever worried 'In case your child might have the same physical handicap as yourself'. Some had already raised this spontaneously, but when it was put directly an even larger proportion (half the cerebral-palsied group and nearly three-quarters of the spina bifida group) were worried about this to some extent. Of the thirty-six cerebral-palsied teenagers who were worried only eight had discussed the question with anyone, all but one with the parents. Of the twenty-two with spina bifida who were worried, only seven had talked about this, three with teachers, two with parents and the rest with relatives or friends. Such fears were realistic in the case of spina bifida teenagers (and we discussed with them the advisability of obtaining genetic counselling at some point). But the fears of the cerebral-palsied teenagers were poorly founded, and we took care to make it clear to the teenager that this was not a likelihood. In some cases the relief on the teenager's face was very marked, and several said they had never raised this worry with anyone before. One boy's face lit up and he said: 'I've been worrying about it for years' (his father had tried to reassure him but the boy hadn't known whether to believe him).

Below we describe some of the reactions of the young people to this question. One cerebral-palsied boy who thought he probably wouldn't have a handicapped child but still worried about it said: 'I'm worried because I've been through it . . . been called names.' Another boy said that he thought it very likely indeed that if he married a handicapped person the child would be handicapped. He added that his parents had said this. A cerebral-palsied girl who thought there was a definite possibility instanced a wheelchair-bound boy she knew, one of whose parents was blind, and one disabled. One intelligent cerebral-palsied boy, who attended an ordinary school, was slightly worried but said it was 'not a strong risk . . . it's not passed on to me genetically so it shouldn't be [handicapped] . . . I've had lessons on genes, and I figured it out for myself.'

As noted before, the spina bifida teenagers were more worried than those with cerebral palsy, but few were well informed about the actual risks. For instance, four boys all had expressed a worry, but when asked how likely they thought it was, one said: 'Maybe it will, maybe it won't', and another, 'around 50–50'. The same sort of variation was found among the spina bifida girls. One, who was *not* worried, said that this was because it was 'not hereditary', and that, if she had a child, the child would have 'the same chance as anyone else of being handicapped'. Another mildly handicapped girl said her mother told her there was no risk, but 'I just think it might happen'. Another girl thought there was a definite possibility. She was worried 'in case it runs in the family', while another had been told that 'most of the time it runs in your family'.

In summary many of the teenagers were already worried about this question, and many were confused. Most of those with cerebral palsy were worrying quite needlessly, while those with spina bifida who were at risk had rarely been given adequate information. Very few teenagers had ever discussed this issue with anyone. Teenagers of course depend heavily upon their parents as well as their schools for information of this kind and so the parents were also asked about their own fears and about whether they had had any genetic counselling.

In the case of the cerebral-palsied group, one-fifth of the parents *were* worried about the risk of handicap – a higher proportion than expected – and three others uncertain. Worrying was not related to the severity of the teenager's handicap. A mother of an athetoid boy, herself a nurse, said that she did worry, even though she said she told herself: 'It's not genetic'; one worried even though she knew her son was handicapped because it was a forceps delivery. A mother of another cerebral-palsied boy said that she thought it was genetic, but nobody had ever talked to her about the causes, while one mother said she had gathered from her GP that cerebral palsy was 'a family problem'. Although the majority of parents knew definitely that cerebral palsy was not hereditary, and went spontaneously into details of the birth and the reasons (anoxia, forceps delivery, prematurity, and so on) which they had been given, the fact that a substantial minority were worried about the genetic risk was a disturbing finding.

Parents of spina bifida children were much more likely to worry – about two-thirds altogether. The small group who 'didn't know' if they were worried or not were mainly mothers who were ignorant of the risks involved. Examples included a mother who said: 'I haven't thought about it . . . to me it was an accident' (she hadn't had any genetic advice). 'I haven't given it any thought'. (This mother went on to say she had had no genetic information – it had been a difficult birth but she just didn't know what caused it.) Most parents, however, did know there was a genetic component and were definitely worried, and some also voiced worries about the risk to their other (non-handicapped) children. Only one mother did know about the risks, but was not worried because she knew her handicapped son (and also her non-handicapped daughters) could have tests.

The parents were also asked whether they had ever discussed the question of the genetic risk to their own child 'with anyone at the hospital or anyone else'. The only parents of cerebral-palsied children who were asked this question were the twenty who were worried or uncertain, whereas all the mothers of spina bifida teenagers were asked, (except two who were so certain that their son and daughter would be unable to have a child that the question was irrelevant). Over half the worried mothers who had cerebral-palsied teenagers, and half the mothers with spina bifida teenagers, had not discussed this question with anyone. In the spina bifida group, the question was least likely to have been discussed if the child was mildly or moderately handicapped. Of the seventeen mothers who had said they were definitely worried, eight had not yet discussed this with anyone. Five had discussed it, and in two cases had been given fairly accurate information, while the other three had been given incorrect information. It may seem unnecessary for parents to think this far ahead when a teenager is only fifteen or sixteen, but many of the parents in the study needed and would have welcomed clear information on this, especially if they realized that the teenagers themselves were already worrying about it.

## (iii) Discussion of aspirations and anxieties with parents

Overall, the findings in this section have shown that many teenagers were worried by questions relating to marriage, sex and parenthood, although, from what they themselves said, only a comparatively small number had discussed these questions with anyone. The parents were therefore asked whether they had ever talked about *any* of these issues

Table 4.7 *Whether parent has discussed with the teenager questions relating to the teenager's personal future*

| | Cerebral palsy | | | | Spina bifida | | | |
|---|---|---|---|---|---|---|---|---|
| | Boys | | Girls | | Boys | | Girls | |
| | N | (%) | N | (%) | N | (%) | N | (%) |
| Haven't discussed as feel no need to | 30 | (67) | 16 | (42) | 8 | (73) | 8 | (42) |
| Haven't as teenager/ parent reluctant to | 4 | (8) | 2 | (5) | 0 | (0) | 1 | (5) |
| Have discussed some, not all of these | 9 | (20) | 18 | (47) | 2 | (18) | 8 | (42) |
| Total | 83 | (100) | 11 | (100) | 19 | (100) | 19 | (100) |

with their children. If they had done so, they were asked for details; and if they had not, they were asked if there were any particular reasons for this, including whether or not it was because of reluctance on the part of the parent or teenager. Their replies are summarized in Table 4.7.

These findings show that the mothers were more likely to discuss these kinds of questions with their daughters than with their sons, probably because mothers find it easier to talk to their daughters about such things, but also because the girls tended to be somewhat more mature than the boys. It was also the case that the spina bifida girls were much more worried than the boys about such matters and were more likely to have expressed their fears. In both groups mothers of moderately and severely handicapped teenagers were more likely to have discussed these questions than were mothers of mildly handicapped children. A large proportion of parents said they had not discussed any of these questions with the teenager as they felt there was no need. They thought he/she was too young, or that their child hadn't really started to think about these things, or was not yet intellectually capable of thinking seriously about them. ('So far he's not really concerned about these things.' 'He's not old enough.' 'These things aren't really relevant to him at the moment.') In some cases they were correct, but in many more, as our conversations with the teenagers showed, the young people were already thinking and worrying about these questions.

In very rare instances, the mother said that she hadn't discussed these questions either because the teenager was reluctant to (five cases) or because she herself was (two cases). For example, the mother of a severely handicapped, cerebral-palsied boy thought it was probably too soon anyway, but she also said that his personal future was a 'touchy subject' as he felt so bitter about being handicapped. A mother of a cerebral-palsied girl thought her daughter 'lives in the present . . . she doesn't want to grow up. I think she's rather afraid of growing up so she shuts all this out of her mind'. Another mother described her cerebral-palsied daughter as only being willing to talk about subjects 'in a jokey way . . . not seriously', although she thought she was very worried underneath.

A minority of mothers had begun to discuss at least some of these questions. Many mothers had talked to their daughters about children and marriage although, as one mother put it, they weren't 'very deep talks as she's more like a twelve or thirteen year old'. One parent mentioned an ASBAH conference for teenagers as being a very useful occasion for the discussion of questions such as these.

The parents were then asked whether they thought their son or daughter had any worries 'about finding a boy- or girlfriend, or the effect of being handicapped on his/her sex life, or on his/her chances of getting married, or of having children or of looking after them or anything else like this'.

The proportion of mothers who considered their children to have *any* worries of these kinds was highest for mothers of spina bifida girls, over 40 per cent of whom said 'Yes', compared with only two parents of spina bifida boys, and around 20 per cent of parents of cerebral-palsied boys and girls. This was further evidence that parents greatly under-estimated the extent of worrying in their children. Again, quite a number of parents said they thought their children still too young to be worrying about these things, and that they didn't 'think ahead', although a number mentioned they thought their son or daughter was 'just beginning' to worry, for example about boy- and girlfriends. Others said they didn't know. One mother said her son, 'likes to keep that part of his life [i.e., girlfriends] secret'. Several did say that although the teenagers didn't say anything, or appear worried, they might be 'worried underneath'. A number of parents thought that the teenager was more worried about whether he or she would get a job than about a future personal life.

However, some parents were well aware of their children's anxieties and raised very similar problems to the ones that teenagers themselves had told us about. The worry which parents were most likely to be aware of was that of finding a boy- or girlfriend (particularly a boyfriend) and about whether or not he or she would get married. The mother and father of a hemiplegic girl in an ordinary school, for example, mentioned how the previous winter it had 'all come out in a rush' that their daughter was self-conscious and felt frustrated and worried because boys never took any notice of her. She hadn't said directly that it was because she was handicapped but that was clearly the reason. Parents were much less likely to be aware that in many cases their sons and daughters had already started to worry about the question of children, including whether they would be able to have any or whether the child would be handicapped.

Finally, the question of how best to discuss such matters with their children was raised. The parents were asked whether they had ever talked to another adult about the best way of discussing these matters with their teenager. The great majority did not feel the need to, and only six mothers said they would like to do so. One said she'd like to know the sort of things to talk to her son about, while another wanted to know about the genetic risks but wasn't sure whom to approach. Only four mothers said that they had actually talked over with another adult how best to approach this. One had talked to other mothers at a meeting her GP ran for mothers of handicapped children, while another said that they had just started to discuss such questions in a parent group at her daughter's school. She thought this was going to be extremely helpful. The school had provided her with leaflets issued by SPOD (the organization set up to give advice on the sexual problems of the disabled: see Appendix B), and hoped to arrange a series of meetings on the sexual problems of handicapped adolescents. In chapter 10 we discuss what the school claimed to be doing with parents on this subject, but from the parents' responses it seemed that it was not really adequate. Experience suggests that, although most parents said they did not feel the need to talk over with anyone how best to discuss these questions with their teenagers, when schools *do* offer advice and set up parent groups, they uncover and help to meet very real anxieties within the parents of which they themselves may not be fully aware.

## Summary

In summary the handicapped teenagers had little experience of relationships with members of the opposite sex, but a large proportion of them worried about such matters. Their concern was often not perceived by their parents, many of whom thought their son or daughter too young to think about this.

While over three-quarters of the control group said that they had 'been out' with a boy or girl, only one-quarter of the disabled teenagers said they had done so, but the great majority, who had not, said they would like to do this. This is also probably an over-estimation of the number of handicapped pupils who actually had experience of a relationship with a member of the opposite sex as we felt that the ordinary and special school pupils interpreted this question rather differently. The lack of opportunity for those in day special schools to form such relationships must also be borne in mind. The handicapped in ordinary schools were much less likely than the controls to have gone out with a boy- or girlfriend (especially the girls, none of whom had ever dated).

Most of the teenagers knew about the facts of life, but the handicapped teenagers in special schools were much less likely to know about contraception. Many were also worried about their capacity for sex or parenthood, which suggests that much more needs to be done in the way of sex education programmes in special schools (see chapter 10).

What is interesting is that similar proportions of the handicapped young people (42 per cent) and the control group (46 per cent) expressed worries about boy- or girlfriends, and it is likely that it would be most beneficial to the handicapped to appreciate that the able-bodied teenagers have many anxieties in this area also. However, the nature of their worries was quite distinct. The great majority of the handicapped teenagers worried about the reaction of a boy or girl to their handicaps and felt that they would be considered unattractive because of their physical handicap, whereas the controls tended to worry about the actual relationship itself.

All of the controls and most of the handicapped teenagers (all but nine) either definitely wanted to marry or thought they would probably want to marry; although when asked if they thought they actually would do so about one-third of the handicapped group (mostly severely handicapped) compared to 12 per cent of the controls were uncertain as to whether they would. Parents' views as to the likelihood of their children marrying were very similar, and tended towards optimism. However, it was clear that here was an area that caused both parents and the young people anxiety. Most parents recognized that their son or daughter would marry only if they could find a partner who could cope with their disabilities, and few spoke of the positive side of the things that their child could offer in a relationship.

The great majority (over 80 per cent) of the handicapped teenagers also said they would like to have children and although many parents recognized this desire, one-third said they didn't know what their son or daughter thought about this, especially if their child was severely handicapped. Some who did know their teenagers wanted children very much, were clearly concerned about this. Many of the teenagers were worried about having children, especially the spina bifida girls. The most common worry was whether their child would be disabled, but many spina bifida and some cerebral-palsied girls also worried about whether they could actually bear children. Few of the teenagers had discussed any of their worries with anyone. Many of the cerebral-palsied teenagers were worrying quite needlessly about genetic risk, while those with spina bifida, who certainly were at risk, had rarely been given adequate information.

Overall, many teenagers and their parents were worried by questions relating to relationships, marriage and sex but very few had discussed these issues between themselves or with anyone else, and even fewer had been given specific advice or counselling. This obviously is a greatly neglected area and counselling on such matters should be made systematically available to teenagers and their families.

# 5
## *Psychological adjustment and problems*

In this chapter we concentrate on psychological problems and psychological adjustment in the young people. As noted already, the few studies which have been made of disabled children and young people suggest that those with neurological impairment (which would include those with cerebral palsy and spina bifida with hydrocephalus) are particularly likely to have emotional or behavioural problems. In this chapter, we look at the adjustment of the young people while in their last year at school, and in chapter 6 at some of the main factors associated with adjustment.

### (i) Terminology: the concepts of 'psychological adjustment' and 'psychological disorder'

When one turns to articles, books, or clinical reports concerned with the mental well-being of children or of adults, one is struck both by the range of terms used, and, more frequently, with the lack of definition and precision about their meaning. Commonly used terms include 'mal-adjustment', 'mental illness', 'psychiatric disorder', 'psychological disorder', 'behavioural and emotional disorders', 'deviant behaviour', and so on. These terms generally carry slightly different connotations, but even when their meanings are clear to those using them, they are often insufficiently well defined for the reader to understand fully what is meant by them.

At the root of the problem is the fact that these concepts are, in contrast to the concept of physical illness, very difficult to define. Ausubel (1961) has defined 'illness' as 'any marked deviations, physical, mental or behavioural, from normally desirable standards of structural and functional integrity'. In physical medicine there is comparatively little disagreement as to what are 'normally desirable standards', and therefore little disagreement about defining illness or health. In psychiatry the notion of 'health' is far less clear; the major problem is always one of deciding where to draw the line between normality and pathology. One of the first and most vocal of the critics of the place of psychiatry within medicine, Thomas Szasz, emphasizes in his article 'The myth of mental illness' (1960) that, 'In contrast to physical medicine, in psychiatry, social norms and values can be of even greater significance than the degree to which the behaviour is statistically unusual', and he therefore suggests that the concept of 'mental illness' should be replaced by that of 'problems in living'. McKay (1975), while recognizing the contribution which the 'medical model' has made to psychiatry, also emphasizes that 'the most important discrepancy between medicine and psychiatry is that whereas medicine is, by and large, an impartial discipline, psychiatry seems inevitably bound up with value systems'.

Additional problems arise when one is investigating the mental well-being of *adolescents*, since it may be very difficult (with the exception of a few clearly recognizable conditions) to differentiate disorder from 'normal' adolescent behaviour and feelings, particularly as very little work has been produced to show what is 'normal' behaviour for this age group. Some of the prevailing stereotypes about what is normal are discussed by Rutter and his colleagues (1976) in an important article, 'Adolescent Turmoil; Fact or Fiction?' They point out that currently prevailing beliefs usually include the following concepts: that adolescence is usually a period of great psychological upheaval and disturbance; that since a central feature of adolescence is, in Erikson's words, the 'identity crisis' (that is, the struggle to achieve personal identity), then this necessarily implies conflict with and increasing estrangement from the family; and that adolescents form a separate culture with different norms from the rest of society.

If these commonly held views are true, then the criteria which one uses in deciding what is and is not normal psychological functioning in adolescence, might well be very different from those applied to other populations. In fact, Rutter's own findings suggest that such assertions are greatly exaggerated. Misleading generalizations have been made which are based on clinical practice rather than on epidemological studies, and these have been taken up by the media and have become part of the folklore of adolescence. Rutter and his colleagues did, however, find that inner turmoil, as represented by feelings of misery and self-depreciation, was quite common in the mid-teens, and one is, therefore, still faced with the question of whether such feelings should or should not be taken as indicators of psychological disorder.

A further problem in defining psychological disorder arises when one's main concern is with physically handicapped adolescents. As we later show, by far the most common way in which the handicapped young people in our study differed from non-handicapped teenagers was in their marked lack of self-confidence and general anxiety and fearfulness, coupled frequently, although not always, with misery and depression. In many cases these are perfectly normal and legitimate reactions to the stress of having to cope day in and day out with a severe disability, such as incontinence, or, in the case of those less handicapped, with the often unsympathetic or inconsiderate reactions of non-handicapped peers. While, in this book, we follow common usage in talking about 'psychological adjustment' or 'emotional and behavioural problems', we want to make it absolutely clear that although we use the same criteria for handicapped and non-handicapped teenagers in defining what is or is not 'adjustment' we would, in the majority of cases, be very hesitant indeed about applying terms such as 'abnormal', 'pathological' or 'maladjusted' to the feelings and behaviour of those striving to cope with the effects of physical disability.

### (ii) Various approaches to the identification of psychological problems

Several different approaches have been adopted generally in defining psychological disorder in the young. First, the administrative one, defining the group thought to be in need of a service. For example, 'maladjustment' is a term which has been in common use since the publication of the *Handicapped Pupils and School Health Service Regulations* (1945), when maladjustment was defined as those 'who show evidence of emotional instability or psychological disturbance and require special educational treatment in order to effect their personal, social or educational readjustment'. The emphasis was therefore on an administrative definition – children who had special educational needs – and this has remained the only real focus for the term 'maladjustment', despite later attempts to define the concept more precisely (e.g., Underwood Committee Report (1955), and its Scottish counterpart (1964)).

The authors of the Isle of Wight Study preferred to use the term 'child psychiatric disorder'. They pointed out that although many of the children in their study with psychiatric disorder 'could reasonably be regarded as maladjusted', the two terms are not synonymous. Their main reason for making the distinction appeared to be that maladjustment includes the concept of the need for treatment, whereas the term psychiatric disorder, as used in the IOW Study, bears 'no connotations that treatment will necessarily benefit a child'. In fact, in common practice, the terms 'psychiatric disorder', 'disturbed behaviour' and 'maladjustment' are often used more or less interchangeably. Teachers and educational psychologists tend to use the term 'maladjusted' more frequently because they are very often concerned with school placement issues; while epidemiologists, child psychiatrists and research psychologists are more likely to use the broader category encompassed by the terms 'psychiatric disorder'.

An approach which seems to us to have gone further than most others in arriving at an assessment of psychiatric disorder was the 'clinical-diagnostic' approach used in the IOW Study. A statistical approach (using behaviour questionnaires with parents and teachers) was used in the first stage as a screening device with the total population. However, since the authors were aware that a behaviour questionnaire or an interview schedule based on observations by others, however carefully worked out, will always be imperfect because it involves a large element of subjectivity, this was followed, in the second stage, by a much more intensive study (involving interviews with teachers, parents and children) of those children whose screening suggested a disorder.

Overall, 'psychiatric disorder was judged to be present when there was an abnormality of behaviour, emotions or relationships which was continuing up to the time of assessment and was sufficiently marked or sufficiently prolonged to cause handicap to the child himself and / or distress or disturbance in the family or community'. This approach is the one which has been the major influence on our study, the main difference being that we used the statistical approach, derived from the questionnaires, as complementary to the clinical / diagnostic approach, rather than as a screening device. (For a more detailed consideration of these various approaches to identifying psychological disorder see Rutter *et al.*, 1970, pp. 148–51.)

### (iii) Criteria to be taken into account in the assessment of disorder

Before describing our own approach, a few general points need to be made about whether or not one assesses a particular child as having a psychological disorder, or psychological problem. First, any difficulty has to be considered in relation to the child's age. As Rutter (1975) emphasizes: 'Since children are developing organisms, assessment needs to be made in the context of a developmental framework. Children behave differently at different ages so it is necessary to know what behaviour should be expected at each age (and sometimes for each sex too). Different stages of development are associated with different stresses and susceptibilities.' As children are not all alike, some knowledge of the range of variability is also needed. Information about 'normative' behaviour in adolescence is still minimal, and this has made the interpretation of data gathered about possible psychological disorders in this age group particularly difficult to interpret.

In deciding whether a child has a disorder one must also consider the cultural and social context of the behaviour, and know what the cultural or sub-cultural norms and values are, as well as taking into account the differences expected at any particular age between the behaviour of boys and of girls. For example, the incidence of disturbed behaviour in primary schoolchildren (as measured by teacher questionnaires) has been found to be significantly higher in boys than in girls. However, a study (Rutter *et al.*, 1974) of children whose parents had been born in the West Indies (the children themselves being born in either the West Indies or in the UK), showed their disorders were less sex-linked, the girls showing rates of disorder, (especially of 'conduct' disorders, as perceived by teachers) much nearer to that in boys. Another recent study (Cochrane, 1979) showed that the presence of psychological disorders (as measured on several indicators) of Indian and Pakistani children living in Britain was significantly lower than in that of British children and children of West Indian parents.

Another aspect of context which makes the identification of disturbed behaviour difficult is that it may be extremely *situation specific* – that is, children may behave very differently in different settings. For example, in Mitchell and Shepherd's study (1966) of behaviour problems in 5–15 year olds in Buckinghamshire, there was a substantial number of children who presented difficulties only at home or only at school, a finding which was replicated in the IOW Study. Consequently, one requires information from different sources to be able to make an adequate rating of psychological well-being.

One must also consider short-term changes which may have occurred in the child's life, for example, if he has recently suffered a bereavement, has had a long period in hospital, has recently changed schools or has been separated from or quarrelled with a close friend. In many cases, these will only result in transient changes in behaviour and an attempt should be made to consider how *persistent* the disturbed behaviour is. Many children are reluctant to go to school, and may go through phases of Monday morning stomach- or headaches; such behaviour only becomes of concern when it persists over months. The extent and severity of the child's problems are clearly of importance in deciding whether or not he has an overall psychological disorder. Isolated symptoms are of little significance unless they are functionally disabling; disorders of real concern are usually characterized by a number of symptoms which are judged to be abnormal either because of their frequency, their patterning or their persistence and also (the other important aspect of severity) because they impair the functioning of the child and/or of other people.

This last point, whether or not the behaviour or feelings are handicapping in terms of functioning, was of particular importance in our consideration as to whether or not a teenager had a problem. Feelings or behaviour could be handicapping to the teenager or others in three main ways: first, it could cause distress to the teenager which may not always be easy to assess. For example, we could not presume in our survey that social isolation necessarily caused suffering since some teenagers were quite content and appeared to have sufficient inner resources to enjoy being alone for much longer periods than is 'normal' for young people of this age group. Aggression too *may* stem from unhappiness, but it may also be an expression of cultural, social and temperamental factors. Conversely, in their assessment of the prevalence of psychiatric disorder in adolescents, Rutter *et al.* (1976) noted that 'many youngsters who appear normal to parents and teachers are diagnosed as showing disorders on the adolescent interview', often on the basis of 'frequently expressed feelings of misery and self-depreciation', which they do not reveal to others without close questioning. Thus, 'regardless of what parents and teachers thought or noticed, the adolescents themselves experienced suffering'. However, the authors also raised the question of 'whether the reported feelings meant clinical depression or whether they represented inner turmoil which is part of adolescent development rather than an indication of psychiatric disorder', and they were unable to arrive at an entirely satisfactory way of deciding what does and does not constitute true psychiatric disorder in adolescence, or just a degree of unhappiness quite normal for that age group.

A second way in which disorder can be handicapping is if it imposes social restrictions on the child. For example, does a physically handicapped teenager's anxiety about going into new situations prevent him from joining clubs and perhaps making new friends? Again, many able-bodied young people may also go through a phase of nervousness in new situations during the teenage years. However, a *prolonged* period of social withdrawal, stemming from a poor self-image and a lack of self-confidence, can be handicapping in the long term if it interferes with the normal processes of social development.

Finally, the disorder may not cause great distress to the child himself, but it may affect his family or peers. For example, irritability may not bother the individual himself as much as those around him. In addition, evidence from Shepherd *et al.* (1966) suggests that behaviour which might be intolerable to one family, given the state of the mother's physical or mental health or because of poor housing and the proximity of neighbours, might be perfectly well tolerated in another.

### (iv) Measuring adjustment or psychological problems in this study

As noted in our introduction, in our study we relied heavily on long interviews with the mother (or both parents) and the teenagers which although highly structured also contained many open-ended questions. These were supplemented by shorter interviews with the teachers, and with completion by the teachers of the Rutter Scale B (Rutter, 1967), which assesses the child's behaviour in school, and also the completion by the teenager and by the mother of the Malaise Inventory (Rutter *et al.*, 1970) which elicits information on a number of items concerned with physical or psychosomatic symptoms or symptoms of distress.

Since they were first devised by Rutter and his colleagues, many researchers have made use of these scales, including those concerned with families with handicapped children, such as Moss and Silver's study (1972) of families with Down's syndrome, studies by Tew and Laurence (1975) and Bradshaw and Lawton (1978) of mothers with spina bifida children, or mothers with very severely disabled children, and by Dorner (1975) in his study of teenagers with spina bifida. The Malaise Inventory and the Rutter Scale B have also been used by Rutter and his colleagues (1976) in a study of 14–15 years old living on the Isle of Wight, and more recently in their study of secondary school children in Inner London (Rutter *et al.*, 1979).

Rutter (1978) makes a strong point that the scales indicate the presence of emotional distress and disturbance rather than psychiatric disorder as such, while Philp (1978) warns that, in the case of parents of handicapped children, some of the items on the Malaise Inventory (such as backache and tiredness) may reflect actual burdens with a real physical cause rather than symptoms of psychosomatic origin. We found the scales a useful complement to the questionnaires given to the parents and teenagers, but found that, by themselves, the scales did miss a proportion of those young people thought to be suffering from stress.

On the basis of all the information available to us from interviews, from the Scale and the Malaise Inventory, we made a judgement about which young people could be described as having 'psychological problems', and which could include problems of emotion or feeling, or problems of behaviour, or both. We found a two-fold classification of those with and without psychological problems misleading and in practice very difficult to apply, and consequently we have made a three-fold rating into those with 'marked psychological problems', those with 'some overt problems', and those with none or only minor overt problems which we have called 'satisfactory adjustment'.

The first category includes mainly young people with long-standing difficulties which have been present for a number of years, plus one or two who were reacting strongly to particular problems present at the time, but who, according to themselves, their parents and their schools had not previously shown marked symptoms of disturbance. The second group really represents a borderline group, whose problems were less evident than those in the first group but who could not be said to be without any symptoms of distress. At some points in the analysis, where we wanted to make comparisons with other studies, we felt that it was more appropriate to include this group with the 'marked problem' group, but when we talk about those with definite difficulties this refers only to those in the first category.

The third category includes mainly young people who appeared truly to have adjusted well to their problems and difficulties, but it did also include some people who were probably as yet too immature to appreciate the difficulties that adult life was likely to present to them, or who, in collusion with their parents, were simply not facing up to the real-life implications of their disabilities. This, of course, is a perfectly valid coping strategy at least in the short term; at any rate it is one which people outside the family should beware of criticizing. But we felt that with some of these young people, difficulties were being ignored which at a later date would inevitably present problems, for example in cases where a young person was content to be very heavily dependent on his parents for company and emotional support, but who was likely later to run into very serious difficulties when his parents became too old to provide for all his needs. However, in terms of his *current* situation the young person could be said to have 'satisfactory adjustment', in that he was content with his present way of life and not unduly worried about the future.

### (v)  The classification of disorders in childhood or adolescence

We should like to refer briefly here to the classification of psychological disorders as defined by Rutter and his colleagues and used in the present study. We would stress again that psychological disorder in childhood and in adolescence is, in the great majority of cases, not equivalent to the presence of an 'illness' or 'disease' which is qualitatively different from normal, while what are termed 'disorders' are, in the words of Rutter *et al.* (1975), 'quantitative rather than qualitative departures from the normal course of development'. Our findings suggest that this is true for most handicapped adolescents we studied, and in only a very small minority of cases (all teenagers with cerebral palsy and epilepsy) could their problems be described as qualitatively different from normal behaviour.

The main categories used by Rutter and his colleagues are 'conduct disorders' (sometimes also referred to in the literature as 'anti-social disorders') such as aggressive behaviour, stealing, lying, bullying, etc., and 'neurotic disorders', such as excessive worrying or fearfulness or frequent and intense misery. If a child's behaviour includes symptoms from both of these categories, he is said to have a 'mixed disorder'. 'Conduct disorders' and 'neurotic disorders' are also differentiated in terms of the child's response to treatment, children with neurotic symptoms being more likely to improve significantly with appropriate help than those with conduct disorders, and follow-up studies carried out by Rutter and his colleagues (1976) also show that the long-term prognosis is better for children with neurotic disorders than for those with conduct disorders.

In the Isle of Wight Study of 10–11 year olds (Rutter *et al.*, 1970), 126 children (about 6 per cent of the total population) were identified as having behavioural problems. These could be broken down into those with 'neurotic disorders' (36 per cent), 'conduct disorders' (36 per cent) and those with 'mixed disorders' (24 per cent); while only about 3 per cent were suffering from 'other disorders', such as childhood psychosis or adult-type neurotic or depressive illness.

No breakdown is yet available into types of disorders found in the Isle of Wight Study of young people aged 14–15 years, but Rutter *et al.* (1976) report that for the most part the type of disorders seen at this age appeared to be 'closely similar' to those seen at 10–11 years, except for two marked differences. First, depression was much more common in adolescence, 'this difference indicating the beginning of a shift to an adult pattern of disorders, although there is not yet the marked female preponderance of neurotic disorders seen in adults . . . Secondly, at age fourteen years, there were fifteen cases of school refusal whereas there had been none at ten years. In many cases, the school refusal formed part of a more widespread anxiety state or affective disorder'.

In our own study we have used Rutter's classification when looking at the nature of the teenagers' disorders, and we included within the 'neurotic disorder' group young people suffering from depression, since this was almost always associated with other problems of the 'neurotic' type, in particular with anxiety and lack of self-confidence.


**Findings from other studies on the extent and nature of psychological disorders in adolescence**

*(i) Findings for non-handicapped adolescents*

Although a great deal of clinical material is available, there have been few epidemiological studies of non-handicapped adolescents. A rare exception was the Isle of Wight Study of 14–15 year olds. In this study, for the total population of over 2000 adolescents, about 300 were identified by the screening procedures described on page 112, as having problems, all of whom were then seen individually for interview by psychiatrists, while their parents and teachers were given individual interviews also. On the basis of all this information an individual psychiatric diagnosis was made of each child thought to have disturbed behaviour. (Graham and Rutter, 1973; Rutter *et al.*, 1976.) The same interview procedures were also applied to a random sample of the general population of teenagers, to see how many had disorders which showed up on interview but not on the screening procedures.

As already indicated, a major problem was the difficulty of deciding what constituted psychiatric disorder in adolescence. This depended to a considerable extent on which source (e.g., the parent or the teenager interview) was used as the main indicator of disorder. If the rating was made on the basis of the parent interview, then the prevalence of disorder was found to be about 13 per cent in both boys and girls. If the interview with the teenager was used, the rating for disorder in the group as a whole rose to about 16 per cent. In addition some children, not picked up by the screening procedures, appeared on interview to have some problems and if the prevalence rate was corrected to allow for this it would rise further to over 20 per cent.

The few other epidemiological studies which have been carried out to estimate psychiatric disorder in adolescence give similar results. A study by Leslie (1974) on 13–14 year old children in Blackburn showed a prevalence rate of psychiatric disorder of 21 per cent in boys and 14 per cent in girls, the information being obtained from interviews with parents and children, and questionnaires from teachers. Another study was carried out in an Australian town (Krupinski *et al.*, 1967; Henderson *et al.*, 1971) where 16 per cent of adolescents were diagnosed as showing some form of psychiatric disorder.

### (ii) Findings for handicapped children and adolescents

Very little is known about the prevalence of psychiatric or psychological disorders in handicapped adolescents, and even for younger children information is scanty. In the Isle of Wight Study, comparisons were made for 10–11 year olds between handicapped children with physical conditions which did not involve the brain, and children with 'neuro-epileptic' conditions (in the great majority of cases those with cerebral palsy or epilespy, or both). Actual prevalence rates depended on the measures used, but if one takes children identified by the screening procedures, the rate of psychiatric disorder for the general population was found to be about 6 per cent, while for the group with physical handicaps but no brain damage it was 9 per cent, and for the neurologically-impaired group the rate was 24 per cent. These figures would of course be somewhat higher if corrected for children missed by the screening procedure, but the main point of interest was that in 10–11 year olds psychiatric disorder was more than four times as likely to occur in children with neurological abnormalities than in the non-handicapped children, and 2–3 times more likely than in children with physical handicaps but no neurological impairments.

Unfortunately, no similar analysis is available from the Isle of Wight Study of 14 year olds, but a study carried out by Seidal *et al.* (1975) of physically handicapped 5–15 year olds living in three London boroughs is of interest. Using the same methods, it confirmed the original Isle of Wight findings and showed a higher rate of disorder in children whose handicap was associated with damage to the central nervous system above the level of the spinal cord (mainly cerebral palsy or hydrocephalus), compared with children with a physical handicap arising from some other cause. 24 per cent of those with an abnormality of the brain were found to have a 'psychiatric disorder with substantial social impairment' compared with only 12 per cent in the other groups. However, while this study is important because it confirms the Isle of Wight findings, since it covers such a wide age range it cannot tell us much about adolescence as such.

Although no epidemiologically-based study exists of the prevalence of psychiatric or psychological disorders in adolescents with cerebral palsy or spina bifida, interesting work has been done which provides valuable qualitative information about the nature of the young people's problems, and as well quantitative data about specific problems, such as depression. For young people with spina bifida, Dorner's work (1975; 1976) is of special interest. His group comprised sixty-three teenagers with myelomeningocele aged 13–19 years (mean age 16.4 years) who had attended the Hospital for Sick Children, Great Ormond Street. It included some children without obvious signs of hydrocephalus, and although a few had IQs of below 70, they were on the whole a rather less handicapped group than ours. Dorner's group also differed from ours in that half had left school at the time of interview. A major finding to emerge from his interview with the young people and with their parents was the high incidence (66 per cent overall) of definite and recurring feelings of misery, especially among the girls, the parents often being unaware of this. In contrast, there was a striking absence of anti-social problems. A study of thirty-five spina bifida adolescents in Melbourne, Australia (McAndrew, 1978) covers, among other things, the psychological problems of those young people with spina bifida. The findings are very similar to those reported by Dorner, with depression a very common feature, together with feelings of low self-esteem.

Other studies which highlight the difficulties and anxieties associated with incontinence are referred to at appropriate points in the text (and are also reviewed in chapter 9 of Anderson and Spain's *The Child with Spina Bifida* (1977)). They include the work of Feinberg *et al.* (1974); Fulthorpe (1974) and Scott *et al.* (1975).

In the case of teenagers with cerebral palsy we were unable to find many relevant studies, and certainly no epidemiological ones. However a useful account, based upon clinical evidence, of the sorts of problem they experience is given in Freeman (1970). A study of the social adjustment of sixty-two young adults, aged 16–35 years, with cerebral palsy was carried out by Brian Rowe (1973). Rowe measured social adjustment in fifty-three of the young adults by administering the Social Adjustment section of the California Test of Personality which covers social standards, social skills, freedom from anti-social tendencies, family relations, occupational relations and community relations. 85 per cent of the group had below average scores (based on American norms), but the findings are difficult to interpret since there was no evidence that the group was in any way representative of cerebral-palsied people, the great majority being attenders at one workshop run by a voluntary society.

In our own study, many cerebral-palsied teenagers had other handicaps such as epilepsy (about one-quarter of the sample) and speech disorders (over half) and a small proportion had a significant hearing loss (about 6 per cent). Thus studies of young people with these as their major handicaps are also of relevance.

Bagley (1971) has looked in detail at the psychological problems of epileptic children, in whom he found a high rate of psychological disorders; and Richardson and Friedman (1974) at the psychosocial problem of American adolescents aged 14–16 years with uncomplicated epilepsy. Theirs was a small in-depth study using interviews with teenagers and their parents, a questionnaire, and group interviews. Of the seventeen teenagers taking part, thirteen were found to have psychosocial problems of some kind. The parents frequently saw behaviour problems as the main difficulty, while problems in peer relationships were the main concern of the young people. As far as we know, no work has been done on the psychological problems of young people in whom speech disorder is their major problem. However, the literature on the psychological problems of children with hearing impairments is extensive (e.g., Rodda, 1970; Reivich and Rothrock, 1972), and shows a high incidence of emotional and social problems in this group.

In this very brief review of research we have concentrated mainly on studies relating specifically to cerebral-palsied and spina bifida adolescents, but research into the psychological problems of young people with other physical handicaps is also very relevant, and Pless and Pinkerton (1975) provide a useful general review of these. Finally, to obtain the feel of what it is like to be disabled three classics in the literature on disability, Goffman's *Stigma* (1963), Wright's *Physical Disability – a psychological approach* (1960) and Hunt's *Stigma: the experience of physical disability* (1966) are highly recommended.

### The present study: extent of psychological problems
### Ratings of overall psychological adjustment: methodology

On the basis of all information available to us, each teenager in the study was placed into one of three categories:

1  those judged to have 'marked' psychological problems, taking into account the criteria discussed earlier (p. 113),
2  those with 'some' problems, less marked than those of the teenagers in the first group, and
3  those whose overall adjustment was considered to be 'satisfactory' – that is, their problems were only minor or there was an absence of any overt symptom.

At the end of each phase of the study when all the teenagers and their parents had been interviewed, the ratings of 'psychological problems' were reviewed by each interviewer separately, and any 'borderline' cases were discussed by the interviewers together before the ratings were finalized.

The ratings of 'overall' adjustment were, as we said above, *clinical* ratings, made on the basis of an overall impression which took into account all available information. This usually consisted of: (i) information derived from the teenager in answer to a structured, detailed and probing questionnaire, the items the young person checked on the Malaise Inventory, plus the interviewer's impression of the young person; (ii) information derived from what the parent(s) said, this was the mother alone in most cases; and (iii) information derived from the school, including the Rutter Teacher Scale B, supplemented in some but not all cases with a discussion of varying length with one or more teachers.

As we pointed out earlier, data derived from several sources may not always be closely correlated. For example, a teenager with a very high (i.e., deviant) score on the Rutter Teacher Scale may have a low score on the Malaise Inventory; or a parent may perceive her child as having no problems of significance, whereas the teenager may reveal at the interview that he or she has been concealing deep feelings of depression, loneliness or anxiety. The reverse may also be true. A very few teenagers had little to say at the interview about problems or even denied that problems existed, yet appeared to the interviewer, as well as to parents and school staff, as miserable or markedly lacking in self-confidence. On the whole, however, data derived from different sources gave a reasonably consistent picture of the teenager's present psychological state. Most of the young people were extremely open and honest about their feelings and behaviour, and the information they gave usually corresponded to that obtained from their parents.

### Findings: extent and nature of overall psychological problems

#### (a) Findings on the overall three-fold rating

In Table 5.1 we consider our ratings of overall adjustment in relation to sex and to whether or not the teenager was handicapped. The findings show that one-third of the handicapped teenagers had 'marked'

Table 5.1 *Overall psychological adjustment in the handicapped and control groups*

| Overall adjustment | Handicapped teenagers | | | | | | Controls | | | | | |
|---|---|---|---|---|---|---|---|---|---|---|---|---|
| | Boys | | Girls | | Total | | Boys | | Girls | | Total | |
| | N | (%) | N | (%) | N | (%) | N | (%) | N | (%) | N | (%) |
| Marked problems | 17 | (28) | 22 | (38) | 39 | (33) | 1 | (7) | 0 | (0) | 1 | (3) |
| Some problems | 13 | (21) | 9 | (15) | 22 | (19) | 2 | (13) | 2 | (11) | 4 | (12) |
| Satisfactory adjustment | 31 | (51) | 27 | (47) | 58 | (49) | 12 | (80) | 16 | (89) | 28 | (85) |
| Total | 61 | (100) | 58 | (100) | 119 | (100) | 15 | (100) | 18 | (100) | 33 | (100) |

Table 5.2 *Overall psychological adjustment, type of handicap and sex*

| Adjustment | Cerebral palsy | | | | | | Spina bifida | | | | | |
|---|---|---|---|---|---|---|---|---|---|---|---|---|
| | Boys | | Girls | | Total | | Boys | | Girls | | Total | |
| | N | (%) | N | (%) | N | (%) | N | (%) | N | (%) | N | (%) |
| Marked problems | 15 | (30) | 14 | (36) | 29 | (33) | 2 | (18) | 8 | (42) | 10 | (34) |
| Some problems | 11 | (22) | 5 | (13) | 16 | (18) | 2 | (18) | 4 | (21) | 6 | (20) |
| Satisfactory adjustment | 24 | (48) | 20 | (51) | 44 | (49) | 7 | (64) | 7 | (37) | 14 | (45) |
| Total | 50 | (100) | 39 | (100) | 89 | (100) | 11 | (100) | 19 | (100) | 30 | (100) |

problems compared with only one control and a further 19 per cent of the handicapped group had 'some' problems, compared with 12 per cent of the controls. Overall, just under half the handicapped group were rated as having 'satisfactory' adjustment, compared with nearly 85 per cent of the controls. Though the control group was small, the overall finding of a disorder rate of 15 per cent is broadly comparable to that of studies (reviewed on p. 115) of non-handicapped adolescents, as was the rather higher rate of problems found in the boys (20 per cent) than in the girls (11 per cent). The very high rate of disorders among the disabled young people also bears out the findings from other studies – that the rate of psychological problems in neurologically-impaired children is 3–4 times as high as it is for non-handicapped children.

Table 5.2 shows the rates of adjustment in the cerebral-palsied group compared with that for spina bifida young people, considering the rates for boys and girls separately within each group. The overall rate of disorders in the cerebral-palsied and spina bifida groups are very similar: about one-third in each group had marked problems, about one-fifth 'some' problems, while just under half were rated as 'satisfactory'. Within the cerebral-palsied group the rates of disorder were fairly similar for both boys and girls; in the spina bifida group, however, there was a difference between the boys and girls, nearly two-thirds of the boys being rated as having 'satisfactory' adjustment, compared to only just over one-third of the girls. Conversely, 42 per cent of the girls had 'marked' problems compared with only 18 per cent of the boys. The findings could not be attributed to differences in severity of handicap between spina bifida boys and girls since very similar proportions in each group were rated as being mildly, moderately or severely handicapped.

Unfortunately, the group of boys was really too small for definite conclusions to be drawn, and also, since many of the anxieties of the spina bifida young people were often closely related to incontinence management (a question discussed later in more detail) it may well have

Table 5.3 *Overall psychological adjustment and severity of handicap (Pultibec ratings)*

| Adjustment | Severity of handicap | | | | | |
|---|---|---|---|---|---|---|
| | Mild | | Moderate | | Severe | |
| | N | (%) | N | (%) | N | (%) |
| Marked problems | 5 | (19) | 18 | (43) | 16 | (31) |
| Some problems | 8 | (31) | 5 | (12) | 9 | (18) |
| Satisfactory adjustment | 13 | (50) | 19 | (45) | 26 | (51) |
| Total | 26 | (100) | 42 | (100) | 51 | (100) |

been that the girls found it easier than did the boys to express their anxieties to women interviewers (both interviewers were female). This seems a strong possibility in view of Dorner's finding that about half the young men in his study (although these were rather older in age than those in Phase I of the current study) admitted to mild, moderate or severe misery or depression, although in his study also, girls were found to be more vulnerable.

Table 5.3 shows the relationship between severity of handicap and the presence of psychological problems, and indicates that while the proportion in each group who were considered to have 'satisfactory adjustment' was very similar (about 50 per cent) there were far fewer judged to have 'marked problems' among the mildly handicapped compared with those who had moderate or severe handicaps. (More will be said about this relationship in chapter 6.)

*(b) Findings on the Rutter Teacher Scale and the Malaise Inventory*

The scores on the Rutter Teacher Scale and the Malaise Inventory were used mainly to supplement the information obtained in the interviews, but are also worth looking at on their own account. Table 5.4 shows the proportion of teenagers with a deviant score on the Rutter Scale (i.e., a score of 9 or more), and compares the cerebral-palsied and spina bifida groups with our own controls and with the fourteen year olds in the Isle of Wight Study. The table shows that the rates for deviance on this

Table 5.4 *The extent of deviant behaviour on the Rutter Teacher Scale (i.e., a score of 9 or more)*

| Group | Total (N) | Total with deviant score | (%) |
|---|---|---|---|
| Cerebral palsy | 87 | 29 | (33) |
| Spina bifida | 30 | 5 | (17) |
| All PH | 117 | 34 | (29) |
| Controls | 33 | 2 | (6) |
| IOW 14 year olds | 2296 | 152 | (7) |

Table 5.5 *Types of disorders on the Rutter Teacher Scale*

| Groups | Total N | Conduct disorders N | (%) | Neurotic disorders N | (%) | Mixed disorders N | (%) |
|---|---|---|---|---|---|---|---|
| Cerebral palsy | 87 | 5 | (6) | 23 | (26) | 1 | (4) |
| Spina bifida | 30 | 0 | (0) | 5 | (17) | 0 | (0) |
| All PH | 117 | 5 | (4) | 28 | (24) | 1 | (1) |
| Controls | 33 | 1 | (3) | 1 | (3) | 0 | (0) |

Scale were very similar for our control group and the Isle of Wight Study group, while the rates for the physically handicapped groups, especially for those with cerebral palsy, were very much higher. These results were also analysed by sex, and showed that all the PH group except the spina bifida boys had a deviance rate much higher than that of the controls.

Table 5.5 shows the breakdown into types of disorder indicated by the Rutter Scale scores and indicates that neurotic disorders were generally more common in the PH group than among the controls (24 per cent overall compared with 3 per cent). Among the controls, the proportion with conduct disorders was also about 3 per cent, but the rate was three times as high among those with cerebral palsy (if those with mixed disorders were included). For the spina bifida group, however, conduct disorders were virtually absent.

A similar analysis was completed for the Malaise Inventory, the mean scores and the proportion in each group with a score of seven or over being shown in Table 5.6. The Malaise Inventory does not discriminate as well between the handicapped and non-handicapped groups as the Rutter Scale, although if the IOW fourteen year olds are taken as more representative of non-handicapped young people than our own control group, then the differences were much more marked. The spina bifida group showed the greatest percentage with high Malaise scores, but it should be remembered that this group contained a number of young people with current physical illness, such as urinary infections, which

Table 5.6 *Findings on the Malaise Inventory as completed by the teenagers*

| Group | Total N | Total scoring seven or more on Malaise Inventory N | (%) |
|---|---|---|---|
| Cerebral palsy | 88 | 20 | (23) |
| Spina bifida | 30 | 9 | (30) |
| Total PH | 118 | 29 | (25) |
| Controls | 33 | 7 | (21) |
| IOW 14 year olds | 175 | 23 | (13) |

would affect their Malaise scores. In all the groups, the girls had very much higher scores than the boys.

## The nature of the teenagers' problems

### (i) General findings: main types of problems

On the basis of all the information gathered about them, the handicapped teenagers with either marked or some psychological problems were placed in one of four groups, using Rutter's classifications (see p. 114).

Teenagers with 'neurotic' type problems usually showed several of the following behaviours: a marked lack of self-confidence, often accompanied by self-consciousness about their handicaps; fearfulness about going into new situations and meeting new people; less frequently by separation anxiety, that is, marked anxiety if separated from their parents, which in a minority of cases took the form of extreme withdrawal; marked worries and anxieties which might be general or specific, for example in relation to incontinence; marked or frequent misery or depression; difficulties in getting on with peers; and occasionally problems of school refusal. The behaviour of those with 'conduct' disorders might include aggression, surliness and disobedience; frequent irritability; in some cases frequent or severe temper tantrums; bullying and fighting; and, rarely, truancy. The group with 'mixed' disorders often presented as conduct disorders, but on close investigation were often also found to be very anxious and lacking in self-confidence. Finally, the 'other' category included three teenagers, all with cerebral palsy and epilepsy, who showed, in addition to problems of the kind described above, behaviour which was sometimes bizarre, usually because they did not appear to be in full control of their attention, with periods when others felt their minds to be 'absent' in some way. These were also young people whom neither the interviewers nor the school staff felt they could really 'get through' to.

The percentage of teenagers falling into each of these categories are shown in Table 5.7. It must be emphasized that in these tables the classification was made on the basis of *all* the information available, and not just on the scores from the Rutter Scale, but they confirm and amplify the trends from the screening tests shown in Table 5.5. In fact, using this method, the proportions thought to have 'marked problems' agreed well with the proportions identified by the teachers as being deviant on the Rutter Scale.

This table shows the overwhelming preponderance of 'neurotic' as compared to 'anti-social' or 'mixed' disorders, regardless of sex, although again anti-social or mixed disorders were more common among boys and neurotic disorders more common in girls. Since only five

Table 5.7 *Percentage of handicapped teenagers with different types of psychological disorder*

| Types of disorder | Marked problems | | | Some problems | | | All teenagers with problems | |
|---|---|---|---|---|---|---|---|---|
| | Boys | Girls | Total | Boys | Girls | Total | N | (%) |
| Neurotic | (65) | (78) | (72) | (54) | (89) | (69) | 43 | (71) |
| Anti-social | (18) | (14) | (15) | (31) | (0) | (18) | 10 | (16) |
| 'Mixed' | (12) | (0) | (5) | (15) | (11) | (14) | 5 | (8) |
| 'Other' | (5) | (8) | (8) | (0) | (0) | (0) | 3 | (5) |
| Total | 17 (100) | 22 (100) | 39 (100) | 13 (100) | 9 (100) | 22 (100) | 61 | (100) |

control group teenagers were judged to have problems (one 'marked' and four 'some' problems) comparisons were not really useful, but it is worth noting that three of the five had neurotic disorders.

The data were also analysed separately for the teenagers with spina bifida and cerebral palsy. As the total numbers were small, especially for the spina bifida teenagers, we included those with 'marked' problems and with 'some' problems in the *total* number with disorders. The findings again confirm those in Table 5.5, that is in both diagnostic groups, regardless of sex, 'neurotic' disorders were by far the most common, while 'conduct' disorders were very rare indeed among the spina bifida group, especially the girls.

## (ii) Specific problems

So far we have talked in rather general terms about the presence or absence of psychological problems. We shall now discuss in more detail the nature of the young people's problems. We start by looking at problems which could be classified as 'emotional' or 'neurotic', in particular at worrying and anxiety in relation to school work and handicaps as well as more general worrying; at lack of self-confidence and fearfulness about going into new situations; and about misery and depression. Finally, we look briefly at anti-social types of disorders. We considered information supplied by the parents as well as by the teenagers themselves, and some interesting similarities and differences were obtained between the two information sources.

*Worrying: its extent and nature.* Information about worrying was obtained from parents, teachers and the teenagers themselves, and we start with the parental replies to the general question about whether they thought their teenager tended to worry much about things. Only a small number of parents in each group (including the control group − about 6−7 per cent) thought that their teenager had a severe problem with worrying, except for the parents of spina bifida girls who reported a rate of about 16 per cent. However, while the handicapped groups' parents frequently reported that their children worried to a moderate degree (nearly half of the parents of cerebral-palsied teenagers, and two-thirds of the parents with spina bifida girls), this was reported by only one-third of the control group parents.

These are some examples of how parents described young people thought to have a marked problem with worrying. One cerebral-palsied boy was described as 'sensitive' and it was said that he had always been a worrier, although he had begun to come to terms with his anxieties over the past year. He worried about his mother's health, his father being a smoker, about cruelty to animals (he had become a vegetarian) and was also very self-conscious about his handicap. Another in this group was a very anxious hemiplegic girl constantly worried, said her mother, about 'the future, boys, everything'. The three spina bifida girls who had marked worries were all in special schools. Not only did they worry about 'life in general', they were also specifically worried by their incontinence problems. In the control group only one teenager was described by his mother as being a frequent worrier. He was always, she said, 'worrying about details, obsessive about little things being done on time . . . his mind is not at rest till he has done them'.

Occasionally, parents mentioned that they felt sure their child was worrying although this was never actually expressed. One mother of a very unforthcoming cerebral-palsied girl of well below average ability felt that 'she bottles up everything'. She thought she had emotions that she might want to let out but had no means of doing so. A mother of a cerebral-palsied boy, minimally handicapped but at a special school, felt the same. 'I'm sure he's bottling up worries which don't come out.' His father added, 'You've only to look at him to know that something is wrong'. In this case family relationships were so disturbed that the boy's reticence was not surprising.

In all groups, a higher proportion of teachers than of parents perceived the youngsters as worriers. Again, the difference between the control and handicapped groups was very marked, and again, it was the spina bifida girls who were perceived by teachers as being the greatest worriers. However, the proportion of teachers of handicapped pupils in ordinary schools who perceived their pupils as worrying was almost identical to that of teachers in special schools, so worrying did not appear to be related to type of school placement (although, as we discuss later, the nature of the worries expressed is often related to some aspect of schooling).

*Teenagers' own reports of worrying.* The general question put to the teenagers about worrying was worded as in the Isle of Wight Study of fourteen year olds: 'I suppose most teenagers worry about some things – apart from the things we've talked about already, what sort of things do you get worried about?' (The main problems already discussed had included feelings about boy/girlfriends, and about marriage; see Chapter 4.) Responses were rated on a three-point scale, results being rather similar to what parents had reported, with a considerably higher incidence of worrying in the handicapped group. Some gave rather general answers to this question (i.e. of the 'everything' type) while others were much more specific, such as school work (which is dealt with in greater detail later) or what would happen to them after leaving school. Fourteen young people raised this issue in terms like, 'What I'm going to do in the future', 'Whether I'll find a job', 'Whether I'll get into college', and so on.

Many of the worries reflected the underlying lack of self-confidence which many parents also commented on. For example, one boy worried because, although he was quite mobile, he was frightened to go anywhere without his mother, while two others, who were quite mildly handicapped, feared being left alone in the house.

It was expected that personal relationships, especially loneliness and peer relationships, would be a great source of anxiety for the adolescent group, but only a small number of them raised this in answer to the general question about worrying. Of those who did, five – all in special schools – mentioned not having friends, two referring particularly to the school holidays. Only two teenagers (one in an ordinary and one in a special school) mentioned teasing as a worry. Seven referred again to relationships with the opposite sex although this had been discussed fully at an earlier point in the interview. However, it should be remembered that since nearly 70 per cent of young people attended special schools they were rarely in situations where they encountered non-handicapped peers. (More questions about relationships with non-handicapped teenagers were included in the follow-up interviews. See Chapter 9.) Another point is that although teenagers often did not state explicitly that they worried about peer relationships, this was implicit in the remarks they made about worries related to being handicapped. For example, three hemiplegic boys (two in special, and one in an ordinary school) said: 'It's my arms . . . I'm embarrassed when people meet me.' '[I worry about] being stared at and talked about in the street . . . I get this every day, especially when I go out on my own.' A boy whose handicap was barely noticeable, and who earlier in the interview denied, quite justifiably, being 'handicapped', worried about 'how I look . . . what people think of me'.

A completely different area of concern was the worry voiced by five boarders about what was happening at home while they were away. Three, whose mothers were unsupported, said they worried, 'about what's happening at home, if Mum's upset. I think about it all night sometimes', or 'whether Mum has enough money'. One spina bifida girl said she constantly worried about 'what's happening at home, to my parents . . . it's always in my mind', while another broke down during the interview because she was so worried about her home, the arguments between her parents, and whether her mother was unhappy. But in general, teenagers very rarely at this point in the interview mentioned worries about family relationships. (This is discussed more fully in chapter 12.)

Only one teenager mentioned here worries about a health problem. However, in answer to item 8 on the Malaise Inventory ('Do you wear yourself out worrying about your health') 5 per cent of the cerebral-palsied group, compared with 3 per cent of the controls replied 'Yes', while 10 per cent of the spina bifida teenagers stated that they had health worries, reflecting the very real differences in the incidence of ill-health between this group, the cerebral-palsied group and the controls.

*School-related worries.*   The great majority of teenagers were happy at school, and the correlation between what they themselves said about this and what their parents said was very close (see Chapter 1). The proportion who said they were 'happy most of the time' was very similar for the control and the handicapped groups. However, when parents were specifically asked whether and how much their children worried about school work, it seemed that the handicapped pupils worried more about this than did the controls (44 per cent compared with 31 per cent), although it is interesting to note that those attending ordinary school did not worry about their work any more than did those attending special schools. The spina bifida children, however, worried rather more about their work (53 per cent) than did those with cerebral palsy (41 per cent) according to their parents.

On the teenagers' own report, only about half as many expressed school work to be a problem as the parents, but again there was no difference between those at ordinary schools and those in special schools. Exams, keeping up with homework, particular lessons, missing work due to absence were all mentioned, and four teenagers reported such worries interfering with their sleep. One spina bifida girl was extremely worried: 'I don't quite grasp the lessons at school, and I don't think I am ever going to grasp them . . . I'm not all that good at reading . . . and spelling . . . and especially Maths . . . I just have a cry. I feel I don't want to go to school . . . but once I'm there I'm all right, they're all so friendly.' Five youngsters in special schools and three in ordinary schools worried about 'getting into trouble' (generally in school). They all lacked confidence and worried about matters which seem small, but loomed large for them, such as 'doing anything wrong' or 'being told off' or 'not being in the right place'.

Another way in which their worries about school was assessed was by asking parents whether their child had, since starting at secondary school, ever gone through a stage of refusing to go to school or making a great deal of fuss about it.

Excluding those who got tearful before going back to boarding school but who were on the whole happy once there, eighteen parents with handicapped children (eleven in special and seven in ordinary schools) and one control said that there had been problems. In most cases these had been resolved during the first two years of secondary school, and only eight parents of handicapped teenagers said there were continuing problems. Five of these were special school pupils (one boy had refused to go back to school) and three were in ordinary schools. Although these three did 'make a fuss' about going to school in no case was the problem a severe one.

The first two years in an ordinary secondary school seems to be a time when handicapped children are especially vulnerable, and four cerebral-palsied children had gone through a stage of school refusal during this time. One boy had been teased so much at his comprehensive school that he refused to go anymore, and his parents had to get the Head to talk to the other pupils. The parents of a hemiplegic girl, also in a comprehensive, said that she had previously made a fuss about going to school especially at the end of the first year when she was 'down-graded' into rather a rough class. 'They were throwing things at her and calling names, even though the teacher was there. She came home in a state.' This girl was moved to another class after the father spoke to the Head. Now, said her mother, 'she seems to be OK once she's there. She likes the teacher . . . but she has a good moan each morning about how she hates school, and if there is any trouble she clams up.'

However, teasing was not found to be a problem only for those in ordinary schools, since six parents of teenagers in special schools reported similar kinds of problems, and it is very important to emphasize that all the disabled pupils in ordinary schools (expect one who was 'uncertain') said they would prefer ordinary to special school placement, despite any problems of this kind. (See chapter 3.)

*Misery and depression.* Misery and depression are commonly experienced among ordinary adolescents as has been reported both by Masterson (1967) and by Rutter *et al.* (1976). The latter found that nearly half of the sample reported 'some appreciable misery and depression and this was almost as common in boys as in girls'. Suicidal thoughts occurred in 8 per cent of their sample. These authors concluded that there could 'be no doubt' that inner experiences of misery were very common, although only a small minority appeared to be clinically depressed.

In his study of spina bifida teenagers, Dorner (1976) found that two-thirds of the group had experienced 'definite and recurring feelings of misery in the past year'. Moreover, 31 per cent of the girls and 15 per cent of the boys 'had had persistent periods of depression and/or suicidal thoughts'. Overall, girls were more likely to feel miserable and depressed than boys, and Dorner considered one reason for this was that the girls in his study had greater mobility problems than the boys, and were more isolated socially.

In our own study, information about misery and depression was obtained from three main sources – the parents, the teachers and the teenagers – who were asked in detail about misery and depression over the past year as well as whether they ever felt that life was 'hopeless or not worth living'. Further information was obtained from the Malaise Inventory.

*Report of parents and teachers.*    Table 5.8 shows that the handicapped adolescents were perceived both by their parents and by their teachers as being considerably more unhappy than were the controls, although only a small proportion of the handicapped group – less than 10 per cent and none of the controls – were perceived by either parents or teachers as having a *severe* problem of misery and depression. The spina bifida group, boys as well as girls (there was very little difference between them in this measure), were thought by both parents and teachers to suffer more from depression than the cerebral-palsied group.

Reports from the parents of the eight teenagers described as being 'frequently miserable', show a great variety of reactions among the young people and did not seem to be linked by a common thread. One mother of an attractive cerebral-palsied girl reported that it was a

Table 5.8 *Misery and depression in teenagers as perceived by their parents and teachers*

| Group | N | Parent interview | | Teachers' report (Rutter Scale) | |
|---|---|---|---|---|---|
| | | Severe problem (%) | Mild/ moderate problem (%) | Definitely miserable/ unhappy (%) | Somewhat miserable/ unhappy (%) |
| Physically handicapped | | | | | |
| Boys | 57 | (5) | (21) | (4) | (30) |
| Girls | 57 | (9) | (36) | (9) | (21) |
| Control | | | | | |
| Boys | 14 | (0) | (7) | (0) | (7) |
| Girls | 18 | (0) | (22) | (0) | (11) |
| IOW 14 year olds | | | | | |
| Boys | 93 | (2) | (5) | Not available | |
| Girls | 87 | (1) | (2) | | |

Table 5.9 *Misery and depression – self-reporting by the teenagers*

| | | Interview with teenager | | Malaise Inventory |
| | | Marked problem (%) | Mild/ moderate problem (%) | Often miserable and depressed (%) |
| Group | N | | | |
|---|---|---|---|---|
| Cerebral palsied | | | | |
| Boys | 48 | (21) | (42) | (24) |
| Girls | 38 | (34) | (53) | (47) |
| Spina bifida | | | | |
| Boys | 11 | (0) | (45) | (18) |
| Girls | 19 | (11) | (68) | (37) |
| Control | | | | |
| Boys | 15 | (0) | (47) | (20) |
| Girls | 18 | (17) | (33) | (17) |
| IOW 14 year olds | | | | |
| Boys | 93 | (9) | (34) | Not available |
| Girls | 87 | (9) | (36) | |

'continuous moan from the time she gets up to the time she gets to bed . . . It's been going on for about nine years . . . she always is miserable . . . just sits and moans all the time . . . I can't get down to why . . . there's always some little thing'. A severely handicapped spina bifida girl who attended a residential special school had had a 'marvellous life' in the past, according to her mother, but now 'sits miserable and vacant all the time'. Even some of the mildly handicapped teenagers were frequently miserable and depressed. One hemiplegic girl who attended an ordinary school was said by her mother to be 'unhappy a lot lately . . . because she's discovering herself.' She thought that boys had 'a lot to do with it'.

Table 5.9 shows the results from questions to the teenagers themselves. As we expected, many teenagers sometimes felt depressed, especially the handicapped teenagers. However, the difference between rates of depression expressed by the handicapped girls compared with the control girls was rather greater than between the boys, except that on self-reports of marked depression, the cerebral-palsied boys confessed to having such problems (21 per cent) whereas none of the spina bifida and control boys did. This may well indicate under-reporting, since the parents' reports indicated that they saw about 10 per cent of spina bifida boys as having marked problems with depression, while in the IOW Study

9 per cent of the non-handicapped boys admitted to having a marked problem. A striking point was that for all groups, including the controls, a very much higher proportion of teenagers reported being miserable or depressed than their parents or their teachers perceived. This too was noted both by Dorner (1976) and in the Isle of Wight Study.

The teenagers were also asked whether life ever felt hopeless or not worth living; those who had felt like this were then questioned further to find out whether they had had suicidal thoughts. Again, it was the cerebral-palsied teenagers who were most likely to be markedly unhappy – 29 per cent sometimes feeling life hopeless, compared with 17 per cent of those with spina bifida and 21 per cent of the controls. Four disabled teenagers and one control reported that at some period in their lives they had taken steps towards suicide, while a further six handicapped teenagers had had suicidal thoughts. Like non-handicapped teenagers, many of the handicapped teenagers felt depressed for no particular reason. As one boy said: 'It comes, then it goes away . . . When I feel really bad I do silly things . . . like riding my bike recklessly.' An epileptic, cerebral-palsied girl who had severe tantrums felt 'miserable most of the time and sometimes wanted to end it all . . . I wish I did end it all sometimes . . . though I don't really know why'.

Many teenagers, however, explicitly referred to depression about being handicapped. This was true of over two-thirds of the girls with spina bifida, although only two were rated as severely depressed. One said she got very emotional and cried a lot 'mostly about people not appreciating you for what you are', and frequently felt like committing suicide. The other said she frequently felt 'just miserable . . . and I make everybody else's life miserable, complaining about being handicapped and not having a boyfriend'. These are, of course, extreme examples but illustrate what many young people in the sample felt, although perhaps not so frequently and with less intensity.

However, in many other cases it was loneliness and boredom which caused the depression, rather than the handicap itself. One cerebral-palsied girl who attended a special school said she had 'nothing to do at home nearly every day and just felt thoroughly miserable about it'. This kind of loneliness and social isolation was described very frequently and it was perhaps the main reason for the unhappiness which so many young people felt. (See chapter 6.)

*Anxieties related to coping with new situations and meeting new people.* The lack of self-confidence of many of the adolescents often showed itself clearly when the youngster was faced with attempting something new or meeting an individual or peer group for the first time. Systematic information on anxiety relating to new situations and/or meeting new people was collected from four sources: (i) the parents' response during the interview to the question 'Would you describe X as the sort of person who tends to be fearful of attempting new situations' (followed up by specific probes); (ii) the teachers' replies to a question in the Rutter Scale as to whether X 'tends to be fearful or afraid of new things or new situations'; and (iii) the question (on the Malaise Inventory) which the teenager had to complete as to whether he or she 'was frightened of going out alone or of meeting people'. A problem with this last question is that it is not directly comparable with the parent or teacher reports since it is very specifically worded, and does not apply to some teenagers who were so heavily handicapped as to find it impossible to go out alone. If this was the case, they responded to the second half only – 'afraid of meeting people'.

The findings from these three different measures are summarized in Table 5.10. The figures for boys and girls are shown together, although the rates were rather higher for spina bifida girls than for the other handicapped groups.

Table 5.10 *Fearfulness in the handicapped and control groups*

| Group | Total N | Parent interview – definitely or somewhat fearful | | Teacher Scale – definitely or somewhat fearful | | Malaise Inventory – teenager report | |
|---|---|---|---|---|---|---|---|
| | | N | (%) | N | (%) | N | (%) |
| Cerebral-palsied | 86 | 36 | (42) | 46 | (53) | 22 | (25) |
| Spina bifida | 30 | 15 | (50) | 12 | (40) | 13 | (43) |
| Controls | 32 | 7 | (22) | 7 | (22) | 6 | (20) |

The findings show that, in general, about twice as many handicapped teenagers than control teenagers were seen to be, or saw themselves as being, fearful in new situations. The most informative measure was the parental report. Parents were required to be very specific and to describe examples of fearfulness during the last year, they were also asked about the amount of encouragement the child needed before attempting something new. Again, our overall impression was that of general rather than situation-specific fearfulness. Responses such as 'he's rather timid', 'he's no confidence', 'he hates new ventures', 'he's anxious . . . afraid of his limitations', were common, regardless of the nature or severity of the handicap. Much smaller numbers of control group parents (mainly with girls) made similar remarks: 'She lacks self-confidence . . . won't go anywhere or on her own', 'she needs a push, has got to have me behind her', 'she's a bit nervous about change'.

Three mothers described, in almost identical words, how strongly their children disliked or feared any sort of change: 'He doesn't like changes . . . likes things as they are . . . even small things.' 'She hates any changes at all . . . When there's a change of class there's always a scene . . . or if there's a new teacher . . . or if we go to a different place for our holiday. She hates any form of change at all.' 'He likes everything to be the same . . . he notices it even if I move things round the room.'

In some cases situations which caused anxiety were those which might well cause apprehension in any teenager – hospital appointments, going off on an assessment course, applying for a job, or going to a job interview. However, the handicapped teenagers were often reported as showing anxiety (in two cases accompanied by nervous rashes) in new situations which appeared to make comparatively small demands on a fifteen or sixteen year old, such as going to a shop, taking the initiative to buy sweets at a PHAB club canteen, or attempting to make toast.

Sometimes the teenagers' apprehension prevented them from trying out a school trip or attending a youth club which would have helped to alleviate their social isolation and loneliness. The following comments were typical: 'I took her to the [local youth] club for the first time . . . but she didn't like it . . . won't go back.' 'There's a tremendous rigmarole before she goes out . . . it's very difficult to persuade her to go anywhere, though she enjoys it when she does.' 'She's a bit of a recluse . . . she's normally anxious . . . I wanted to take her to try a youth club but she said, What will they think of me because I'm in a wheelchair?' 'She's definitely fearful . . . when we were on holiday she didn't even want to go out [of the caravan] . . . there was a youth club on the camp site . . . she wouldn't go . . . she won't walk into a roomful of strangers . . . I don't force her.'

While it was often the case that those teenagers who were most fearful of attempting new situations tended also to be those who lacked friends outside school, this was not always so. One attractive, moderately handicapped, cerebral-palsied boy, for example, who had many real friends, both handicapped and non-handicapped, was fearful about attempting new situations. He wouldn't join a PHAB club or a swimming club although he enjoyed swimming. On several occasions he had put his name down for a school outing or school holiday, but had withdrawn at the last moment, and he was adamant that he would not go away to college. His mother said that she couldn't understand what was behind it except that she thought he must just be 'unsure about whether he'll be able to cope'. Sometimes he gets 'a horrible feeling that he won't see me again'. So far 'I haven't pushed him', however she was now beginning to think that she should 'be forceful getting him over these things. It's no use letting him have his own way'.

When the teenagers were asked about fearfulness in meeting new people or going out alone, their responses again demonstrated a general lack of self-confidence and many handicapped young people gave examples of this. One girl said, 'Yes . . . I get hot and bothered . . . for instance, I was very worried about meeting you, and I panic when it's time to get back to [boarding] school, though I don't talk about it'.

Another replied, 'I get panicky . . . about meeting new people or doing new things'. Very few of the control group said they were frightened of meeting people or going somewhere they didn't know.

### Worries about specific aspects of the handicapping condition

(a) Anxieties about incontinence and its management.   In chapter 2 problems of incontinence management, especially of those with urinary bags were discussed, but we did not then consider specifically the teenagers' anxieties. However, after mothers had been asked how their children coped with their incontinence, they were then asked, 'How does . . . feel about his/her bladder problem – do you think he/she worries about it or that it gets him/her down?' Of the twenty-four young people with urinary bags there were only seven (29 per cent) whose mothers thought that they did not worry. Twelve (50 per cent) thought their children worried to some degree, and five (21 per cent) said that they were severely worried. One mother said, 'There are frequent accidents . . . she's very embarrassed . . . often in tears about it'. Another said, 'Lately she's been very depressed . . . she's worried about being smelly and that other people will know'. Several mentioned that their children worried about this much more now that they were older. One said, 'She's embarrassed about the bag being emptied, is anxious when we go out about whether there will be anywhere for her to go . . . she won't do it in front of other people. She's only been like this since she's older'. Another mother said she noticed her daughter's anxiety when 'you watch her putting on clothes . . . I see her eyes . . . she notices if the bag's showing at all . . . there's a great to-do in case anyone sees it. When it's being changed she often says why did I have to have this as well as my back'. Several mothers spoke of the young people's anxieties about having to tell a boy- or girlfriend about their incontinence, and this was confirmed in the discussion with teenagers themselves.

In some cases the teenager wouldn't talk much about it, but the mother felt there was underlying anxiety. 'It's hard to say . . . she won't put herself out for anyone . . . but it worries her that she can't wear nice clothes . . . it's on her mind all the time . . . I can see her feel it occasionally.' One boy never spoke directly to his mother about it, but she said: 'I know he's worried when he pulls faces . . . grumbles at the TV . . . he doesn't want others [peers] to know about it . . . he's always been like this.' No teenager had been actually teased or rejected on account of their incontinence, although the *fear* of this was clearly always present.

Another way of examining the extent of anxiety about incontinence was to ask both the teenagers and their parents which aspects of their handicap worried them most. All the young people with urinary appliances also had mobility problems which were severe in many cases, while some had additional problems such as epilepsy. The mothers themselves usually saw the incontinence as the greatest problem (almost 60 per cent), and only 25 per cent saw mobility as the major difficulty. However, although half the teenagers were more worried about their incontinence, half saw their impaired mobility as their primary difficulty. When parents were asked what they thought the teenager was most worried about, although they were generally correct, they tended to underestimate the extent to which the young people were worried about both incontinence and poor mobility.

This raised the question of the extent to which teenagers confided in parents about their incontinence problems. Eighteen parents said that their children were able to discuss these anxieties at least with one parent – the girls being more likely to discuss it with their mother only. However, two mothers said that there was 'nothing to discuss', and in four other cases the question hadn't been discussed, although each of these teenagers (all boys) had said that they felt incontinence to be their greatest problem. Two of these mothers said that their sons 'didn't give much away', although they were aware that they were worried. Another said her son used to talk about it, but had 'clammed up' in recent years.

*(b) Anxieties about speech defects.*   As noted in chapter 1, over half the cerebral-palsied teenagers had speech defects. In twenty-one cases the defects were comparatively mild, but twenty-eight teenagers (one-third of the group) had defects ranging from moderate to profound. The parents were not asked directly about the extent to which the young people felt upset and frustrated because of their difficulties in communication, but twenty of the twenty-eight parents whose teenagers had moderate or profound defects said quite spontaneously, in response to a question about peer relationships, that they experienced some anxiety or frustration in this respect. Many mothers mentioned that their teenagers became upset because other people hadn't the patience to listen to them. Typical comments were: 'People often can't understand her . . . she hasn't met the neighbours . . . she's still very nervous about it, especially meeting new people.' 'It's not only his speech but he dribbles too. He gets embarrassed . . . it's worse if he's concentrating. He's grown up with the children in his area but they only play with him if there's no one else around.' 'The majority of local children are scared of him . . . they're not being unkind, they just don't want to know.' 'The local kids stare and he gets very frustrated . . . his brother's friends are OK . . . when he's with strange people or in a strange place he's reluctant to talk in case they don't understand. Once he knows he's understood it makes his day.'

Many young people with moderate or severe defects had adjusted well to their difficulties, so these problems were not inevitable. For example, the mother of one athetoid boy with a severe speech defect said that he had accepted this very well and had got to know several local children, some of whom 'seem to understand more of his speech than adults . . . he's very good repeating what he says and saying it in a different way . . . he's very persistent about trying'. However, the majority definitely needed advice about how to cope with strangers, and this seems a group for whom social skills training, including role-playing, might be valuable.

*(c) Anxieties about epilepsy.* Mothers were asked whether their children felt worried or depressed about their fits, if so what exactly it was that worried them, and also if they thought their child's epilepsy made it more difficult for him or her to make friends. Most parents, especially those whose children had only occasional fits, said that they were not worried about this, but nine parents (out of a total of twenty-three with fits) said that their children did worry. In two cases the anxiety was mild, and in seven cases more marked. Only two parents thought their child's fits (in one case both frequent and severe) had affected peer relationships.

The seven who definitely worried included one boy who tended to get depressed because his frequent major fits (at least once and sometimes several times daily) meant that he couldn't go out unaccompanied. This made him angry and jealous of his seventeen year old sister. His recent move to a residential special school had given him a much fuller social life than had been possible at home. While at an ordinary school his fits had affected his relationships with his peers, not because he was teased about them, but because he could not go out with them. However, according to her mother, one girl had become more worried about her fits since going to a school for cerebral-palsied teenagers since she often saw others having fits and was frightened about what happened to her when she had one. When asked the general question about worries this girl had referred specifically to epilepsy because the fit 'lasts so long . . . can last fifteen minutes . . . my mind goes blank and I can't hear anything they're saying.' Another boy was also worried about the fit itself, for example of falling and hurting himself, or of having a fit while using public transport, and his mother said that 'he panics if he's not taken his pill'. She thought that his condition might have affected his relationships with his peers in his special school. One girl in an ordinary school also worried about her fits, even though they were infrequent (once a year or less), and had never occurred at school. She was worried about what her peers would think if they knew. After her last fit (a major one) she was adamant that the school not be told the reason for her three-day absence from school.

## Aggressive and anti-social behaviour

Although the teenagers were much more likely to have problems of an 'emotional' type than to show overt anti-social behaviour, this did occur in all of the groups, and showed itself most frequently in general irritability or, in a minority of cases, actual temper tantrums. Apart from irritability other types of conduct disorders were relatively uncommon. For example, lying was reported in only about 10 per cent of all groups, while only one handicapped pupil and one control habitually truanted.

The parents were specifically asked whether the teenager 'ever has moods of being cross or irritable, or temper tantrums'. In all groups a substantial proportion of teenagers – generally from 40–60 per cent, (although less for the control boys) – showed some degree of irritability, but in comparatively few (only 11 per cent of handicapped and one control) was there a severe problem. It was the cerebral-palsied teenagers who seemed to have the most intense problems, some giving vent to severe tantrums or rages on occasions. The spina bifida teenagers were more likely to be described as being very irritable rather than as having rages. Looking at the information given by parents alongside that given by the teachers on the Rutter Scale suggested that irritability and temper tantrums tended to be present either at school or at home, but not in both; thus of the fifteen teenagers reported by parents as being very irritable at home, only four were reported by teachers as being very irritable at school.

The teenagers themselves were also asked during the interview whether they sometimes found that they got irritable and bad-tempered, and further probes were made to ascertain the severity of the problem. Only eight said that they were irritable or bad-tempered and, in contrast to depression, self-reporting was lower for irritability than from parental reports. One boy said he became very irritable whenever his handicap prevented him from doing something (e.g., buttoning clothes). Another got irritable in school (a special school) when other children 'boss me around'. Then he said, 'I do really flare at them – more or less every day'. Only one spina bifida teenager, a boy, reported frequently getting irritable. This happened at his special school when other pupils said things that were not true, or made fun about his getting into trouble, when he would 'let rip'.

Among the controls, the three girls who said that they got irritable were all very frank about this. One had a difficult relationship with her mother and got particularly irritable as she felt her mother didn't understand that she needed time to herself to study. Another described herself as 'moody and snappy' most of the day. The third said she frequently got annoyed by 'other people' at school and would take it out on them or on her mother.

## Summary and conclusions

Overall the findings in this study on the extent of psychological problems confirm previous work in that the rates for the physically handicapped teenagers, all of whom suffered from conditions associated with cortical malfunctioning, was three to four times higher than for the controls. It must be emphasized that a difference of this order would not be expected for handicapped young people where the condition did not involve neurological impairment. The overall rate of problems shown by our control group (15 per cent) was also very similar to that reported by others.

Severity of handicap was related to the proportion of *marked* problems shown, but approximately half the teenagers were without overt problems regardless of the degree of handicap. However, even the mildly handicapped showed a much higher rate of problems overall and of 'marked' problems than did the controls.

Within the handicapped group, the spina bifida boys seemed to have fewer overt problems than did the spina bifida girls or the cerebral-palsied boys and girls. However, it seems possible that this difference may not be reliable (the numbers being quite small) since the proportion of spina bifida boys showing problems was much higher in Dorner's study (1976). The fact that both interviewers were female may also have affected the rate of reporting by spina bifida boys of problems arising with the presence of urinary appliances. In general, however, the spina bifida girls appeared to present more problems than any other group.

Looking at the types of disorder shown, we found that most disorders were of the neurotic type, and that conduct disorders were relatively infrequent, especially among the spina bifida group. As one might expect, the rates for conduct disorders in boys were rather higher than in girls. Findings from the Rutter Teacher's Scale and the Malaise Inventory (as completed by the teenagers) generally agreed with the overall pattern shown by the clinical ratings, that is, the difference in the rate of disorder between the control and physically handicapped teenagers and the preponderance of neurotic rather than conduct disorders.

The main problems shown were depression, fearfulness and worrying with specific anxieties related to schooling and to particular aspects of handicap. About 60 per cent of the physically handicapped were said to worry, compared with 40 per cent of controls, although the proportion regarded by parents as severe worriers was about the same in each group (6 per cent). Whereas the control parents reported only 15 per cent of their teenagers as getting depressed, all of whom were thought to have a mild problem only, 30 per cent of parents of handicapped children thought they got depressed, including 7 per cent who had a severe problem. Depression was also more common among girls than boys. If self-reports were used, then the rates for depression rise to 70 per cent for the handicapped group and 50 per cent for the controls, with about twice as many of the handicapped reporting a marked problem as the controls. Anxiety in coping with new situations or in meeting new people was about twice as common among the physically handicapped teenagers than the controls, whether parents, teachers or self-reports were considered.

The only conduct disorder reported at all frequently was irritability – 11 per cent for handicapped teenagers compared with 3 per cent for controls. Among the spina bifida group, where the behaviour described was not really extreme, this may well have been the overt expression of general tension and depression, while among the cerebral-palsied group really violent rages were sometimes reported, which seemed to be quite different in kind and possibly were related to neurological disorders of some kind.

In general, the handicapped group presented frequently as lacking in self-confidence, having low self-esteem, and worrying about their handicaps and lack of skills, and in consequence very often showing signs of real misery and depression. However, it should also be remembered that about half of the handicapped young people were rated as having 'satisfactory adjustment', and only about one-third were thought to have marked problems.

The questions which arise next are, what were the factors associated with the presence of psychological problems or adjustment, and is there any pattern which might explain why some handicapped young people are very worried and concerned about their situation while others are not? The next chapter will attempt to throw some light on these questions.

# 6

## Factors associated with teenagers' psychological problems

### Introduction

Our aim in this study was not only to decide the prevalence and nature of the psychological problems of the young people with cerebral palsy and spina bifida, but also to examine a range of factors which might be associated with the presence of these problems. Can we give any indication as to why some disabled young people were relatively free from marked psychological problems, often despite severe physical disabilities, while others, sometimes less disabled, had severe problems? Why was it that the spina bifida girls seemed more likely than the other groups to suffer from depression and anxiety?

These are important questions since, if we can elucidate even some of the factors which are strongly associated with the presence of problems (we have deliberately chosen the term 'associated' rather than 'caused') then we are in a better position to do two things. First, we can alert teachers, doctors, social workers, psychologists and others as to which young people (and indeed children) are most vulnerable to anxiety and depression so that they can keep a closer eye on these youngsters and provide extra support before the problems become acute. Secondly, if we have clues about the origins of these problems we are in a better position to suggest the nature of the support and practical help which is required by teenagers and their families. In Section A we look at the approaches and some of the findings of other studies, and in Section B at our own findings. The studies discussed in Section A are mainly of non-handicapped young people, but it seems likely that factors which influence the adjustment of ordinary teenagers will have equal relevance for those who are disabled. In chapter 5 many of the additional stresses imposed by and specific to disability were discussed. In this chapter we do not neglect 'handicap' factors, but also wish to draw attention to the ordinary adverse factors which affect the psychological adjustment of *all* young people.

### Section A: Findings from other studies

#### Clinical Studies

Most studies of psychological disorders in both non-handicapped and handicapped children have been clinically rather than epidemiologically based, and most of the suggestions made as to the possible origin of the disorders have been made on the basis of clinical experience rather than systematically gathered statistical evidence. Examples in the case of non-handicapped young people are the books by Weiner (1970) and Masterson (1967) and a more recent article by Framrose (1977). We have already referred to a number of clinical studies of disabled young people – Freeman's article (1970) on cerebral palsy, the studies by Bagley (1971), by Goldin *et al.* (1971), and Richardson and Friedman (1974) of epileptics, and Volpe's study (1976) of Canadian orthopaedically handicapped children. These and other general accounts, such as Mattson's discussion (1972) of the effects of long-term illness in childhood, are referred to in Pless and Pinkerton's review (1975) of recent studies on adjustment in chronically disabled children and young people.

In most clinical studies, the influence of parental attitudes upon the development of the handicapped child's self-concept, and the dangers of parental over-protection or, to a much lesser extent, rejection, e.g., Kogan and Tyler's work (1973), are emphasized. Adverse family and social factors which might equally well operate in families with non-handicapped children are also discussed. Such studies are also concerned with the specific characteristics of disability upon adjustment, for example the type or site of the lesion, its visibility, the extent to which it is or is not socially acceptable and so on. Clinical studies can provide valuable insights into the processes which may give rise to disorders in individual non-handicapped or handicapped adolescents. However, conditions such as cerebral palsy and spina bifida are comparatively rare, and very few clinicians have extensive experience of a group with specific problems, such as teenagers with spina bifida (an exception is Dorner, 1975; 1976).

*Epidemiological studies: factors associated with disorders in ordinary adolescents*

Three main groups of factors have been investigated on an epidemio-logical basis in 'normal' children and young people. These are, 'person-ality' factors, family factors, and school factors.

*'Personality' factors.*   'Personality' factors refer to attributes within the child, rather than within his family or environment, which influence the development of his psychological problems. The two most important in non-handicapped children are *sex* and *age*. Rutter and his colleagues (1970; 1976) have found that rates of childhood psychiatric disorder are different between boys and girls, and to some extent between adolescence and childhood, as we have already indicated in chapter 5.

Much less well researched is the relationship between psychological disorders and what have sometimes been called 'temperamental' factors, that is relatively persistent dispositional traits which are established very early in life and are probably partly innate and partly determined by very early environmental factors. The classic work on such traits was done in America by Thomas, Chess and Birch (1968). Their New York long-itudinal study, suggested that a wide range of personality characteristics measurable in infants (including activity levels, adaptability, intensity, persistence and distractability) may predict later behaviour disorders.

Their work has in part been confirmed by Graham et al.'s study (1973) of adverse temperamental characteristics (ATC). They suggest that while it 'seems improbable that ATC lead directly to psychiatric disorders . . . it appears that particular ATC renders the child more vulnerable to the adverse effects of family discord and other "stress factors".' The effects of ATC on other people are likely to be influential. 'The very difficult infant [e.g., the highly irregular, unadaptable child with pre-ponderantly negative mood] may be more likely to elicit critical feelings from his mother and more liable to generate discord between his parents. Similarly, parents are sure to be more intolerant when diffi-culties arise later in such unattractive or less lovable children.' Such characteristics may be modified by organic dysfunction. A comparative study of ATC in infants with a diagnosis of cerebral palsy or hydro-cephalus would be exceedingly valuable, although there would be very large methodological problems to overcome. But it is highly likely that some of the young people in our study, because of personality traits noticeable to parents from an early age, may have been more vulnerable to stress or to adverse parental reactions although this was not something we could measure.

*Family factors.* The second group of factors which may be associated with psychological disorders are family factors. Rutter *et al.* (1975) found that psychiatric disorders were twice as common in 10–11 year old children attending school in an Inner London borough than they were in 10–11 year olds in the Isle of Wight. In attempting to account for this difference they identified four sets of variables which were associated with disorder and deviance in both areas, but were much more common in London families. Three were family factors – 'family discord, parental deviance and social disadvantage'. 'Family discord' included marital discord producing 'unhappy disruptive quarrelsome homes', and 'a broken home', that is, where the child was not living with both natural parents. These factors have been frequently referred to in clinical studies of disorder.

'Parental deviance' included families in which the father had been convicted of some offence and/or had been in prison, but a more common type of parental deviance was psychiatric disorder in the mother. Another study of Rutter's (1966) shows that children of mentally ill parents were particularly at risk of developing psychiatric disorders. In the IOW Study, psychiatric disorder in the mothers, usually comprising 'mild chronic or recurrent depressive or neurotic conditions' (Rutter, 1970), was present in half of the mothers of children with psychiatric disorder, but in only 10 per cent of the mothers of 'normal' children. The same association of disorder between mother and child was not, however, found in London 'largely because of the very high rates of disorders in the mothers of normal children'.

A factor examined in the IOW Study of fourteen year olds was 'alienation' between the teenagers and one or both parents. Teenagers in the 'psychiatric disorder' group were more likely than those in the non-disorder group to quarrel with their parents, show physical or emotional withdrawal or communication difficulties, and fewer went out with their parents. However, most parents said that this alienation had begun when the child was much younger: only in a very few cases did it arise in adolescence. Also it was more common in children with persistent disorders than with new disorders. Thus, alienation *arising for the first time* in adolescence was not, the authors concluded, a common causal factor in adolescent disorder, although long-term estrangement between parents and children was.

Other factors associated with the presence of psychiatric disorders in the children were related to social class (children with fathers in semi-skilled or unskilled jobs were more likely to show disorders), overcrowding (more than one person per useable room), and family size, 'four or more children living in the household' being the best discriminator in the Isle of Wight families, and 'five or more children born to the mother' in the London families.

*School factors.* What of the impact of the environment outside the home upon the child or adolescent? Rutter *et al.* (1979) introduce their important study of secondary schools and their effects on children with these words:

> For almost a dozen years during a formative period of their development children spend almost as much of their waking life at school as at home. Altogether this works out at some *15,000 hours* during which schools and teachers may have an impact on the development of the children in their care. Does a child's experience at school have any effect; does it matter which school he goes to; and which are the features of the school that matter?

One of the main conclusions was that the 'children's observed behaviour in the school was strongly associated with school process variables' that is, with some of the factors which discriminated between individual schools. The authors go on to say that there are 'other aspects of children's behaviour which may be strongly influenced by . . . personal, family and social variables. But for the behaviours we considered it seemed that to a very large extent they developed as the child's response to the school environment he encountered.'

Earlier work by Rutter and his colleagues (1975) had already shown that among 10–11 year olds there was a significant association between psychiatric disorder and certain school features, that is, children in schools with a higher turnover of teachers and/or children showing high deviance rates, such as delinquency and truancy.

## Factors associated with disorders in neurologically impaired young people

The studies described above were all of non-handicapped children and adolescents. The only large-scale study of disorders among those with neurological dysfunction, in which an attempt was made to examine factors associated with disorder, was the study of 'neuro-epileptic' 10–11 year olds (those with cerebral palsy or epilepsy) on the Isle of Wight, already referred to in chapter 5. Rutter, Graham and Yule (1970) point out that while the rate of disorder was about four times higher in this group than in non-handicapped children, many of the associated factors were similar in both groups. Psychiatric disorder did not correlate with social class or family size but it was 'considerably and signficantly' more common in youngsters from an overcrowded household, a broken home, a family in which there was marital discord, and in children whose mothers themselves had psychiatric disorders.

## Section B: Factors associated with disorders in our own study

### (i) Clinical impressions of factors associated with the presence of psychological disorders

Before finalizing our 'overall adjustment' rating for each teenager, we wrote concise summaries for all sixty-one teenagers whom we considered to have either 'marked' problems (N = 39) or 'some' problems (N = 22), including our impressions of the factors in the child, the family and the school which appeared to be related to the presence of the disorder. Many if not most of the teenagers' problems had their origins prior to the teens, and although we made no attempt to obtain data relating to the pre-school or primary school period, parents sometimes raised this spontaneously. In the majority of cases several causal factors were at work, including interactions too complicated to disentangle between the teenager's reaction to his handicap and that of his parents.

Clearly, this cross-sectional approach has great limitations but we believe we were able to identify at least some of the main factors which, at the time of interview and in the year preceding it, had given rise to or were maintaining the teenager's problems. In about one-half of the cases (thirty) one factor appeared to be of particular importance, for example the mother's mental health, or the teenager's anxiety about incontinence, or the presence of epilepsy and in the other half (twenty-seven) two major factors were present. In four of our cases we had no definite idea about the origins of the disorder. In *all* cases, however, there were many interactions between the factors we considered as of particular importance and other factors in the teenager, the family and society, and especially the school. These are listed in Table 6.1.

The table speaks for itself and we only wish to add two points. The first is that we were constantly struck by the association between problems in the teenagers and adverse family factors. These appeared to play an important part in the disorder in forty-one of the sixty-one teenagers with 'marked' or 'some' problems and (except for c and e) were factors which have been found to affect the well-being of non-handicapped youngsters. There is no clear evidence to suggest that a higher proportion of handicapped than of non-handicapped teenagers come from such pathogenic families. However, the effect of depression in a mother, or of a family too burdened to be able to give much time to any one member, is more likely to be damaging to a handicapped teenager simply because he or she is more likely to feel insecure, vulnerable and in need of support.

The second point is that where factors in the teenager were concerned, there were only four definite and three possible cases (group a) where the clinical evidence indicated a clear link between the *neurological* impairment as such and the disturbed behaviour. All the other factors recorded here were related to the handicap itself rather than to 'personality', although where the parents thought the child had always been shy (that is, a 'temperamental' factor) this might have been entirely unrelated to the handicap.

*(ii) Statistical associations between these factors and the presence of psychological problems*

*(1) Factors in the young people – severity of handicap and overall adjustment.* In chapter 5 we found that there was a much higher incidence of psychological problems among the cerebral-palsied and spina bifida teenagers than among the non-handicapped adolescents, whether these were the 14–15 year olds surveyed on the Isle of Wight, or our own small control group (see Table 5.1). In our study, it was the spina bifida girls who showed the highest rates of disorders.

When the incidence of psychological problems was considered in relation to severity of handicap, the results show that although the proportion in each group whose adjustment was rated as satisfactory did not differ greatly (about a half in each group), differences were apparent

Table 6.1 *Clinical impressions of particularly important factors associated with the presence of psychological problems*

| *Teenagers with 'some' or 'marked' problems* | *N = 61* |
| --- | --- |

*Factors in the teenagers*
a) Organic damage: problems secondary to epilepsy in six cases and undiagnosed 'turns' in one. Four seemed definitely related to organic damage, and three possibly. ... 7
b) Constitutional/temperamental factors, e.g. mother reports child has always been anxious and over-reacted to stress. ... 5
c) Frustration because of communication problem (i.e. hearing or speech defect). ... 5
d) Anxiety related to the social consequnces of incontinence. ... 6
e) Self-consciousness about handicap and resentment about being handicapped (i.e., handicap has come to dominate teenager's thoughts and to have marked effect on behaviour). ... 7

*Factors in the family*
a) Mother's mental health affects her ability to give teenager the necessary support (e.g., severe depression, agoraphobia, other neurotic problems). ... 8
b) Poor marital relationship, and evidence that teenager worried about this. ... 5
c) Other disturbance in family relationships affecting the teenager. Either overt or covert rejection by one or other parent (in three cases by mother, in three by father) or general disturbance of intra-family relationships (two cases), or upbringing in institution (one case). ... 9
d) Generally unsupportive family. No evidence of rejection related to handicap. These included large, disorganized families or overburdened families (e.g. many young children or single working parent and/or low income) and included one family where both parents were disabled. ... 12
e) Families which gave too much support. We have tried to avoid the misused term 'over-protection', but in these cases it was marked. Four of the seven teenagers concerned were in ordinary schools. ... 7

*Factors in the environment*
a) Disorder related to unhappy/inappropriate school placement now or in past. This group included three hearing-impaired CP children who had had constant changes of school, one who hated his current boarding school, and two whose problems were attributed in part by parents to previous unhappy school placements. ... 6
b) Rejection/teasing by peers. All these teenagers were at ordinary schools. ... 4
c) Social isolation. Teenager goes out very little, especially in the school holidays, and feels depressed and unconfident most of the time. Has no really close friends even at school. ... 12

Table 6.2 *Psychological problems related to sex and degree of handicap*

| | Mild handicap | | | | Moderate or severe handicap | | | |
|---|---|---|---|---|---|---|---|---|
| | Boys | | Girls | | Boys | | Girls | |
| | N | (%) | N | (%) | N | (%) | N | (%) |
| Marked problems | 3 | (19) | 2 | (20) | 14 | (30) | 20 | (42) |
| Some problems | 7 | (44) | 1 | (10) | 6 | (13) | 8 | (16) |
| Satisfactory adjustment | 6 | (37) | 7 | (70) | 25 | (56) | 20 | (42) |
| Total | 16 | (100) | 10 | (100) | 45 | (100) | 48 | (100) |

between those with mild handicaps and those with moderate or severe handicaps if the incidence of marked problems only was considered. Among the mildly handicapped fewer than 20 per cent had marked problems compared with between 30–40 per cent for those with more severe handicaps (see Table 6.2). These differences were not related to type of handicap since in the cerebral-palsied and the spina bifida groups there were similar proportions of boys and of girls with mild, moderate and severe handicaps. However, since many studies of disorder show sex to be an important variable, we looked at sex differences among the mildly handicapped and among those with moderate and severe handicaps in relation to overall ratings of problems. The results are shown in Table 6.2. These findings show that, contrary to expectation, there was no clear relationship between sex and the incidence of problems in those with moderate or severe handicap, while in the case of the mildly handicapped teenagers, fewer girls had problems (though the numbers here were very small).

*The presence of specific disabilities and overall adjustment.* The relationship between overall adjustment and particular disabilities such as incontinence, epilepsy and speech disorders, is examined next. First we looked at presence of a urinary appliance, since this is a source of great anxiety to young people. We compared the presence of problems in those with and without appliances, considering only those teenagers who were severely handicapped, since it seemed important to hold this factor constant (see Table 6.3). In fact, all but two of those with appliances were rated as severely handicapped. Of the twenty-two young people with appliances, fourteen (twelve girls and two boys) had urinary diversions, and eight penile bags.

As expected, a much higher rate of disorder was found in the group with urinary appliances, twice as many of whom had marked problems or problems overall. It is reasonable to assume that this can be attributed to

Table 6.3 *Overall adjustment and presence of a urinary appliance*

| Group | Total N | Overall adjustment | | | | | |
|---|---|---|---|---|---|---|---|
| | | Marked problems | | Some problems | | Satisfactory adjustment | |
| | | N | (%) | N | (%) | N | (%) |
| Severely handicapped teenagers who have urinary appliances | 22 | 9 | (41) | 5 | (23) | 8 | (36) |
| Severely handicapped teenagers who do not have urinary appliances | 29 | 7 | (24) | 4 | (14) | 18 | (62) |

the teenagers' constant anxiety about incontinence management, or about the possible reaction of others to their incontinence.

Many studies, some of which were referred to in chapter 5, have shown that children and young people with epilepsy are particularly likely to develop psychological problems. As noted in chapter 1, we did not find it possible to differentiate between the teenager's type of epilepsy, although it is well known that there are particularly strong associations between behaviour disorders and certain types of epilepsy, in particular temporal lobe epilepsy. In our own analysis we simply made a comparison of adjustment in those cerebral-palsied teenagers with and without a diagnosis of epilepsy, regardless of how well controlled this was. The results are shown in Table 6.4.

The findings show a marked difference between those with and without epilepsy both in the proportion with marked problems and in the proportion with satisfactory adjustment. Over two-thirds of the teenagers with a diagnosis of epilepsy had marked problems compared with only one-fifth of those with no such diagnosis, while only 21 per cent of those with epilepsy were judged to be 'adjusted', compared with almost 60 per cent of those without. This was despite the fact that fits were generally well controlled, and that there were only seven teenagers who were fitting at least monthly.

Table 6.4 *Overall adjustment and epilepsy*

| Group | Total N | Overall adjustment | | | | | |
|---|---|---|---|---|---|---|---|
| | | Marked problems | | Some problems | | Satisfactory adjustment | |
| | | N | (%) | N | (%) | N | (%) |
| CP teenagers with epilepsy | 19 | 13 | (68) | 2 | (11) | 4 | (21) |
| CP teenagers without epilepsy | 64 | 13 | (20) | 14 | (22) | 37 | (58) |

Table 6.5 *Adjustment and the presence of a speech defect*

| | | Overall adjustment | | | | | |
|---|---|---|---|---|---|---|---|
| Group | Total N | Marked problems N | (%) | Some problems N | (%) | Satisfactory adjustment N | (%) |
| CP teenagers with marked speech disorders | 17 | 2 | (12) | 3 | (18) | 12 | (71) |
| CP teenagers with slight speech disorders | 18 | 5 | (28) | 2 | (11) | 11 | (61) |
| CP teenagers without speech disorder | 24 | 6 | (25) | 7 | (29) | 11 | (46) |

Next we looked at those cerebral-palsied young people who had no speech defects and compared them with those who had a mild defect and those who had moderate or severe defects. We omitted from this analysis young people with epilepsy or with 'other' types of seizures, and those with a hearing loss. This left us with seventeen whose speech defects were marked, eighteen with mild defects, and twenty-four with normal speech. The findings (shown in Table 6.5) show that there was no evidence to suggest that a speech defect of itself led to psychological problems, which is surprising in view of the fact that many parents spoke of the difficulties and frustrations which the young people experienced in communicating with people outside the family.

The numbers were small so that the finding cannot be taken as conclusive, but it is of considerable interest. One possibility is that teenagers with marked defects had inadequate means of communicating the extent of their anxieties either to their parents or to the interviewers, and were in fact a less well-adjusted group than they appeared to be. However, we do not believe this was so in most cases, and many of those with severe speech defects, who were almost always athetoids, appeared both to us and to their parents genuinely to have come to terms with their disabilities compared with many of the other cerebral-palsied teenagers. However, the whole issue of coping with a severe speech defect (in those whose hearing is normal) requires further investigation.

The last group we consider briefly were the five cerebral-palsied teenagers with marked hearing impairments. This is too small a number to make any reliable comparison of their adjustment with that of the other young people. Also, two of the five, both of whose adjustment was rated as satisfactory, came from Indian families and received a great deal of support from a large extended family network and for this reason cannot be considered representative of hearing-impaired cerebral-palsied teenagers (especially in view of Cochrane's recent findings (1979) on the lower rates of psychiatric disorder in Asian families).

Of the other three teenagers with a hearing impairment, two rated as having 'marked' problems. One, a severely handicapped girl, attended a PH school which her mother felt was not really meeting her needs, and the staff there reported anti-social behaviour. She found both her hearing impairment and her poor mobility (she depended on a wheelchair outside the home) hard to adjust to. At home she sometimes got into violent tempers and hit people if she was unable to express herself or if other people could not understand her. The other was a boy who, after a long series of unsatisfactory school placements, had recently entered a residential school for children with hearing impairments and other handicaps. Both he and his parents felt this was the first appropriate placement he had ever had. Problems noted by the school included anti-social and aggressive behaviour, although this was less evident now than formerly. He was still a 'loner', didn't mix well, and was 'immature' in his behaviour compared to his peers; he also showed much attention-seeking behaviour. At home he had no friends, and when he could not understand what was going on his behaviour was extremely demanding.

*IQ and overall adjustment.* The last main factor in the teenagers which was looked at in relation to overall adjustment was IQ. The teenagers were not tested by the researchers, but all the data already available, including teachers' ratings, were used to assign them to one of two main groups: those with IQs of 85 or above, and those with IQs of below 85. Sixty-seven of the handicapped teenagers (56 per cent) fell into the IQ 85+ category. Within the cerebral-palsied group, forty-nine (55 per cent) fell into the 85+ range, compared with eighteen (60 per cent) of the spina bifida group. In Table 6.6 overall psychological adjustment is looked at in relation to IQ, taking into account severity of handicap.

These findings show a most marked and consistent trend: irrespective of severity of handicap, a much higher proportion of teenagers with IQs below 85 were likely to have marked psychological problems, and a much lower proportion to be in the 'satisfactory adjustment' group.

*(2) Family factors.* At the beginning of this chapter some of the family

Table 6.6 *IQ and overall adjustment, taking into account severity of handicap*

| Overall adjustment | Mildly handicapped | | | | Moderately handicapped | | | | Severely handicapped | | | |
| | IQ 85+ | | IQ below 85 | | IQ 85+ | | IQ below 85 | | IQ 85+ | | IQ below 85 | |
| | N | (%) | N | (%) | N | (%) | N | (%) | N | (%) | N | (%) |
|---|---|---|---|---|---|---|---|---|---|---|---|---|
| Marked probems | 2 | (11) | 3 | (43) | 8 | (29) | 10 | (67) | 4 | (19) | 12 | (40) |
| Some problems | 5 | (28) | 2 | (29) | 3 | (11) | 3 | (20) | 3 | (14) | 6 | (20) |
| Satisfactory adjustment | 11 | (61) | 2 | (29) | 17 | (60) | 2 | (13) | 14 | (67) | 12 | (40) |
| Total | 18 | (100) | 7 | (100) | 28 | (100) | 15 | (100) | 21 | (100) | 30 | (100) |

factors which have been found to be associated with psychological disorders in non-handicapped adolescents were discussed. It was possible to examine some of these in the present study in two main groups; first, those we term 'psychosocial factors', including the physical and mental health of the parents; a report by the mother herself on over-protection of the teenagers; marital discord; membership of a one-parent family, family size. The other group consisted of socio-economic factors including social class, overcrowding and poverty.

*Physical health of parents and adjustment in the teenagers.* The ability of parents to offer teenagers support will to some extent be determined by their own physical and mental health. Although we focused almost entirely on the mothers, we did also ask them whether their husbands had 'a health problem or handicap'. Our main purpose in asking this question was to find out whether the health of the parents of the disabled teenagers differed in any significant way from that of the control group, and also whether the parents' state of health was related to the young person's adjustment.

The proportion of fathers with physical and/or mental health problems as reported by their spouses was almost identical for all three groups. Sixty-seven per cent of fathers of cerebral-palsied teenagers, 65 per cent of spina bifida teenagers and 69 per cent of control group fathers were said to be in good health, and only three fathers (two of controls, one of a cerebral-palsied boy) had severe health problems. We had no evidence that the father's state of health was related to the overall adjustment of the teenagers.

The mothers were asked a series of detailed questions designed to elicit information about the nature and extent of any current physical and/or mental health problems. On physical health, they were asked how their health was at the moment, whether, during the past twelve months they had had any problems or had been to their doctors, a clinic or a hospital, whether they had been prescribed any medication for their health and if so whether they were still taking it now. Each question was followed by very detailed probes related to when the problem had occurred, its frequency and severity, precipitating factors, and the effect of the problem on the mother's functioning and relationships. On the basis of all information obtained an overall rating was made of the mother's present *physical* health. There was no difference in the incidence of physical ill-health between the mothers of controls or handicapped teenagers, a finding similar to Gath's (1977) in her study of children with Down's Syndrome. Half the mothers in each group had mild or moderate problems, and only three had severe health problems, (two with a cerebral-palsied teenager, and one with a spina bifida teenager). No relationship was found between mothers' physical ill-health and the presence of problems in the teenager.

*Mothers' mental health and adjustment in the teenagers.* In relation to mothers' mental health, one question which differentiated between the controls and those with a handicapped child was whether the mother had 'been to a clinic or hospital in the past twelve months to see a specialist about a problem with tiredness . . . headaches . . . poor sleep . . . depression . . . any pains . . . nerves?' Only 13 per cent of mothers of controls had been to a clinic or hospital compared to nearly twice as many mothers of handicapped teenagers. This is very similar to the proportion (27 per cent) of mothers of spina bifida adolescents reported by Dorner (1975) as having been to the doctor in the last year with psychiatric symptoms. In terms of severity of handicap 30 per cent of those with severely handicapped teenagers had been to a hospital or clinic, compared with 21 per cent of those with moderately handicapped teenagers, and 27 per cent of those with mildly handicapped young people, that is, irrespective of severity of handicap, the difference between these mothers and the control group mothers was still marked.

Table 6.7 *Whether mother worries much*

| | Cerebral palsy | | Spina bifida | | Controls | |
|---|---|---|---|---|---|---|
| | N | (%) | N | (%) | N | (%) |
| Never/rarely worries (less than once a week) | 18 | (21) | 6 | (20) | 14 | (45) |
| Sometimes (once a week or more) | 41 | (49) | 9 | (30) | 10 | (32) |
| Daily (marked problems) | 25 | (30) | 15 | (50) | 7 | (23) |
| Total | 84 | (100) | 30 | (100) | 31 | (100) |

In Table 6.7 we consider the relationship of type of handicap to self-ratings of mother's worries. Here again, there was a very marked difference between mothers of controls and handicapped teenagers. Nearly half of the control group mothers said they never or rarely worried, compared to only one-fifth of mothers of handicapped teenagers. When it came to the proportion who had a *marked* problem of worrying, the main difference was that while half the mothers of the spina bifida teenagers worried frequently, less than 30 per cent of the mothers of the controls and of the cerebral-palsied teenagers did so. Looked at in relation to severity of handicap, nearly one-quarter of mothers of mildly handicapped young people had a marked problem of worrying, about the same as in the control group, while the rate for those with a moderately or severely handicapped teenager was about 40 per cent.

The Malaise Inventory gave another indication of the level of stress currently experienced by the mothers. This inventory has been used in other studies with mothers of handicapped and non-handicapped children, although in most cases the children were younger than those in our study. Rutter, Graham and Yule (1970) compared 160 mothers of 10–11 year olds who had neurological problems (mostly cerebral palsy and epilepsy) or severe intellectual retardation, with a control group of 162 mothers and found generally non-significant differences. Tew and Laurence (1975) compared forty-one mothers of spina bifida children with mothers of a control group. The mean Malaise score for the mothers of the spina bifida children was 7.1 compared to 4.7 for the controls, mothers of severely handicapped children having significantly higher Malaise scores (9.2), as did mothers of incontinent children and those with children with an IQ below 80. Dorner (1975) looked at sixty-three mothers of adolescents with spina bifida, and found that 32 per cent of mothers had a score of 7 or more on the Malaise Inventory, whereas Rutter found that in the general population only 11 per cent of mothers had scores this high. The very high mean Malaise scores (9.0) have also been recorded for mothers of very severely disabled children all meeting the requirements of the Family Fund and described by Bradshaw and Lawton (1978).

In our own study, the mean Malaise score was highest, as the findings reviewed above might suggest, for the mothers of the spina bifida teenagers (6.3) while there was little difference between the scores of mothers with cerebral-palsied teenagers and the control group mothers (both about 5.0). The mothers' Malaise score was also looked at in relation to the severity of the teenagers' handicaps. The mean score for the mothers of mildly or moderately handicapped teenagers was just over 4.3, while for those with severe handicaps it was 6.1. The mothers who were most likely to show symptoms of stress, therefore, were mothers of spina bifida teenagers and mothers of severely handicapped teenagers (regardless of type of handicap).

One problem with the Malaise Inventory is that although a high score may be given, for example, through an interview, the Inventory misses a high proportion of those suffering from considerable stress, and a low score does not necessarily indicate an absence of stress. In order to obtain an overall rating of the mothers' mental health we relied more heavily on interview data than on the Malaise Inventory. A three-fold rating (no problems, mild or moderate problems, and severe problems) was made on the basis of all our information, and the findings are shown in Table 6.8.

Table 6.8 *Mothers' present mental health*

|  | Handicapped | | Controls | |
| --- | --- | --- | --- | --- |
|  | N | (%) | N | (%) |
| No problem | 51 | (44) | 22 | (71) |
| Mild/moderate problem | 52 | (45) | 8 | (26) |
| Severe problem | 12 | (11) | 1 | (3) |
| Total | 115 | (100) | 31 | (100) |

Mothers of handicapped teenagers were nearly twice as likely as mothers of controls to be rated as having a mental health problem of some kind. Those who were most likely to have problems of mental health were the mothers of spina bifida teenagers. Although the numbers with *severe* mental health problems were small, they were twice as high (16 per cent) for mothers of spina bifida than of cerebral-palsied teenagers, while the rate for the control group mothers was very low (3 per cent).

Further analysis showed that mothers with severe mental health problems were more likely to be mothers of severely handicapped young people than of moderately or mildly handicapped youngsters. Of the twelve mothers with severe problems no less than 75 per cent were mothers of severely handicapped young people. However, over 40 per cent of mothers were thought to have no problems, regardless of severity of handicap.

Brown and Harris (1978) have shown that women who have a confidant are much less prone to depression, and the mothers were therefore asked who, if anyone, they usually talked over their worries with. The differences between the groups were not marked, although a slightly higher proportion of mothers of handicapped teenagers (about 43 per cent) said they confided in their husbands, compared with the control group mothers (about one-third). Overall just under one-quarter of all mothers appeared to have no one in whom they confided but this was not clearly related to distress. The majority of those mothers who did talk over their worries said that they found this helpful, this being equally true for mothers of non-handicapped and handicapped teenagers.

Information about the mental health of the mother of a disabled teenager is important since, as chapter 12 shows, these young people rely primarily on their mothers for support, and a worried and depressed mother will find it very difficult to give consistent support to an anxious, depressed and lonely teenager. This point becomes even more important when, in investigating the relationship between the mother's mental health and the teenager's overall adjustment, it was found that these two factors were strongly associated.

In Table 6.9 we have selected two groups of mothers: those who had *either* a severe mental health problem as rated in the way described above *or* a score of 10 or more on the Malaise Inventory, and those who had no major problems. We have then related these findings to the adjustment of the teenagers, and the results show that nearly half the teenagers whose mothers had a marked mental health problem themselves had 'marked' problems, compared to only one-quarter of those whose mothers had no mental health problems. However, the proportion of teenagers with satisfactory adjustment was approximately the same in both groups.

It is difficult to reach conclusions about the nature of the relationship between mothers' and teenagers' psychological problems. A mother

Table 6.9 *Mothers' mental health related to overall adjustment in the handicapped teenagers*

| Teenagers' adjustment | Mothers' mental health | | | |
|---|---|---|---|---|
| | No major problems | | Severe problem and/or score 10+ on Malaise Inventory | |
| | N | (%) | N | (%) |
| Marked problems | 17 | (25) | 10 | (48) |
| Some problems | 15 | (22) | 1 | (5) |
| Satisfactory adjustment | 36 | (53) | 10 | (48) |
| Total | 68 | (100) | 21 | (100) |

may have worried more because of her teenager's problems, or the teenager's problems may have been exacerbated by the mother's personality. The latter explanation seems the more likely, since mothers who worried frequently did not, in general, worry only or mainly about the teenager, but in their own words about 'everything'. These seem likely to be mothers who found it harder to give their handicapped children the confidence they needed to cope with their difficulties.

*Relationship between teenager's adjustment and personal independence.*  Another family factor which was examined was the relationship between the teenager's overall adjustment and the extent to which the mother herself reported that she gave him or her too much help. (See Table 6.10.) Mothers who said they were satisfied with the independence the child had already achieved (sixteen), or that they were inconsistent in their behaviour (seven) have been omitted. The findings suggest that teenagers were less likely to show problems if their mothers encouraged independence. The findings may well be distorted by differences in severity of handicap, but it is one worth further exploration. Perhaps teenagers feel more self-confident if they are doing more for themselves,

Table 6.10 *Overall adjustment related to encouragement of independence by mother*

| Adjustment | Mother usually encourages independence | | Mother tends to give too much help | |
|---|---|---|---|---|
| | N | (%) | N | (%) |
| Marked problems | 17 } | (44) | 9 } | (70) |
| Some problems | 8 } | | 10 } | |
| Satisfactory adjustment | 32 | (56) | 27 | (30) |
| Total | 57 | (100) | 27 | (100) |

and if so this is something that could be encouraged in schools and colleges.

*Marital discord, single parents and large families.*    Many studies have shown a relationship between marital discord and the incidence of psychological problems in children. We made no systematic attempt to measure marital discord, although we did touch on this area. However, it is worth recording that in the six families with handicapped teenagers in whom marital discord was overt, four of the teenagers had marked problems, whereas in the eighty-nine families where there were two parents and no marked discord only 32 per cent had marked problems.

Other factors looked at were the effect of being in either a single-parent or a large family. Neither factor appeared to be related to adjustment in our study. Twenty teenagers came from broken homes, one-quarter of whom had marked problems compared with one-third having marked problems where the handicapped teenager was being brought up by both parents. Fourteen teenagers came from families with five or more children, but again the proportions who had problems or satisfactory adjustment differed little from the proportion of those with families of four or fewer children.

*Socio-economic factors.*    Social class, overcrowding and household income were also found not to be related to ratings of adjustment, at least in so far as we were able to measure these variables. The number of teenagers from social classes IV and V were very small so perhaps it is not surprising that no relationships were formed. However, there were twenty-one teenagers from overcrowded homes (that is, where the ratio of people to useable rooms was greater than 1:1), but they were no more likely to show psychological problems than those living in less crowded homes. There were also fourteen children whose parents were at the time of the study either in receipt of supplementary benefit or on very low incomes. Again, these teenagers were no more likely to be poorly adjusted than the teenagers in better-off homes.

This suggests that the socio-economic factors which are associated with psychological disorder in non-handicapped young people do not have the same significance in teenagers who are disabled, although of course the numbers in this study are too small to provide a conclusive answer to this question.

### (iii) School and other environment factors

Teenagers attending ordinary schools are exposed to many more potential stresses than those attending special schools, in particular to the reactions of non-handicapped peers including the possibility of overt rejection (teasing or being ignored) or covert rejection (failure to make close friends). They also had to cope with their own feelings about being

Table 6.11 *Type of school (ordinary or special) related to overall psychological adjustment*

| Adjustment | Controls | | Physically handicapped | | | | | | | |
|---|---|---|---|---|---|---|---|---|---|---|
| | | | Ordinary school | | Day special school | | Residential school | | All special schools | |
| | N | (%) | N | (%) | N | (%) | N | (%) | N | (%) |
| Marked problems | 1 | (3) | 7 | (19) | 19 | (35) | 13 | (46) | 32 | (39) |
| Some problems | 4 | (12) | 10 | (27) | 7 | (13) | 5 | (18) | 12 | (15) |
| Satisfactory adjustment | 28 | (85) | 20 | (54) | 28 | (52) | 10 | (36) | 38 | (46) |
| Total | 33 | (100) | 37 | (100) | 54 | (100) | 28 | (100) | 82 | (100) |

'different'. Many pupils in ordinary schools were self-conscious about their handicaps, often being somewhat withdrawn and timid in their behaviour. It must be remembered, however, that many pupils in special schools showed a very similar or even more marked pattern of fearfulness, self-consciousness and lack of self-confidence, and as shown in chapter 3 they also suffered from greater social isolation, particularly in the school holidays.

Table 6.11 shows the incidence of psychological problems in relation to the type of school attended, and shows that although the handicapped teenagers in ordinary schools had a much higher rate of 'marked problems' (and problems in general) than did the controls, they also had a much lower rate of 'marked problems' than did the handicapped children attending special schools. The rates for 'satisfactory adjustment' however, were very similar for the handicapped children in ordinary schools and those in special day schools.

Earlier we showed that there was an association between the presence of marked problems and a moderate or severe handicap. It was difficult to disentangle this factor from the 'type of school' factor since relatively few moderately and severely handicapped pupils attended ordinary schools compared with the proportion in special schools (50 per cent compared with 91 per cent). However, this finding at least indicates that children with a mild or moderate handicap attending a normal school do not appear to suffer greatly from the problems that this causes for them.

When comparing the teenagers in special day schools with those in residential schools it was found that a rather higher proportion of the latter had marked problems (46 per cent compared to 35 per cent) while a lower proportion had satisfactory adjustment (36 per cent compared to 52 per cent). This finding is not surprising since it is well known that the decision to place a child in a residential special school is often closely related to problems in the child's home environment, or in some cases to

Table 6.12 *Relationship between social life and psychological adjustment*

| Social life | Marked problems | | Some problems | | Satisfactory adjustment | |
|---|---|---|---|---|---|---|
| | N | (%) | N | (%) | N | (%) |
| Good | 11 | (20) | 6 | (20) | 3 | (9) |
| Satisfactory | 25 | (46) | 13 | (43) | 11 | (35) |
| Poor | 19 | (34) | 11 | (37) | 18 | (56) |
| Total | 55 | (100) | 30 | (100) | 32 | (100) |

the fact that the child's emotional and behavioural problems are such that the family finds it difficult to cope.

*Social isolation.*   Many teenagers talked about the depression they felt because of their poor social life and lack of social intercourse outside school hours, especially when left at home day after day during the school holidays. Consequently, we looked at the relationship between psychological adjustment and overall ratings of social life to see if these factors are related. The results are shown in Table 6.12 and indicate that those with 'marked' psychological problems were much more likely to have a poor social life than were those with 'satisfactory adjustment' (56 per cent compared with 34 per cent), while those with 'good adjustment' were twice as likely as those with 'marked' problems to have a good social life (20 per cent compared with 9 per cent).

These findings are difficult to interpret for two reasons. First, as already discussed, those who were severely handicapped were much more likely to have 'marked' problems and were also less likely to have a full social life, so this result may simply be re-stating the relationship established earlier between severity of handicap and psychological problems. Secondly, it is difficult to distinguish between cause and effect. This result may indicate that teenagers with 'marked' problems were less likely than those with good adjustment to attract friends and social invitations, rather than that a poor social life resulted in greater psychological stress. However, our impression was that the quality of the young person's social life was a contributory factor to adjustment in at least some cases, and there were certainly instances where having an active social life outside the home appeared to protect the teenager from the effects of other difficulties which he was experiencing.

*Summary of the main factors associated with the presence of psychological problems*

*Factors in the teenager.*   As would be expected from previous research findings on children with handicaps associated with cortical damage, the rate of problems among the handicapped group was three to four times higher overall than the rate among the control teenagers, about half the handicapped teenagers showing overt problems of some kind. The rate was highest of all for the spina bifida girls, over 60 per cent of whom were rated as having problems. Severity of handicap was important in that the incidence of marked problems was highest in the group with severe handicaps and lowest in those rated as mildly handicapped on the Pultibec Scale. However, an equally important finding was that about half of all handicapped young people did not currently have any overt psychological problems, regardles of the degree of handicap. What is most important to understand is what factors were associated with an absence of overt problems among those with moderate or severe handicap, and what made some of those with a mild handicap more vulnerable to distress than others.

Looking at specific disabilities (controlling for overall severity of handicap) the presence of epilepsy, a urinary appliance or low ability (IQ estimated to be below 85) were all associated with higher rates of marked problems and lower rates of 'satisfactory adjustment'. However, the presence of a speech disorder did not of itself appear in our study to be related to psychological adjustment. There was a suggestion that whether or not the teenagers had been encouraged to be independent was an important factor and these findings need further investigation.

*Factors in the family.* While in terms of physical health there appeared to be no difference between the control mothers and the mothers of handicapped teenagers, on various measures of mental health the mothers with handicapped teenagers appeared to have a higher rate of overt problems; more mothers with handicapped children had seen a doctor in the previous twelve months for a psychosomatic problem, more worried regularly, and more were rated as having mild or marked problems in mental health. However, the differences between the control and handicapped group was not so clear when comparing scores on the Malaise Inventory.

Furthermore, mothers who were rated overall as having a marked mental health problem or who had a very high score on the Malaise Inventory (over 10) were more likely to have a son or daughter with marked psychological problems. Also mothers who saw themselves as severe worriers were more likely to have a teenager with a marked disorder. However, about half the teenagers did not appear to have overt problems regardless of the presence or absence of severe mental health problems in the mother. It was impossible to say whether difficulties in the teenager were caused by the mother's psychological problems, or whether the latter were the result of disturbances in the teenager, but the interviewers' impression was that these were mothers whose problems were general rather than specific to the handicap. They found it harder to give their handicapped children the support they needed, and their children were more vulnerable to distress than those with mothers who were emotionally more stable.

No other specific family factors were found to be of significance in themselves, but families who were judged to be unsupportive for some reason (because the marital relationship was poor, family relationships generally poor, or because of poverty, overcrowding or disorganization) did predominate among the teenagers with poor adjustment, and it is likely that these factors worked in some cumulative fashion which we were unable to demonstrate statistically given the small sample size.

*Other factors.*   Children who attended ordinary school (a higher proportion of whom were mildly handicapped) were less likely to show overt problems than those attending special schools, although the proportion with problems was higher for handicapped children attending ordinary schools than for the controls. Because of the differences in degree of handicap, it was difficult to interpret this finding. However, it does seem reasonable to assume, on the basis of this result, that attending an ordinary school does not impose severe stresses on those with mild or moderate handicaps, particularly since all those attending ordinary schools stated that they preferred this despite any difficulties they had encountered. It appeared that the quality of social life was related to psychological adjustment, those with a poor social life being much more likely to have a poor adjustment and vice versa. Although it is difficult to distinguish between cause and effect here, it is at least likely that leading an active social life can act as a factor protecting against psychological stress.

# II
# The transition from school to adult life

# 7
# *Post-school placements of the follow-up group*

## Introduction

In chapters 7, 8 and 9 we consider the fifty-one young people from the original sample of 119 whom we were able to follow up approximately one year after they had left school. Chapter 7 falls into two main sections: in Section A we look at the general situation facing disabled school leavers in England and Wales at the end of the 1970s, taking into account other relevant research findings; in Section B we give a straightforward description of our own follow-up group, and of the situation in which they found themselves about a year after leaving school.

## Section A: Opportunities open to disabled school leavers: the present situation

On leaving school most disabled young people will have the option of following one of three broad avenues. The first is to obtain a job in open or sheltered employment; the second is to obtain some type of higher or further education, or of vocational training, preceded perhaps by a period of assessment, the expectation both for disabled and able-bodied young people who follow the second path being usually that at the end of this period they will be better equipped to obtain a job, though in the case of the handicapped, this is not always possible. But there are some disabled youngsters who are so severely handicapped that they may not be able to follow either of these paths, or they may not wish to do so if, for example, training involves leaving home. A third option available for these young people is some other type of day (or less frequently residential) provision run by a social services department or a voluntary body. Additionally, there are a number of young people who, for a variety of reasons, are following none of these paths and spend most of the working week at home – and it must be hoped that this is only temporary.

In the first part of this chapter we shall look at current trends affecting the three main types of placements. Research findings from the other studies are referred to where relevant, although these are in fact very few, which throws much light on the current situation of physically handicapped leavers.

## (1) Employment: trends and prospects for disabled leavers

*Employment as the goal of most disabled school leavers.* Our own findings and the experience of others point conclusively to the fact that most disabled young people are no different from able-bodied leavers in being quite definite about wanting paid employment, either immediately after leaving school or after a period of further education or training. This is hardly surprising in a society such as our own which is still so thoroughly imbued with the work ethic – an ethic which pervades society and its institutions, including both our ordinary and most of our special schools. The reasons for this strong desire to work are both material and, perhaps especially in the case of disabled leavers, psychological. The material (financial) incentives to work are obvious. Most young people in employment can usually expect an adult wage by the age of eighteen years, and this will have a considerable effect on the quality of their social lives. Those who are earning will have money to spend on clothes, records, a deposit for a motor-cycle or a car, entertainment, girlfriends and so on, while those who are not must depend on benefits which are simply not comparable to even the minimum adult wage. For example, a recent (1978) Royal Commission on the distribution of income and wealth has shown in a background paper, *The Causes of Poverty*, that there is a very high incidence of financial hardship among the disabled, especially those with severe physical handicaps. For example, 32 per cent of disabled men had family incomes which were at or below the official UK poverty line. The situation was even worse for single disabled women.

For most disabled school leavers, however, the psychological significance of obtaining employment is likely to be even greater than the financial incentive. A job provides a sense of personal identity, self-esteem, responsibility and dignity, and the feeling that the young person has been accepted as an adult member of society. People are, more often than not, categorized and valued in terms of what they 'do'. For an unemployed disabled young adult who is not studying or training for eventual employment it can be very difficult to answer the question, 'What do you do?' without having a sense of being 'different', and without suffering an even greater loss of self-confidence. Having a job enables an individual to feel that he or she is making an active contribution to the community, either because the end-product is seen as useful, or, at the very least, because he is supporting himself.

Another psychological or social function of work is that it gives the young disabled person the chance to widen his horizons. Work provides a change of environment, which is desirable for everybody, but which may be of particular importance to those whose opportunities for social contacts are limited by their immobility. Work provides the individual with a whole new range of social contacts and, for handicapped young people, perhaps their first real opportunity for mixing with and making friends with the non-handicapped. It can both assist their social development and add to the sheer enjoyment of and interest in life, especially for those whose leisure activities are restricted and who lack friends.

The need of handicapped young people to find companionship through work or an equivalent 'alternative' is of course shared by other groups in the community. It is one of the main reasons given by retired people – especially women – for wanting part-time work, and it helps to explain why large numbers of women with young children either go out to work, or wish to do so. An important study carried out by Brown and Harris (1978) on the social origins of depression concludes that one of the main factors protecting susceptible women from depression was having a job. One way in which the authors explain the mechanisms at work is that having a job provides a sense of self-esteem and also increases the chances of making new social contacts and developing new interests.

Yet another psychological function of work is that even when it is boring and repetitive, it provides a structure and a regular routine to the day. Most people, whether or not they are disabled, need this framework; and young people who have attended special schools and institutions, where the day is often highly structured for them and where little thought has been given to teaching them how to organize their own lives, particularly feel the lack of a structured routine.

Although most people, including disabled school leavers, would be unlikely to articulate their reasons for wanting a job in quite these terms, these are all very cogent reasons for trying to ensure that everything possible is done to widen employment opportunities for disabled young people.

*Reasons for pessimism.* Nevertheless it is becoming increasingly apparent to young people and their parents that there are many reasons at present for pessimism about the prospects of paid employment for those leaving school or colleges of further education or training, and that certain groups in the community, including the disabled, are particularly vulnerable. These have been discussed in more detail elsewhere (Anderson and Tizard, 1979; Jackson, 1978). First, long-term trends in mechanization are steadily reducing the total number of jobs – or at least the labour time – needed by society to maintain or increase its standard of living. Secondly, the number of unskilled and semi-skilled jobs – the only ones which slow learning young people are qualified to do – is shrinking. These trends have been marked over the last decade and are likely to be accentuated in the future by further technological advances, especially by the application of microtechnology to industry and commerce. In the UK, the Central Policy Review Staff (1978) and the Department of Employment (DE) (1978) have been attempting to predict the long-term social and employment effects of microtechnology, and there can be no doubt that it will have a major job displacement effect. Jobs likely to be particularly affected are those which are repetitive, but require precision and reliability, as well as telecommunications and clerical work which in the past have provided sources of employment to many handicapped young people.

There is clear evidence that youth unemployment has been increasing over the last decade. In 1973 the Holland Report (Manpower Services Commission) pointed out that between 1972 and 1977 unemployment among young people rose 'three times as fast as unemployment among the working population as a whole', with an even greater increase in unemployment among 'special groups', which included disabled young people. This was true in spite of growing attempts to encourage employers to take on more disabled people. Disabled young people were not only more likely to be out of work than the able-bodied, but to be without work for longer periods.

There have been three recent studies of the employment prospects of young handicapped people. First, the Tuckey Survey (1973) sponsored by the DHSS, DES and DE 'to investigate the range, availability and suitability of the facilities for further education, training and employment of handicapped school leavers'. From over 7000 children, covering the whole range of handicaps, expected to leave special schools in the year 1968–9, a sample of 1700 was selected for further study about whom basic information was obtained from the schools; 788 of these were included in the follow-up study carried out in 1971, of whom 247 were physically handicapped. Information about this group was obtained from careers officers, the young people themselves, their parents and, where applicable, their employers.

The findings at that time were reasonably optimistic: 64 per cent of the leavers interviewed had done some paid work since leaving school 18–24 months earlier, three-quarters of these in open and the rest in sheltered employment. Some had gone straight into employment and some had had some training or further education first. However, these figures conceal the fact that many leavers underwent a long and anxious period before finding employment and also that periods of employment are often interspersed with long periods of unemployment. The principal reasons for leaving a job – especially the first job – appeared to be either that the work was too demanding or, in a number of cases, because the pay was poor.

Secondly, a useful Report sponsored by the Scottish Education Department (1975) of physically handicapped pupils leaving special schools in Scotland showed figures very similar to those of the Tuckey Report: 51 per cent went straight into employment, 21 per cent into sheltered workshops and work centres, 11 per cent into training courses and 2 per cent only to colleges of further education. At the time of the survey 13 per cent were unemployed and 2 per cent were in hospital.

The authors comment on the surprisingly high proportion of those who found jobs immediately after leaving special school.

More recently, in 1976–7, the National Children's Bureau carried out a survey for the Warnock Committee of the employment status of handicapped school leavers. Their sample was drawn from the eighteen year olds taking part in the National Child Development Study, and included all handicapped young people, including ESN(M) leavers, as well as the physically handicapped. The main finding (Rowan, 1979) was that unemployment was four times more common in this group than among non-handicapped young people. Whereas 66 per cent of non-handicapped eighteen year olds were employed, this was true of only 48 per cent of the handicapped group.

*New opportunities in employment.*   Although it would be foolish to ignore the major trends which will make it much harder for disabled young people to find work, there are at least some encouraging pointers in the direction of finding better solutions to this problem. First, the fact that employment prospects are today much poorer for *all* young people has meant that in the UK, as in other countries, new programmes are being introduced to alleviate unemployment among school leavers as a whole. These programmes, particularly the Youth Opportunities Programme (YOP) could, if exploited in an imaginative way, be of particular benefit to handicapped leavers. In fact this has not been the case so far, and the most recent DE estimate (Rowan, unpublished paper) was that only about 1 per cent of those taking part in the YOP scheme were youngsters registered as disabled.

The YOP (funded by the Manpower Services Commission, but organized on a local basis) came fully into operation in September 1978. Its aim was 'to help unemployed young people to prepare for work and improve their chances of getting and keeping jobs'. It was intended to help 'those school leavers and other unemployed young people under the age of nineteen who have most difficulty in obtaining employment, usually those with low formal academic attainments, some with additional difficulties'. Its main elements include work experience on employers' premises, project-based work experience (in particular, work involving environmental improvements), community service schemes, and work preparation schemes of various kinds. The participants receive a standard tax-free allowance of £25 per week. Handicapped leavers can be admitted to the scheme immediately on leaving school, and can stay on it for more than twelve months if this is considered desirable. It has also been recognized by the MSC that the scheme should be helping more of those with moderate or severe handicaps than has been the case up to now, and greater efforts will be made to include them in the second phase of the programme. A recent Working Party Report to the MSC, *Special Programmes, Special Needs*, suggests how YOP and other schemes can be adapted to include the handicapped, and lists examples of good practice throughout the country, including both voluntary and statutory schemes.

A second encouraging development is that public attitudes towards the employment of disabled people are changing, albeit slowly, and it is beginning to be recognized (as, for example, in the Warnock Report, paras. 10.76–83) that there are many hitherto untapped opportunities for handicapped people in open employment. Already, in a number of countries, important new legislation has been passed to help disadvantaged people to obtain employment. A discussion of these issues, and a summary of the steps taken in selected countries belonging to the Organization of Economic Co-operation and Development has been prepared by the Manpower and Social Affairs Committee of OECD (MAS (78) 1: *Disadvantaged Workers in the Labour Market in Selected Member Countries*, 30 January 1978) and there is no doubt that much more will be done in the future to provide 'positive discrimination' in favour of the handicapped. In the UK the Quota Scheme* is now under discussion, and the Manpower Services Commission and National Advisory Council for the Employment of Disabled People have recently suggested in their document *Positive Policies* to employers how to give full and fair consideration to disabled young people.

Earlier we spoke of technological change as likely to have an adverse effect on the employment prospects of many handicapped people. This is more likely to be true of those who are mentally rather than physically disabled. Developments in microelectronics may open new job opportunities as well as superseding some of the older ones, but these new jobs will probably demand a higher level of education than did the jobs which will be lost; for example, there will be greater opportunities for those with skills in mathematics, the physical sciences, and craft, design and technology. Unfortunately, most of these subjects are ones young people with neurological abnormalities find particularly difficult. However, for those who have reached the required educational level, it should be increasingly possible for those in clerical, professional and managerial occupations to work from home at least part of the week. Another potential advantage, to those living outside the major conurbations, is that 'the growth of distributed rather than centralized data processing will offer organizations greater flexibility in allocating work to different locations'. This opportunity to work at home will be particularly welcomed by many severely physically disabled people, although there is of course the danger that they will be socially isolated in this way.

---

* The Quota Scheme refers to current legislation whereby employers with workforces over a certain size are required to take 3 per cent of their employees from those registered as disabled. Outside the public sector it has never been successfully enforced.

The last encouraging new development is that within special education there is an increased emphasis on helping young people to make the
transition from school to adult life by the provision of courses to prepare
them for work either at school or after school leaving, through improved
social and vocational training, and through work experience of various
kinds. Hitherto schemes of these kinds have, in most parts of Britain,
tended to be organized for and geared more towards the needs of
mentally rather than physically handicapped young people, but this
situation is beginning to change.

*Sheltered work.*   Before moving on to look at trends in further education, the question of the provision of sheltered work must be raised.
Three main types of sheltered workshops exist in the UK – those sponsored by local authorities; those sponsored by voluntary organizations;
and the Government-backed Remploy, which is an independent, non-
profit making company aimed at providing work under sheltered conditions for those so severely disabled that it is unlikely that they would be
able to otherwise obtain employment. In the UK about 94 Remploy
factories employ around 8500 people. Those attending Remploy factories must be registered as disabled, be able to get to the factory by themselves and work a normal day, and must be capable of producing at least
one-third of an able-bodied person's output (or two-thirds in agriculture
and horticulture).

The main point to be made, however, is that there is a great shortage
of sheltered workshops, that the existing ones tend to be dominated by
older people who become disabled through accident or illness, and that
comparatively few vacancies occur each year since, by definition, few
members are ever able to move into open employment. Because sheltered workshops are so anxious to meet production targets and reduce
operating losses, they do very little in the way of rehabilitation or
training to help their employees to progress to open employment as
Warnock recommends. Consequently, it is extremely difficult for handicapped school leavers to get places. It is sometimes said that it is more
difficult for a young person with any significant degree of physical
disability to get into a sheltered workshop than it is to get an ordinary
job.

### (2) Further education and vocational training

Studies of handicapped leavers suggest that at least half from special
schools could benefit from some sort of further education or training. In
our own study, we included under this umbrella phrase those in higher
education, placement in ordinary colleges of further education (which
might include both non-vocational and vocational courses), placement
in special colleges of further education and/or vocational training, and

places in centres designed primarily to give long-term assessment, while at the same time providing a further education or training element. Trends in each of these sorts of placement will be considered briefly below.

*Higher education.*   The National Bureau for Handicapped Students has taken a major initiative in trying to make all establishments of higher and of further education more aware of the needs of handicapped students. It also provides useful information on the facilities available for handicapped students in various institutions. The Warnock report recommends that all establishments of higher education 'should formulate and publicize a policy on the admission of students with disabilities . . . and should make systematic arrangements to meet [their] welfare and special needs, including careers counselling' (DES, 1978).

Apart from problems of access and inability to meet special needs, the main reason at present for the relatively small numbers of handicapped students in establishments of higher education is that few young people have left special schools with the requisite entry qualifications, even among those who might have the ability to cope with the demands of higher education, a point discussed in more detail in the Snowdon Report (1976).

*Ordinary further education colleges.*   While few handicapped school leavers go on to higher education, many more go on to further education, and developments in ordinary further education colleges have been described as a 'growth area' in the field of the education of those with special needs. This has only recently become the case. The 1976–7 survey of eighteen year olds carried out by the National Children's Bureau for the Warnock Committee showed that only 5.6 per cent of handicapped eighteen year olds were still at school or in further education, compared with 29 per cent of the non-handicapped group.

Earlier surveys of handicapped leavers, for example the Tuckey Report, pointed out that many more young people are considered able to to benefit from further education than actually go on to do it. There is no doubt that one problem has been the lack of suitable courses, arising either from a lack of initiatives, finance, or of trained staff and, in the case of the physically handicapped, accessible premises. Warnock has drawn attention to the duty of LEAs 'to provide for all young people who want continued full-time education between the ages of sixteen and nineteen, either in schools or in establishments of further education . . . it is essential that they should . . . ensure that an adequate number of places in schools and establishments of further education are available to and taken up by young people with special educational needs'. In practice, a flexible range of provision is required.

Warnock emphasizes that wherever possible young people with special needs should be given the necessary support to enable them to attend ordinary courses of further education (para. 10.37). Frequently cerebral-palsied and spina bifida school leavers have reached only a low level of educational achievement and social competence by the age of sixteen, and many will therefore need or benefit from an extension of their general education. However, it is becoming more widely recognized that many of these young people will find an ordinary college of further education 'a more appropriate setting than a school in which to continue their general education'. These should aim not merely to improve literacy and numerary skills. Handicapped young people, because of their more limited experience, are frequently more immature and more lacking in social skills than their non-handicapped peers, and further education courses must recognize and cater for these needs also, as well as providing suitable courses for the multiply handicapped whose learning capacity is limited, and who will never be able to move into open employment. Warnock of course makes recommendations on both these issues (paras 10.38 and 10.39).

Most of the innovations in ordinary further education colleges have so far been in setting up work preparation courses, usually designed for those with mental or social handicaps, or only mild physical handicaps, rather than for young people with moderate or severe handicaps (that is, the majority in our own study). Only a few ordinary further education colleges have set up courses specifically aimed to cater for the needs of more severely disabled young people. Examples of these are the Work Orientation Unit at the North Nottinghamshire Further Education College, Airedale and Wharfedale Further Education College, Bourneville College, Birmingham and Trowbridge Technical College, Wiltshire. The Bridgend College of Technology provides courses and also has a purpose-built hostel attached mainly for the disabled, but taking some non-disabled students. A good deal of published material exists about the North Nottinghamshire Work Orientation Unit (e.g., Hutchinson and Clegg, 1975; see also the description in Anderson and Spain, 1977, p. 278).

Although all ordinary establishments of further education should, as Warnock recommends (para. 10.42), designate a member of staff as responsible for the welfare of students with special needs in the college, and for briefing other members of staff, few ordinary colleges will have the resources needed to take severely disabled young students. Since the numbers of this group are comparatively small, some sort of regional planning is therefore necessary, and one of the main recommendations of the Warnock Report was that: 'within each region there should be at least one special unit providing special courses for young people with more severe disabilities or difficulties which would be based in an establishment of further education (para. 10.40). This will require a co-ordinated approach to further education provision on the part of the LEAs within each region.'

*Special national colleges of further education and/or training.* With one exception, all the national colleges which provide further education and/or vocational courses exclusively for the physically handicapped are run by voluntary or private organizations. The one exception is Hereward College in Coventry (See Lowe, 1977) which is administered by a local authority and provides a year's foundation course with the opportunity for further academic vocational courses. In fact most colleges began by providing only vocational training, but have found that, because many prospective students could not meet their minimum entrance qualifications, they had to provide basic academic courses also, and many students spend the first year in further education before they are considered to have reached a level needed for entry into one of the vocational training courses.

The standards in terms of the training provided, the facilities available and the accommodation offered in these colleges vary considerably. They also draw from very wide catchment areas so that the students can only visit their homes infrequently and at considerable expense to the local authority or to parents. Consequently, some severely handicapped young people who might have been willing to attend a residential college if it were near enough to their homes for them to be able to return home at weekends, or fortnightly, turn down places because of anxiety about leaving home. Another disadvantage to having a national catchment area means that it is impossible for colleges to follow up students adequately when they leave to ensure that they do go into suitable placements, or to help them with family or residential problems if these arise.

In the Warnock Report it is suggested that these colleges could eventually provide a more useful function as part of the pattern of further education provision in their region rather than as national centres catering for particular areas of disability, and it is therefore recommended (para. 10.44) that they 'should in time all become part of the regional patterns of further education for students with special needs'. This recommendation would, we think, be very much in line with the preferences of the young people and parents taking part in this study.

However, one advantage which a voluntary society has, is that it can pioneer developments for a group with very special needs and there may be a case for exceptions being made to the recommendation above. For example, one of the newest colleges of further education is Beaumont College in Lancaster. This college, run by the Spastics Society and opened in September 1977, offers a day and residential education for seventy students. It was set up for a very specific purpose: to provide for cerebral-palsied young people in the lower ability range whose needs were not being met elsewhere. It is described as an 'educational experiment' whose justification will lie in the design, organization and implementation of an entirely new curriculum which is 'planned residentially and based firmly on the handicapped young person's needs and abilities'. The aim is to provide 'continued education . . . conceived in terms of extra time and as a "bridge" into society'. The curriculum (also referred to in chapter 10), which is described as a 'social learning curriculum based on individual assessment of students' educational needs', covers the following areas: basic literacy and language development, basic numeracy, interpersonal, social and communication skills, activities of daily living, vocational and personal development, craft studies, and environmental and community studies.

*Colleges with a central emphasis on assessment.*   One other college requires a brief individual description. This is Banstead Place, a residential college for the assessment and further education of physically handicapped school leavers with severe or multiple handicaps. It aims to provide 'total assessment educational, personal, medical, vocational and social', with the aim of producing a positive recommendation for each client's future, in terms of his occupational and residential needs. The programmes usually last about a year, and include education, training in independence and mobility, vocational assessment, work experience, social activities and use of leisure, learning to drive and use of public transport.

*(3) Day centres and equivalent forms of provision.*   There are two groups of physically handicapped leavers whose problems are especially acute. First there are those who have such severe physical difficulties (for example athetosis) that it seems highly unlikely that they would ever find open or sheltered employment, even after special vocational training. Secondly, there are young people who are less severely physically disabled but whose level of attainments or ability are such that they have little chance either of getting employment or of entry into most existing further education or vocational courses (with the exception of Beaumont). Young people in these two groups can usually be offered places in local authority day centres or, for those of lower ability, adult training centres, while a few may be placed in the Spastics Society's day work centres. These centres, which have been surveyed by Schlesinger (1977), provide for young cerebral-palsied people who are considered 'unemployable'. They differ from the typical day centre in being totally work orientated, but we have not classed them as a form of sheltered employment, since the clients are not paid a wage, but rather a small weekly sum on the same basis as some day centres and Adult Training Centres (up to a maximum of £4 if full welfare benefits are to be retained).

Day centres, with some notable exceptions, have been and probably still are the Cinderellas of the post-school provision available to disabled leavers. Recent research into provision for those unable to find employment has centred on Adult Training Centres, much of the work stemming from the Hester Adrian Research Centre in Manchester, for example Young Persons' Work Preparation courses, Speake and Whelan (MSC, 1979), and the publications from the National Development Group. In contrast, virtually no research has been carried out on day centres, although a National Institute of Social Work survey (unpublished) should throw some light on the problems of their clients and their staff.

Even without such research, however, it is clear that the main problem for handicapped young people is the fact that the number of potential users within the younger age range is comparatively small, and most of those who are disabled and living in the community are elderly. Consequently, most attenders at centres are over fifty years old while the number of young disabled people may be very small. An associated problem is that the users vary enormously in terms of intellect and interests so that it is difficult to plan a programme which caters for the needs of all. Some centres are understaffed, or the staff have little training, and they often feel very isolated. The centres are usually run by social services departments and often there is little contact with the education authority. The Warnock Report has little to say about day centres (perhaps because so little research on them exists) but the committee was clearly concerned about the lack of education input and recommends (para. 10.53) that 'there should be a specifically educational element in every adult training centre and day centre, and the education service should be responsible for its provision'. Indeed, it was felt that this should be a statutory responsibility of the education service. Yet another difficulty is that centres generally provide no training so that there is no clear means of progression open to users (for example to sheltered work), and furthermore there is generally no mechanism for *reassessment* of their clients' abilities and potential, which may change quite rapidly during the late teens and early twenties.

There are some signs that local authorities are beginning to take a more imaginative approach towards provision for their younger clients, or potential clients of day centres. For example the recently opened Michael Flanders Day Centre in Ealing has a special course with about twelve places for a 'School leavers' group' (maximum age twenty-five). It was difficult at first to fill the places, even when these were offered to neighbouring boroughs, which illustrates the difficulty both in making special provision for a group whose numbers are so small, and of reaching those young people currently in unsuitable placements who could benefit, since there is no adequate system for ensuring that information about such a centre gets to parents or to the young people themselves.

Another approach is that pioneered by the Tuckeys at the Stone House in Corby, a centre of heavy industry with a population of about 50,000 (Tuckey and Tuckey, 1979). Although the Centre is outside the area in which our research was carried out, we describe it in some detail to give an idea of an alternative approach to the usual kind of day centre provision.

Originally planned as a 'day centre for the handicapped and elderly', the Tuckeys were able to develop what was in effect a community centre. While concentrating its attention on the needs of disabled people, the Centre had an open door policy to others in the community, for example relatives and friends of the users, as well as the parents of handicapped children, and other people with special needs provided that they were under fifty years old on arrival, and 'intellectually capable of organizing their own lives' within the context of the Centre. Users were given as much independence as possible within the limits of their disabilities, and a minimum of organized help, in order to encourage self-help and foster a community spirit. At the end of five years there were about 100 people using the Centre in the course of a week (some came daily, others much less frequently) of whom about sixty were disabled. Most users were under forty-five years, and some were in their late teens and early twenties.

When considering the activities of the Centre, the organizers rejected the possibility of sub-contract work, which, since it involves deadlines, is difficult to combine with other activities. They thought rather of 'meaningful and pleasurable activity' but had no highly structured programme, aiming rather to 'create a social ambience in which people felt confident enough to try a wide range of activities and to help each other achieve certain goals'. Some activities had an element of 'volunteering'; users might do toy repairs for the toy library, make something for the play-group, build a piece of equipment for the Centre, help an aphasic user practise his speech or reading, or help prepare the midday snack. Other activities were more purely recreational. Regular activities which some of the disabled users helped to run, but which benefited or involved other members of the local community, included a telephone information service on disability, a toy library for handicapped children, a mixed play-group and a youth club. The disabled users were encouraged to make a life for themselves outside the Centre and enabled them to do so by a flexible system of transport. The managers were more concerned if a user had no social life outside the Centre than if he or she was an occasional user only.

The two main developments which the scheme's organizers thought were most needed in the future were first, an expansion of adult education, through improved links with the local Adult Education Department and the addition of a craft instructor and an adult education tutor, who could divide their time between the Stone House and domiciliary visits. Classes and groups could be held on the Centre's premises (possibly run by some disabled users who had special skills) but open to anyone who was interested. The second development thought necessary was the setting up of an assessment unit at the Centre, to look at the everyday needs and problems of an individual and his family, together with an appraisal of the resources available to them.

*Research on spina bifida and cerebral-palsied school leavers*

Although many research studies have been carried out into the post-school placement of ESN(M) school leavers (reviewed, for example, by Rodgers, 1979), and although severely mentally handicapped young people are being followed up in research carried out at the Hester Adrian Centre (Mittler, personal communication, 1979) much less is known about what happens to physically handicapped leavers in general, and cerebral-palsied and spina bifida leavers in particular.

An account of studies conducted on the placement of leavers with spina bifida was given in an earlier book (Anderson and Spain, 1977) which referred to data available from Dorner's study (1975) and from a small-scale survey carried out by ASBAH, the Association for Spina Bifida and Hydrocephalus (1975). The findings from these studies are summarized in Table 7.1 and highlight the disturbing fact that one-quarter of the leavers in both studies had no employment or occupation of any kind when they were interviewed.

Table 7.1 *Placement of leavers with spina bifida (from Dorner, 1975 and ASBAH, 1976)*

| Type of placement | ASBAH survey | | Dorner's study | |
|---|---|---|---|---|
| | N | (%) | N | (%) |
| Open employment | 17 | (20.4) | 13 | (39.4) |
| Full-time FE/training | 13 | (15.7) | 7 | (21.2) |
| Sheltered employment | 14 | (16.9) ⎫ | | |
| Day centres | 17 | (20.4) ⎬ | 5 | (15.2) |
| Not working | 22* | (26.5) | 8 | (24.2) |
| Total | 83 | (100.0) | 33 | (100.0) |

* Four of these were not working because of illness

The only other relevant findings are from two studies of adults with spina bifida cystica. This group, however, comprise a somewhat different population from today's spina bifida school leavers, both in the nature of their handicaps and their school and training experiences. In particular, a much smaller proportion of them are severely disabled or have hydrocephalus than today's teenagers, while fewer of those with severe disabilities had an adequate education (many only had home tuition) or any sort of vocational training, compared with young people today. The larger of the two studies (Evans *et al.*, 1974) was of 202 adults with spina bifida cystica who had attended the Hospital for Sick Children, Great Ormond Street, London before 1954. Nearly half (mostly with uncomplicated meningocele) had no serious disability and were leading normal lives, but there were forty-seven men and fifty-eight women with a serious disability. Although about half of this group were working regularly, or were active housewives, one-third of the men and about one-quarter of the women had never worked at all.

In the other study (Beresford and Laurence, 1975) the present placement of fifty-one adults living in South Wales was investigated. Of particular interest was the placement of twenty people with 'moderate' handicaps (walking with aids and partially continent or continent after operation) and sixteen with 'severe' handicaps, (chairbound, and/or totally incontinent). Sixteen of those with moderate handicaps and eight with severe handicaps were in 'normal occupations' (twenty in open employment, three were housewives and one a full-time student). As in the Evans *et al.* study half of those employed were in office jobs.

Among the encouraging points to emerge from these studies were first, the fact that a substantial number of those with moderate and severe handicaps were coping well in open employment, and secondly, that office work of some kind offered reasonable prospects for employment to many of those without severe hydrocephalus. However, a disturbing finding was that quite large numbers of young people had frequent periods of unemployment, and even worse, in the Evans study about one-third of the group had never been employed and would 'never be able to lead independent lives in the sense of being able to be both financially self-supporting and to care for their own physical needs'.

No recent studies on the post-school placement of cerebral-palsied young people are available. However, a survey published by the Spastics Society in 1964 reported on the results of an investigation of fifty-four young people born between 1940 and 1944, and who had attended schools within the London County Council area. All were over eighteen at the time of interview. It was found that thirty-three (over 60 per cent) were in employment, though many had had long periods of unemployment since leaving school, and there had been much trial and error before a suitable job was found. Most of those without jobs were in various day centres (N = 10), six others had been admitted for long-term residential care (mostly those with severe mental handicap), one was a housewife, one in training and three were unoccupied at home.

Although the study was small and is now out of date, the findings suggest that the prospects for employment for cerebral-palsied young people, at least those who do not have severe retardation, is considerably better than for those with spina bifida, perhaps mainly because a higher proportion are mobile, and so access is not a problem. However, a more depressing picture is given from a survey of 209 pupils leaving five Spastics Society residential schools between 1966 and 1970. By mid-1971, only one-quarter of leavers were in open or sheltered employment, 15 per cent were in further education or training, 19 per cent were in day centres and 7 per cent in Adult Training Centres. Only 14 per cent were classed as unemployed, but 20 per cent were in residential homes and no comment was made about their employment (Spastics Society, 1971).

## Section B: Findings from the post-school follow up

This section discusses the placement of the fifty-one young people from the original sample of 119 who had left school in the year following the Phase I interview and who were available for study. The findings generally suggest that the young people would benefit from a frank discussion of their situation and of the things likely to help them deal with their difficulties. Encouraging closer relationships with their peers to help them develop skills in confiding is one obvious way in which the teenagers' situation could be improved, together with encouragement to develop interests of any kind, both as an end in itself and as a basis for friendships with people of similar interests.

All those young people from the original sample who were no longer attending school by the end of the summer term (July) 1978 were seen in the follow-up study, the interviews taking place 12–15 months after the teenagers had left school. In all, fifty-six young people from the original sample had left school within this period, of whom fifty-one were available for study. In two cases, only the mother could be interviewed, and in another case only the teenager. This section describes the situation of the young people in each of the four main placement groups, that is, work, further education or training, day centre, or no employment. It also discusses the overall satisfaction of the school leavers and their families with their present situation and with what had happened to them over the previous year.

Interviews were conducted with the teenagers themselves, and also separately with one or both parents, usually the mother. Most of the young people were interviewed alone in their homes, but in a few cases, for reasons of timing and/or privacy, the interview was carried out at the teenager's college or day/work centre. Because the sample was so small, results are quoted in a mainly anecdotal way, illustrating the kinds of issues which arise in practice in the post-school experience of young handicapped people.

### Comparison between the follow-up sample and the original sample

Table 7.2 shows the numbers in the follow-up sample from each diagnostic group, compared with the original sample. The proportions within each group was almost identical to that of the original group and the follow-up group, although all five eligible for inclusion but not available for study were cerebral-palsied.

*Age, sex and social class.* The mean age of the group at follow up was 17 years 9 months and, as in the original sample, just over half the group (55 per cent) were male. Comparisons between the original sample and the follow-up group on type and severity of handicap, type of school

Table 7.2 *Diagnostic groups*

| | Total in original sample | | Eligible and followed up | | Eligible but not available | | Not eligible* | |
|---|---|---|---|---|---|---|---|---|
| | N | (%) | N | (%) | N | (%) | N | (%) |
| Cerebral palsy | 89 | (75) | 38 | (74) | 5 | (4) | 46 | (73) |
| Spina bifida | 30 | (25) | 13 | (26) | 0 | (0) | 17 | (27) |
| Total | 119 | (100) | 51 | (100) | 5 | (4) | 63 | (100) |

* i.e., had not left school by July 1978

attended, and social class, reveal that there were no substantial differences between the Phase I and Phase II samples, so that although our numbers in the follow-up were small, they are likely to be fairly representative.

*General situation of the follow-up group as a whole during the post-school year.* Just over half of the teenagers (N = 26) in the follow-up group left school at sixteen years, twenty (39 per cent) left at seventeen years, and five (10 per cent) left at eighteen or over. There was no difference between those in ordinary and special schools in this respect. Over three-quarters left school at the end of the summer term.

It is interesting and somewhat surprising to note that there was also little difference between those attending the two types of school in age at leaving, about half in each case (50 per cent in special and 58 per cent in ordinary schools) leaving at sixteen years. Until the school leaving age was raised to sixteen in 1972, of course, children attending special schools were required to spend an additional year in school, on the grounds that they were usually retarded scholastically and needed an extra year in school to catch up with their peers. One might have expected that this tradition of staying on beyond the statutory leaving age would have continued, but from our discussions with the teenagers it appears that many could see no value in remaining at school because in many cases no special curriculum was provided for the post-sixteen year olds and they considered it a waste of time.

Nearly one-quarter of the follow-up sample had attended ordinary schools, and 76 per cent had been to special schools including twelve pupils (24 per cent of the total group) who went to residential schools. The majority were rather poorly qualified on leaving school as Table 7.3 shows, particularly those leaving special schools, who of course tended to have more learning difficulties than did those in ordinary schools, (although it must be remembered that all had been selected as having IQs of 75 or over). Additional evidence that this difference in ability does not account for all the differences observed is that several young people

Table 7.3 *Summary of formal qualifications on leaving school*

|  | Group from ordinary schools | | Group from special schools | | Total | |
|  | N | (%) | N | (%) | N | (%) |
|---|---|---|---|---|---|---|
| None | 2 | (17) | 22 | (56) | 24 | (47) |
| 1–3 CSEs | 4 | (33) | 11 | (28) | 15 | (24) |
| 4 or more CSEs and/ or 1–3 O levels | 4 | (33) | 5 | (13) | 9 | (18) |
| One or more A levels | 1 | (8) | 0 | (0) | 1 | (2) |
| Other | 1 | (8) | 1 | (3) | 2 | (4) |

leaving special schools with poor qualifications subsequently went on to further education and were successful in examinations. Perhaps the main reason for the difference was the small size of the special schools (discussed in chapter 1), and their consequent inability to offer the range of subjects and the stimulation that the more able students required.

Over half of those leaving special schools (56 per cent) had no qualifications at all compared with 17 per cent of those in ordinary schools, while in ordinary schools over 40 per cent had at least four CSEs, compared with 20 per cent of those in special schools.

*Living arrangements.*   Over two-thirds of the young people were living at home full-time at the time of the follow-up interview, while all but two of the rest were in residential college and living away, for a short period, during term-time only. Only two young people were living permanently away from home. One very severely handicapped girl was living in a residential home while learning to become more independent and to ease the strain on her mother following a divorce. One boy had been placed in residential care because his mother, although not completely rejecting him, was unable to offer him a home due to his illness combined with a number of other problems, which will be described later. In four other cases there was a change in the marital status of the mother, two having divorced in the previous year and two having remarried, but this did not affect living arrangements. However, it was apparent that in several cases either the young person or the parent or both were already thinking about alternative accommodation, and that in a few cases this was becoming an urgent problem as we shall explain in chapter 8.

*Main placements of the follow-up group.*   The majority of the young people had been in the same placement for all or most of the post-school year, although a few had very complex histories indeed, and they were classified according to their main placement throughout the year or to

Table 7.4 *Main placements of the follow-up group*

| Group | Placement at time of Phase II interview | | Placement at most recent contact (6–12 months later) | |
|---|---|---|---|---|
| | N | (%) | N | (%) |
| Employment | 9 | (17) | 17 | (33) |
| Ordinary further education | 8 | (16) | 13 | (26) |
| Special further education | 17 | (33) | | |
| Day centre (or equivalent) | 12 | (24) | 10 | (20) |
| At home | 5 | (10) | 11 | (22) |
| Total | 51 | (100) | 51 | (100) |

their current placement if this had been of long standing. Four broad groupings were chosen: employment (including sheltered employment); education and training (including higher education, further education, assessment and vocational training, subdivided according to whether they were attending an ordinary or a special college); day centres of any kind; and an 'At home' group, who were without a placement of any kind and had been so for a substantial period before the interview took place. (Those who had left college within the previous six weeks and who were without a placement at the time of the interview were *not* included in this group, but were coded as if they were still at college.) These findings are summarized in Table 7.4, which indicates that nearly half of the school leavers had gone on to further education or training of some kind, while about one-quarter were in day centres, and less than 20 per cent were employed. Just under 10 per cent had had no occupation for all or most of the first year after leaving school, but this figure based on the situation current at the time of the interview masks the very long periods at home spent by eight young people from the other groups. For example, four in the day centre group were at home for 6–8 months before being placed, and four in the employment group had either taken several months to get a job, or had lost a lot of time from work due to illness or difficulty in getting a second job when the first failed.

Because over 60 per cent of the sample were in further education at the time of interview – usually on one-year courses – we thought it would be useful to contact the sample again at the time of writing (6–12 months after the Phase II interview) particularly to see what had happened to those who had left full-time education. The results in the second column of Table 7.4 show that at this point the number in open employment had risen to one-third, while the proportion in full-time education or training had dropped to one-quarter (the proportion in day centres was approximately unchanged). However, the most disturbing result of this inquiry was the discovery that almost twice as many young people were then unoccupied, including three of the original 'at home' group who were still without occupation eighteen months or more after leaving school. The group included four teenagers unoccupied due to illness, one who had left his day centre without having an alternative placement, while three had left further education eight months earlier, but had been unable so far to secure an acceptable long-term alternative.

*Placement in relation to type of school attended.*   Of the twelve young people in the follow-up survey who had attended ordinary schools, half were in open employment, three in ordinary colleges of further education and only three were in special facilities of any kind, all taking courses at residential colleges with a view to open employment. Of those who attended special schools, only seven (less than 20 per cent) were in ordinary placements, two in open employment and five in ordinary further education, while one boy was in a Remploy establishment. All the rest were in special facilities of some kind or were without a placement at all.

*Employed group.*   Of the nine young people in employment, only one was rated as severely handicapped; she used a wheelchair outdoors, was incontinent, and could not use public transport. All the rest were rated as mildly handicapped (all walking well and using public transport). Three had no visible handicaps, apart from slight limps or clumsiness, but five had impaired control of at least one upper limb. All had 'average' or 'low-average' IQs, and seven had obtained some GCEs. One boy had a Remploy placement although his disabilities were very slight compared with the rest of this group. It seemed likely that if he'd been to an ordinary rather than to a special school, open employment would have been tried for (it was not even considered in his case). At our most recent contact, he had still not moved into open employment.

Of the eight in open employment, five had office / clerical jobs of some kind, mostly very junior, but one carried quite a lot of responsibility (by the end of the first six months he was actually managing the small office in the section of the firm where he was working). The remaining three young people in this group had unskilled manual jobs, two as labourers and one as a messenger.

Only one school leaver had got his first job through the careers service, although two others used the careers officer for their second job when their first placement had failed. In both cases the careers officers concerned secured good placements and really helped the young people to regain their confidence. The Remploy job was obtained via the local Disablement Resettlement Officer, although this was only achieved after a great deal of chasing up by a very determined mother. Many of the young people in fact made disparaging remarks about how little preparation for work or help in finding a job had been provided by their school or the careers service. A few had been involved in linked further education courses or work experience courses in their final year at school which had been helpful to some extent. Only one had been on an assessment course, but she was not at all pleased with the advice given and had ignored it. Most felt in retrospect that their last year at school had not been beneficial, and none wished that they'd stayed on an extra year. One boy, who had been to an ordinary school, was very explicit about his feelings that school 'gives you a wrong impression of the world', and described his disappointment on discovering that 'I couldn't get a job [the job he wanted] with the qualifications I had' (three CSEs). Two young people stated that they definitely missed friendships at school and hadn't been able to replace these.

However, all the teenagers in this group definitely enjoyed being part of the adult world of work despite any difficulties they were encountering. With the exception of two who had severe health problems, the stresses that they had encountered during the year in connection with work were little different from those frequently encountered by able-bodied young people in their first year after leaving school, and the experience had matured them. However, it was a cause for concern that many of the young people had not succeeded in making friends at work and that in one placement serious problems had arisen about how much help to accept from work colleagues. It seems likely that some kind of social skills training would have been beneficial to these young people had it been available.

*Further education group.* Nearly half of the young people seen in the follow-up had entered some form of further education (FE), vocational training or assessment. Eight had taken up places in ordinary FE or higher education establishments (only one being residential), and seventeen had gone to special colleges for the disabled, all but two of which involved a residential placement. Only one of the young people in special further education was in a Unit attached to an ordinary FE college. In fact this was for less able rather than disabled school leavers, and it is unlikely that the teenager in question would have been able to attend had she had anything other than a slight locomotor handicap. The only other special provision which was not residential was a small unit attached to a special school.

Although the majority of teenagers and their parents were generally satisfied with their college placement, there was quite a high level of dissatisfaction among both those in ordinary and special FE with the information made available to them about the range of possible options. Only one-quarter expressed themselves 'fully satisfied' on that score. Some complained that they were 'given no advice at all' or that 'you had to do it all yourself' [that is, get the information]. One said,

'The school didn't suggest any alternatives; they just agreed with us.' Although pleased, in general, with the advice given to those who went on assessment courses, some parents and teenagers complained about the lack of detailed feedback. 'No one told us what she really could do, only which college to go to.' Another said, 'We didn't hear the results of the assessment and we would have liked a wider range of possibilities in case . . . [the recommended placement] fell through'. It was this feeling of lack of control over one's own future that bothered the teenagers most, rather than the choice of placement itself. The common feeling of parents that all was not being revealed was summed up by one who said she believed that 'the school reports they send you give quite a different picture from the ones locked up in the office'.

### Ordinary FE group

*Characteristics of the group.* Surprisingly, in terms of severity of handicap, this group of eight young people were by no means without considerable problems. On the Pultibec Scale only one was rated as minimally handicapped, five were rated as moderately handicapped, and two as severely handicapped. Six were cerebral-palsied and two had spina bifida. However, what is probably most significant is that while all in this group had some locomotor impairments, none was in a wheel-chair or heavily calipered, and although some had difficulty negotiating stairs, all but one were able to use public transport unassisted. In terms of upper limb problems three young people had quite marked problems, two having poor control of both upper limbs. A third boy had one severely affected limb, though he could use the other quite normally. Three others were rather clumsy. None suffered from epilepsy, but two had speech impairments, one quite marked, while the two spina bifida teenagers were incontinent of urine, one having rather unreliable bowel control also. It is interesting to note that only three young people in this group had been to an ordinary school, while two had been to day PH schools and three to residential PH schools. All were estimated to be of at least low average ability.

*Type of placement and any special help required.* One young man was at Cambridge University and was the only one in this group who lived away from home; one boy was attending an art college and one a college of commerce. The remaining five were in colleges of further education – usually the one nearest to home. All the young people in this group were pursuing ordinary courses alongside non-handicapped students. Only three had needed any special arrangements made for them at college (all minimal) such as permission to use a typewriter in class or for examinations, or extra classes. The student at Cambridge was given a ground floor room in college, with a telephone installed, and was allowed to have a car (a privilege denied other students) and he also got a lot of help from his college neighbour. All the students said how helpful the staff had been in general, and felt confident that if a difficulty arose they could consult and receive assistance; two mentioned informal help they'd received from fellow students (for example, one helped with note-taking during class time).

Three students walked to college, two were taken in the family car, and two had taxis (paid for by the local authority) since the alternative was a complicated journey by public transport. One mother had a transfer arranged for her son because of a difficult journey. However, one young man, admittedly with only a minimal locomotor handicap, made a daily journey to college taking $1\frac{1}{4}$ hours, using a combination of moped, train and walking.

Four young people said they had some difficulties with their courses. The boy at art college hadn't done well in his exams at the end of the first year, and only gained a place in the second year following a special interview. This boy has managed to continue at the college, however, and appeared to be doing quite well 18 months later. One young man, who had previously attended a residential PH school, found the pressure of work quite hard because the pace was faster than at school, and his slow writing made for particular difficulties, but he was managing by working long hours at home. The Cambridge student could manage his courses well except for the quality of his draughtsmanship (he was taking an engineering degree), and he was worried about being forced eventually to change courses because of this. The fourth teenager found the shorthand part of her two-year course so difficult that she left at the end of the first year, however she immediately got herself a job using the other skills acquired and was still working at our last contact.

Apart from these difficulties, none spoke of any serious problems, either when first starting or at the time of the interview. Neither of the two people who were incontinent had had serious difficulties, although both had had some problems in managing without special facilities.

*Course content, why chosen and future plans.*   Apart from the students at art college and university, all students were on courses which were aimed at office work of some kind and included academic studies. Except for the girl who left her course early, all the students were very satisfied indeed. They liked their teachers and some gave them very high praise for the quality of teaching and their general helpfulness and understanding of the students' problems. All the young people in this group were clearly aiming for open employment and although sometimes a little apprehensive, were fairly confident that they would be able to manage this if they could master the qualifications. A few had very specific ideas about what kind of job they wanted, but most were fairly open to ideas because they were a year or more from completing their courses.

*Friendships.* The one aspect of college life where these students as a group were not particularly successful was the social side, although they found the other students generally friendly, and some offered particular help where necessary. Indeed three students said that they were offered too much help at first and had to learn ways of turning this down. However, only two of the young people claimed to have made many friends whom they saw regularly outside college, and this included the Cambridge student whose circumstances were different in any case because he was residential. The other boy said he'd made 'tons' of friends whom he saw at pubs and discos (although his mother thought that these were all acquaintances rather than real friends).

One girl was very disappointed indeed with the attitude of the other students towards her. She had come from a residential special school where she had been one of the least handicapped students, had few visible handicaps and had been very popular. She was looking forward to going to college and mixing with non-handicapped people but found her fellow students, though not unfriendly, too preoccupied with themselves to have time for her. She said: 'They're all right in class but outside class it's "hello" that's all'. She missed her former school friends greatly and the warm, supportive atmosphere of the school; she had found the past year when she had to fend entirely for herself very hard going.

The other five young people, while not complaining about their fellow students' attitudes, all wished that they had more contact with them outside college. Two said this wasn't possible because they lived a distance from their colleges and no other students lived nearby; in one case, this seemed a genuine problem, but in the other it was more doubtful. No clear reason was given by the others, although one said that 'some handicapped people, not me, find it difficult to go out and meet normal people in case they laugh at you'. Another who did not use public transport unassisted (although it's likely in fact that she could have done so) made the excuse that she couldn't get out much on her own.

The impression gained was that these young people on the whole were rather tentative in their approach to their able-bodied peers, and were not able to make the extra effort needed to bridge the gap of embarrassment which so often acts as a barrier to relationships between the handicapped and the able-bodied. In fact, most of the teenagers in this group denied feeling nervous of mixing with the able-bodied, and only one admitted to having real problems in this respect. But this is not the same thing as having the self-confidence needed to make the very positive overtures which the handicapped need to make, certainly at this age, if they are to make real contact with the able-bodied. This was particularly difficult for those who had been to special schools and had had little practice in how best to make approaches to the non-disabled.

At present, while handicap is still a social stigma and schooling for the disabled is still largely segregated, the able-bodied have little opportunity to learn at a young age to mix easily with the handicapped, and the onus, unfortunately, must be on the handicapped person to make the first overtures and find ways of minimizing the embarrassment in their company that most able-bodied people feel. As with those in employment, the evidence here suggests that even the most courageous who are prepared to take the plunge into integrated education still need some help and preparation if they are to handle social situations successfully; especially perhaps at this age when all young people have a heightened awareness of themselves physically, and generally tend to be somewhat gauche and ill-at-ease in social situations.

*Likes and dislikes generally.*   Despite the difficulties which the young people had encountered (none very serious but all requiring some effort to overcome), all but one were enthusiastic about their placements, few offering any reservations at all. Some were very effusive, saying how friendly the teachers were, or that the students were 'a continuous laugh'. One of the boys whose social life within college was quite successful was exceedingly enthusiastic, saying that 'it proved to me that I could mix – I've got to know so many people it's unbelievable – I found I had more friends there . . . than ever I had at D—.' (His special school.)

The only student who liked college less than school was the girl already described who found the change in atmosphere from her special school so great, and even she described her feelings as 'mixed' rather than saying she wholly disliked it. In fact this girl was having a rather unhappy time at home as a result of the mother's remarriage, which had caused a rift between herself and her mother. With more support and a more settled home atmosphere she might not have found the difficulties with friendships at college so distressing.

The picture which emerges was of a fairly handicapped group of young people who had accepted the challenge of competing on equal terms with their peers in ordinary education establishments and have done exceedingly well. The goodwill of the staff in their colleges seemed to be universal; special arrangements of a discreet and sensible kind were made where necessary, and in general the staff seemed to have inspired the students with the confidence that if any problems arose they would be sympathetically dealt with.

Of the five categories of post-school activity we have defined, the young people in this group were by far the most contented. Their parents were also without any complaints and most were very positive about how helpful the college had been and the way the experience had matured and given confidence to their children. While it is true that this group did tend to be rather more able academically and to have fewer loco-motor problems than did the other groups, some were quite markedly handicapped in other ways, so their success cannot be accounted for entirely in terms of minimal disability.

The very positive experience of this group is a great encouragement to those who are pressing for greater integration of the handicapped within ordinary further education, especially when it is remembered that no special facilities or staff were allocated to these students. The main improvement one would suggest which would have made their experience even more enjoyable and rewarding, would be the provision of counselling to help with the social aspects of college life for those who were not gaining the maximum benefit from the potential social opportunities.

*The group in special education or training*

There were seventeen young people in some kind of special education, training or assessment, in nine different establishments altogether, which varied very widely in course content and general aim. Only two students were living at home, another came home most weekends, and one visited his family every Saturday. The other thirteen were in full-time residential colleges and only came home in vacations.

*Characteristics of the group.*  On the whole this was a fairly handicapped group, although two young people were rated as 'mild' on the Pultibec Scale, and eight were rated as moderately handicapped. However the remaining seven were severely handicapped, including four with serious multiple handicaps. In terms of locomotor function, surprisingly only four were confined to wheelchairs, while four others walked indoors but usually used a wheelchair outdoors. Over half the group, nine in all, walked well either with a limp or an abnormal gait and could use public transport.

Again, in upper limb function, the number with severe problems was surprisingly small; three had a problem with both upper limbs (two of these having very poor control) while two had a severe disability, and two minor problems in one limb only. Eight had no upper limb problems, although one was rather clumsy. Only four had severe speech defects, one of whom had no intelligible speech and used a 'Possum' for communication. Another had a less marked problem, his speech being perfectly intelligible, while a third had slow speech with some words mispronounced. Only two students had a serious learning difficulty (probably borderline ESN). In addition, two teenagers had epilepsy, and three wore appliances for incontinence.

Three young people in this group had attended ordinary day school, and one had attended a residential school for the maladjusted (her handicap was very mild and were it not for her behaviour problems she could have attended an ordinary school, and indeed did so at the primary level). Eight had been to day schools for the physically handicapped and the remaining five to residential special schools of some kind.

*Type of placement and course content.* Two young people were attending one year courses in colleges specifically aimed at assessment. One was being assessed for office or clerical work, and when interviewed at the end of the course was hoping to get work in open employment. The other was a very severely handicapped boy, unlikely even to get sheltered employment. Two other teenagers were attending purely vocational establishments which they enjoyed greatly, while six were in colleges offering basic education plus vocational courses in commerce or office skills. These courses varied in length from six months to three years.

Five students, including some of the most severely handicapped, were attending the same college, Beaumont, which offers a one or two year course to less able students covering a wide range of skills including further education, independence training (cookery, needlework, etc.), drama, art, crafts, typing and environmental studies, with some work experience available if appropriate. The general aim of the course is to make the young person as independent as possible, to widen his experience and to assess his capabilities and interests in both work and leisure activities.

The remaining two young people were in rather experimental situations; one was attending a newly established FE Unit attached to a special school, offering a 2–3 year course with, in principle, the same range of activities and with the same aim as Beaumont's, but being limited currently by the small number of students (six) and staff (three). The other was in a Work Experience Unit attached to an ordinary college of further education, designed for less able school leavers. The survey student was the first with a physical handicap (very slight indeed) who had been accepted there. The unit offered some further education and independence training, such as cooking, and a 'world of work' course, including some work experience; it was intended to last one year.

*Why the course was chosen.* In contrast to the group in ordinary further education, the majority of young people in this group hadn't actually chosen their course or college, but had merely followed the advice offered by professionals, over two-thirds as a result of a Spastics Society assessment course. Even where the students were very satisfied with the placement there was often a feeling that the decision had been presented to them as a *fait accompli* and parents also complained about the lack of consultation.

Again, the impression came through very strongly that these young people did not feel in control of their own lives. People examined them, discussed them behind closed doors, and announced a decision, which was usually passively accepted, but there was no general discussion of the alternatives available or opportunity for the teenager to participate fully in the decision making himself. In no instance had a placement in an ordinary college of further education been discussed with the student, even when this was patently a real possibility.

*Any difficulties with the course or college.*   None of the young people found their courses really difficult. Seven said there were minor difficulties with some things, such as fine manipulative tasks, but all were coping. Except for minor complaints about particular subjects they didn't like, most students were fairly satisfied with their courses. Only two had serious complaints, both because they felt they were not offered enough variety of subjects, and were therefore bored. All but two travelled to college by public transport, often with a train escort. None expressed any difficulty about travel arrangements, although some journeys lasted 4–5 hours.

The majority said that the greatest difficulty was in learning to live away from home and manage more for oneself. Many were homesick at first and took a while to settle in, while others had continual difficulties over matters such as handling pocket money. One athetoid boy with no speech found it very hard to live away from home, but he had matured over the year and become more resigned to the idea that ultimately he would need a permanent residential placement. The girl who had attended the maladjusted school had particular difficulties at first in getting on with her peers. None of these problems was severe, and where help was needed it was usually forthcoming from fellow students or staff, especially care staff and social trainers who were often mentioned as being particularly understanding. However, it should be noted in this context that three teenagers in the 'at home' group, whose histories will be described later, had left their special colleges because the placement had broken down in some respect. This represents a failure rate of 15 per cent and given the bleak outcome for the young people involved, is a serious cause for concern, since it appeared that there was no system for monitoring students who dropped out of college to ensure that some suitable alternative was provided. In addition, several young people wished they had had more discussions with staff about how they were doing and felt ill-informed generally about their progress. For example, one boy said his college held case conferences every eight weeks and felt that he should have been told the outcome of these.

As for coping with incontinence, the four spina bifida teenagers concerned were very satisfied. Two were fully independent before leaving home and had no problems at college, while two on entering college had frequent problems with leaking bags, but this had greatly improved as a result of their increased competence due to the advice received at college. Two cerebral-palsied boys needed help with toileting but found all the arrangements satisfactory. Two of the 'at home' group, however, had left their colleges partly because of incontinence difficulties. One boy had attended a residential college (not one of those attended by any other survey pupils) where the staff had not been competent to deal with his incontinence problems and more particularly his pressure sores. Consequently, he had been sent home after three months, and the neglect had led to serious medical complications. Another girl left college partly because she wasn't independent enough in appliance care. Since similar cases have been drawn to our attention it seems appropriate to emphasize that any special residential college accepting students with incontinence should have competent members of staff or readily available outside help for students in need. The consequences of not doing so are not only weeks or months of immobilization and the disappointment of the student, but possibly the more serious one of permanent damage to the kidneys.

*Parents' feelings about the placements.* The majority of parents were satisfied with the placement itself and with the course (there were only three with definite complaints). However, like the students, many parents complained that they didn't receive enough information and didn't really know what progress their children were making. All but four of the parents had visited the college before the student was admitted, and only three had not visited since; most visited their children regularly to go to open days, or to pick them up at the end of term. Nevertheless, they felt starved of information. The parents of the two placed in non-residential establishments and the weekly boarder were the most satisfied because, being closer to home, they were able themselves to keep in regular contact with the college.

Of the residential establishments only Beaumont seemed to make an effort to keep the parents informed, although even then a full report came only when the student was leaving. One parent said, 'I don't know what the course is . . . I can see he's become a young adult, but I would like to have more information'. Others made similar comments, such as 'they don't keep in touch', or 'I'm happy he's doing what makes him happy, but I don't feel I know what's going on'. The lack of written or 'phone communication was a very real problem, making personal contact difficult, as most of the colleges were distant.

Again, here is a picture of professionals working actively, and successfully in most cases, to help the young people in their charge, but frequently not communicating the knowledge they had gained to the parents, nor to the young person himself, to help them understand the limitations and the potential of the young people. It would seem reasonable to expect colleges to produce a report at the end of the first term to inform parents and students of progress or problems to date, which could form the basis for a discussion at least with the students if not the parents, to be followed by another at the end of the first year, on the lines of the Beaumont comprehensive reports.

*Friendships.* In contrast to the group in ordinary colleges, most of the students in this group, being residential, had a very active social life while at college which they enjoyed greatly. Only four young people appeared to have had any difficulties. A couple had not made any special friends although they both said that the other students were generally friendly. One, an Asian, said he'd prefer to be at home where he knew people, while the boy with the very severe speech impairment hadn't made friends, although the staff claimed this was more due to a lack of effort on his part to communicate than to an unwillingness on the part of the other students. The girl in the very small Unit attached to a special school definitely missed the variety of people available for friendships at school. She had made only one friend in the Unit but didn't see her outside and went back to school and to her youth clubs to see her 'real friends'. The girl who had attended the maladjusted school, while initially having considerable difficulty with friendships, eventually made several friends, though she too rarely saw them outside because they lived too far away. However, she was very pleased with the eventual success of her social life in college. She said, 'I certainly enjoyed myself with the boys there', and speaking of her relationship with her boyfriend she said, 'It was lovely.'

All the others claimed to have made friends, including some close friendships. One said with pride, 'I seem to be popular.' He had made friends outside the college as well as inside and thought of moving to that part of the country when his course was over. Many said how much they appreciated the variety of leisure facilities available both within the college and outside, and the freedom to go outside college that was allowed them in the evenings and at the weekend. One girl said: 'It's changed my life being here, going out more, travelling, freedom.' She went out regularly to the local leisure centre as well as taking part in many college activities.

However, very few felt that they would be able to maintain these friendships once they'd left college because of the distances involved and problems with transport. Two with boyfriends had exchanged visits to each other's homes for a weekend and one had been to stay the weekend with another college friend. Only one other student said she was making arrangements to see friends after the course finished. Apart from some 'phone calls, most seemed resigned to the fact that the friendships couldn't be pursued outside college. For some teenagers it would indeed be difficult to do so, but having learnt to travel by taxi and train to get to college, even those in wheelchairs would have been able to visit their friends for the day or overnight, at least occasionally. It did not seem as if anyone at college had discussed this with the students or helped them to find ways of maintaining the friendships begun at college, at least until other more local friendships had taken their place.

In contrast to the activity at college, within their home environment only two of the young people in this group were rated as having a satisfactory social life, while eleven were considered to have very restricted social intercourse. In fact the social situation at home had tended to deteriorate somewhat from the previous year when they were at school. In only two cases did there appear to be any improvement in social life at home between the two interviews (one was a student at a day college and the other lived near enough to college to be able to visit it easily after he had left).

The contrast for these young people between the liveliness and variety of activities available to them at college and the boredom and restrictions of life at home depressed them greatly, and this perhaps accounts for their passiveness and failure to maintain the contacts made at college. It would also seem that even the best of the residential colleges had not discussed this problem of loneliness in the home and how best to take steps to broaden social contacts in some way, once the students had left college.

*Likes and dislikes generally.*   There were six young people who only liked college 'on the whole' or who had 'mixed feelings', including some already mentioned who didn't like their courses particularly, and the girl in the very small day unit who missed her school friends. Others who weren't very enthusiastic about college missed home and took a long time to settle in, or would have preferred a job, or were worried about the future.

Eleven of the young people in special colleges were wholeheartedly pleased with their placement, mostly because of the general atmosphere and the social life, rather than because of the course itself. Four talked about the friendliness and the opportunities for leisure activities, and the others, while mentioning this, spoke more about the greater freedom given to them and how much they appreciated this. Typical comments were, 'The staff treated us like students not like at school', 'You could do what you wanted without people breathing down you', 'You can stay out late – at weekends till what time you like . . . it's freedom.'

When considering what the objective situation must have been, since any residential college – especially for people in this age group – must inevitably have a number of irksome regulations and a fair degree of supervision, one can only conclude that what the young people were responding to was the contrast between the college atmosphere, which fostered responsibility and independent decision making, and what they'd been used to previously at school and at home. It highlights the desire these young people had to be given more independence and to be allowed to take decisions and some risks, and suggests that they really appreciated the opportunities given them at college to do this.

*Teenagers' future plans at the time of the interview and subsequent outcome.* At the time of the Phase II interview, a high proportion of the students in special colleges had no clear plans for the future. On the basis of their handicaps and abilities, only six were clearly eligible for work and knew what they wanted to do, while two others hoped to get some kind of work, though they weren't sure what they wanted. Three young people were hoping to go on to a special industrial training college and two others to do further office training, but in no instance were the plans definite, and this was a cause of anxiety. The remaining four students, all severely handicapped, had no idea what they would do on leaving college. Though realistically the most likely outcome was a day centre, it did not appear that this had been discussed to help them think through the implications, or to decide what additional activities they might be able to organize for themselves in terms of leisure or education.

At the time of our most recent contact, eighteen months or more after leaving school, five of the teenagers were still in further education while four were in employment. All the remaining students had left college and were in unsatisfactory situations. Two had been in hospital but hoped to be able to go back to college eventually, while one girl had been at home for nearly a year awaiting another training placement; three were in day centres which they didn't like, and two were at home without any occupation, the prospects for both being pretty bleak. The most distressing aspect was the failure of services to provide any adequate follow up for those who left college to help them find a placement, discuss possible alternatives, or make a satisfactory life for themselves in some way at home.

### Day centre group

A higher proportion of young people studied were in day centres or their equivalent than were in open employment (N = 12, i.e. 24 per cent). In a few cases this was intended as a temporary expedient while awaiting another type of placement, but for most it was clear that no other provision was being planned. In addition, several who were in further education at the time of the interview but who on completion of their courses had no other placement to go to, eventually ended up or would end up in day centres.

*Characteristics of the groups.* Half the group were rated as severely handicapped, and on the whole these teenagers were very disabled indeed; all were in wheelchairs and all had an upper limb problem to some degree (one having little control in both arms). Three had marked learning disabilities (borderline ESN), three had severe communication problems, one was partially sighted and two were incontinent. Six young people were rated as moderately handicapped but only one needed to use a wheelchair and even she could walk a little indoors. The other five did not even need appliances, walking with an abnormal gait or with a limp, and all but one of these used public transport without assistance. Three had poor control in one upper limb only and one was clumsy. Two had mild speech defects, one had frequent epileptic fits, and three were of poor ability (borderline ESN).

*General arrangements.* Ten of the young people attended their Centres full-time, while one went to another Centre on the one day his regular Centre didn't operate. Only one attended for four days a week with no alternative arrangement for the fifth day. All but two spent at least six hours a day at the Centre (including the lunch break) but of course the journey to the Centre, usually by special transport, sometimes lengthened the day considerably.

The activities undertaken at the Centres varied so widely that no generalizations are possible. Six primarily concentrated on industrial contract work of various kinds, which was very repetitive and limited in scope, and included making up cardboard boxes, while craft or leisure activities were the main occupations in three other Centres. One did half craft and half industrial work, and only two offered a wide range of activities including further education, craft, typing, outside visits, cookery, dressmaking and general self-care skills. Only three teenagers were engaged in further education of any kind. Four Centres did not offer any opportunities for continuing education, and the rest could only offer basic literacy.

*Satisfaction with placement.* The most striking fact about those in day centre placements was the very high level of dissatisfaction expressed by the young people and their parents. The two main criticisms which were voiced repeatedly were first, that the activities in the Centres were boring, repetitive and generally insufficiently demanding, and secondly, that the majority of other attenders in the Centres were elderly. Most of the young people in this group wanted some kind of alternative and this should have been possible, at least in the short run, even for those whose level of disability was high. Only three were so grossly handicapped that a further education or training placement would have been very difficult to obtain, the remainder being no more handicapped than others who were at college, and at least two were less handicapped even than some of those in open employment.

Only one young man was fully satisfied with his placement. He was very severly handicapped indeed, and fully accepted the limitations that this entailed and his expectations were low compared with the others in the group. However, he was also very lucky in that he was a member of a new Centre for younger people and had been given the opportunity to be involved in running it and in choosing the activities. He had been placed for the first seven months after leaving school in a day centre for the elderly which had distressed him very much, and he had really hated going there, although he had tried hard to adjust to it.

Three of the young people were very unhappy in their day centre and could see no benefit from it at all, except as a preferable alternative to sitting at home. One of these, a bright and not too handicapped young man was placed 'temporarily' in a Spastics Society centre while waiting for a place at a training college, although this never materialized. Most of the other members at the centre were very severely handicapped and he found that both depressing and isolating. He had made no real friends and he thought the machine work he did very boring and repetitive. Another girl, awaiting a place in a college although nothing definite had been arranged, was very disappointed with the activities at the Centre. She said, 'I'd like to have it all changed. We don't do intelligent things. We just sit around and I find it boring'. She found the other members, most of whom were elderly, 'not very quick in the mind', and wanted to be with more people of her own age and more 'ordinary people'. The third young man had been rejected by the training college where he'd hoped to go and felt very bitter about this, especially as no alternative placement was offered. He wanted more interesting work and found it 'depressing that handicapped people are put all in one place'.

The remaining eight young people in day centres, while having similar criticisms, did not feel as strongly as this, and the general impression was that the placement was tolerable, *provided* that it was not the end of the road. As one said, 'I like it . . . but I don't fancy spending the rest of my life here.' Four young people who entered the day centre after many months at home doing nothing accepted it because 'anything's better than being at home.' However, the young people had no clear ideas about what else they wanted to do, and some talked about 'a job' without any real notion of what might be possible. Two were so severely handicapped that they recognized that a job was impossible but still wanted something more engaging than their current situation. This included an intelligent girl with no speech and very poor hand control who did virtually nothing at the Centre all day, the staff there being quite unused to catering for someone with this degree of handicap.

The main problem with day centres seems to be that the pace of work and the type of activities chosen are geared mainly for the benefit of the older members, the aim being to provide relatively undemanding activities to keep the elderly members active but not stressed. This is not unreasonable in that the majority of the disabled in society *are* middle-aged or elderly, but the consequence is that the pace and type of activity offered is quite unsuitable for young people leaving school who are in fact anticipating, as do most school leavers, an environment which will demand more of them than school. The desultory atmosphere of these Centres was evoked by many of the teenagers who explicitly wanted more pressure to be put upon them. 'I would like it more organized . . . you can do what you like . . . I don't want to just pass the time.' 'Unless a new job comes through you just get on with it [the work] or not as you like. They've just got to keep you occupied, that's all.' 'I can't see it [the work] going anywhere; there's no future.' Sometimes the young people had very clear ideas about what activities they wanted to pursue, for example one wanted more typing and another wanted to paint, but they didn't seem to have been given choices or encouraged to make decisions like this for themselves.

Of course it is probably true that the activities undertaken at the Centres were no more boring than the repetitive industrial or office routines which would be the only possible *paid* work that these young people could be offered, and which in fact is the lot of the majority of the able-bodied working population. It is perhaps worth considering why such work is tolerable to many normal people but intolerable for these youngsters. Three factors may be important: first, a prime function of work is to provide self-esteem – a feeling of being useful to society in some way. However, much of the work at the Centres seemed pointless to the young attenders in that the goods produced were not saleable (not being of a high quality) or considered 'useful' or 'wanted' commercially, while the industrial contract work usually involved making items like cardboard boxes which do not have high status. These activities were not respected by the teenagers' families either, who tended to see them as time-wasters rather than as work. One girl reported that her mother had said, 'It's all right for you, you don't do anything all day'.

A second point is that drudgery, bearable in itself if the remuneration is good, or at least adequate to allow the worker financial independence, becomes intolerable if it is poorly paid. In fact the main source of income for most young people at the day centres was supplementary benefit, though some were also receiving the mobility allowance and the attendance allowance. If a centre is organized to produce saleable items, then up to £4 may be paid to the clients without loss of benefit, although only five people in the group were earning this supplement. The average total weekly income for this group was £22, even if the mobility and the attendance allowances were included (the latter is really a payment to the mother for her work as care person, although nominally paid to the handicapped person after the age of sixteen) and £18 if the attendance allowances were not included (compared with £30 average for those in employment).

Thirdly, boring jobs are tolerable to many people because of the comradeship provided by their workmates. Going to work produces social if not intellectual stimulation, and many of the friendships which people pursue outside working hours are initiated at or through work. Most of the day centres could not serve this function for the younger clients because of the age of the other attenders; indeed, according to the parents, the majority were over retirement age. Most of the young people had made one or two friends, but the choice of friends of a similar age group was very restricted and it was unusual for friendships to be close or to be pursued outside the Centre, partly for this reason, but also because distance and transport problems made contact difficult.

When parents were asked about their satisfaction with the Centres, only three had no complaints – in each case the young person himself was fully or quite satisfied. Most parents felt the placement was unsuitable because the other attenders were too old or much lower in ability. In fact half the parents didn't wish their child to be in a day centre at all, while three others did not disagree with the principle, but thought the teenager should be doing different activities or should be in a different kind of day centre.

*How placements came about.*   Given such a high level of dissatisfaction it is interesting to note how and why these placements came about. Three of the young people were so handicapped that an alternative placement would have been difficult to arrange; four had been placed in Centres intended as a temporary expedient while the authorities investigated the possibilities of a college placement; three had turned down the offer of residential college because either they themselves, or their parents hadn't wanted them to go away from home, while two had been rejected by the college where they had hoped to go and no alternative had been arranged.

The three very severely handicapped young people had had the Centre placement arranged for them before they left school. One boy, a severe athetoid with a very marked speech defect but of normal ability, had rejected the idea of residential college because he couldn't see the point given that he obviously would never be able to hold down even sheltered employment. He liked his Centre which specially catered for young people. One very severe athetoid girl with no speech had elderly parents who could no longer care for her physically, since she was totally dependent and needed two attenders constantly. Her parents were looking for a residential placement, and meanwhile the day centre gave the mother some daily relief but offered little to the girl, since she couldn't participate in the activities of the Centre and no special arrangements had been made for her. She was of average ability and got very bored; both she and her parents felt she'd be better off with more younger people. The third boy liked some things about the Centre but some elements he described as 'babyish' and generally felt there was not enough pressure to work. He had especial difficulty in making contact with the elderly attenders because of his speech defect; he felt they 'couldn't be bothered . . . I try to make friends with them but they won't make friends with me . . . because I can't speak well. They haven't enough time.'

None of the other nine attenders was so severely handicapped that alternative placements would have been impossible to arrange, at least for one or two years, and they were not physically different from the group who were in further education or training. The three who had turned down the offer of a residential college had been left rather high and dry by the services, and were at home for long periods (six months or more) before a Centre place was arranged. It seemed very likely that if the offer of residential college had been repeated a year later the young people or their parents' attitudes might have been quite different.

Apart from the severe athetoid boy and two who were awaiting definite college places, one had the impression that most people in the day centres had fallen between services in some way, and had ended up in their particular Centre not because it was really thought to be the most appropriate place, but because no one had given sufficient thought to discovering whether there might be a better alternative, or whether the Centre's activities could be adapted in order to meet their needs. These weren't planned placements in any kind of overall programme to help the young people gain more experience, become more independent or achieve a particular goal, other than avoiding the distress of being at home doing nothing. Three placements had been arranged by a social worker primarily to help the family out of a difficult dilemma ('What to do with him now he's left school') and in three cases the placement was found following the initiative of a family or neighbour because nothing else had been suggested.

For the four young people who had been at home for a long period after leaving school, the day centre did offer some kind of relief both to them and to their families. Two had become so depressed at being at home that they had become really ill. One stopped eating and lost three stones in weight over a couple of months. She said: 'I felt like ending it all . . . I thought I'm gonna die and not eat anything because I felt hopeless and didn't want to live.' The other said, 'I got very depressed . . . cracked up really. I felt useless'. For such people the day centre was at least a release from that ordeal, but hardly a real choice.

*Lack of information and of autonomy.* Once again, most of the young people and their parents were critical about how little information they'd been given on possible placement, or on what the day centre could and could not offer, and even where there were no strong dissatisfactions with the Centre, there was still a feeling that without full knowledge of the alternatives no real choice had been possible. This feeling of lack of autonomy by parents and teenagers came across very strongly. 'They just put me here, I couldn't say nothing.' 'You only have the choice of going away [to college], with no certainty of a job after, or of coming here.' 'You just get put in one of these places.' One father said: 'You're in other people's hands . . . I wasn't told there are these possibilities – x, y, z – I was only told *their* opinions of where he should go.' Another parent said, 'We weren't given any idea at all of what J. can do or where she would go.' One girl who resisted strongly the idea of going to a day centre said she felt, 'they were going to take me over. I started getting defiant . . . said I was ill, not going, I wouldn't accept it.' It seems that the very least one can offer these young people is a dignified discussion of the options available (or lack of them) given the level of their handicap and the reasons why, if the day centre is recommended, this is seen to be the preferred option, despite the limitations of the placement.

*Day centre staff.* One positive note, however, which came through without exception, was the fact that the day centre staff were seen to be sympathetic, friendly people with whom the young people could and often did discuss their feelings and difficulties. One had the impression, therefore, that the day centres needn't have been such an unrewarding experience if the staff had been helped to design programmes for the younger members, utilizing outside resources to supplement what could be offered in the Centres, and making sure they had contact on at least some days with other young people.

*Links between day centres and schools and the quality of social life.* Two further points should be made about the day centres, although these were not complained of by the teenagers themselves. First, contacts did not appear to have been established between the Centres and the young people's schools and this lack of continuity must have hindered the development of any training programme for the attenders. For example, in the case of the severe athetoid girl, who could not participate in the centre activities at all because of the severity of her handicaps, her previous school had arranged special assistance for her, and her school attender had clearly developed skills in helping her to communicate and participate which could have been passed on to the Centre's staff to everyone's satisfaction and benefit.

Secondly, only one Centre appeared to organize any social events outside normal hours and none of the others seemed to have seen the need to help their clients improve their social life at home. Only two members of this group were rated as having satisfactory social lives and, given the very poor work satisfaction, it was especially important that they receive help in broadening their social contacts. It is probably significant that the only Centre which did have a club and where the members appeared to meet each other socially in the evenings or weekends was an adult training centre for the mentally handicapped. There appears to be a much better appreciation by those concerned with the care of the young mentally handicapped of the need to help develop social contacts, and this point will come out more clearly in the discussion in chapter 10 of the social skills programmes available in schools to help handicapped young people in the transition to adult life.

*Was the young people's dissatisfaction justified?*   A point of view which is sometimes voiced is that the young people's dissatisfaction with the day centres represents their failure to come to terms with their own limitations. Two points can be made in answer to this. First, there was clear evidence from the young people that the Centres were not geared to their particular needs, and where attempts had been made to design programmes with younger clients in mind, and especially where the clients themselves were involved in the programme organization, then the level of satisfaction changed dramatically. It is obviously difficult to design a special programme for younger people in Centres where the clients are predominantly elderly, but it should be feasible to discuss possible activities with the client, his family and his school to discover his potential and preferences and to arrange that he spend at least part of his time doing things of his own choice. Links with local schools, further education colleges and adult education institutes would facilitate this, as well as perhaps providing the young people with additional opportunities for meeting others of their age group.

Secondly, perhaps the main problem in the attitude of the young people themselves was the failure of many to recognize their very slender chances of gaining employment. However, this is largely the product of the false expectations raised in them by their schools, and also by others, rather than a failure in the young people themselves. It did not appear that any had had a real opportunity to discuss the whole issue of employment – or its lack, the demands of the market, their chances of gaining work, how best to deal with permanent unemployment. (This is equally important of course for those who had gone on to further education, the majority of whom were unlikely to find open employment, but whose expectations were certainly oriented towards this.)

This failure to prepare the young people for the realities of life after leaving school was probably in part a natural, but nonetheless regrettable, reluctance by the adults in contact with them to raise this depressing issue (although of course alternatives to work can be very rewarding if planned with imagination), and partly a failure by the adults to recognize the capacity of the young people themselves to appreciate their own situation, and to enter into a sensible dialogue about the choices available. It was very striking in the interviews that even children rated by their schools as borderline ESN or low average could be very perceptive about their situation, and indeed extremely eloquent about their feelings and responses. One girl in a day centre after seven months at home, who had been described as borderline ESN by her teachers, summed up her situation very vividly: 'When I left school I felt I wasn't in control of anything, not even my own mind . . . I wanted to be independent, get a job . . . I had great hopes at first when I left school but they were all knocked down one by one.' The school staff and the careers service must have appreciated that a day centre was the most likely placement for this young person. An opportunity to discuss this fully before leaving school as well as afterwards and to decide how best to make use of her time both in the day centre and out of it, would have helped minimize her distress and approach adult life with a more positive and less victimized attitude.

### 'At home' group

The number of young people without any occupation at all was quite small at the time of the Phase II interview, and consisted of five teenagers (10 per cent of the total group). They had spent all or most of their time since leaving school without a placement, and three were still without any prospects of any kind at the time of the interview. However, at our most recent contact with them, 12–18 months after they had left school, the number without occupation had more than doubled, because many who left special further education after one year found themselves unable to get a placement (see Table 7.4). It is obviously important to look at the experience of this group in detail, therefore, both because this situation was very distressing to the young people and their families, and because their histories illustrate very clearly what the deficiences are in services which created this situation.

*Characteristics of the group.*   Three of the five teenagers were rated as severely handicapped on the Pultibec Scale – all three were in wheelchairs including two spina bifida young people with incontinence. The other two were rated as moderately handicapped and were both athetoid, but quite mobile and could use public transport unassisted. All three cerebral-palsied young people in this group had upper limb problems although none was very severe, one being merely awkward at fine manual tasks. All the young people in this group were average or low-average in ability, and none had marked learning problems which would make it difficult for an able-bodied teenager to find a job or a training placement, although one had quite a marked speech impairment. All had been to special schools, two of them residential.

*Immediate post-school experience.*   Three of the young people had been placed, on leaving school, in a special residential college for further education. Two left college within a few weeks of placement because they couldn't settle in. One girl who had attended residential school for many years nevertheless got very homesick at college, partly because she was not independent in handling her urinary appliance and this had caused problems. However, it is probable that worries about home were a more important cause (though not stated), since her parents had separated during the year and the girl, an only child, was exceptionally close to her mother. She very emphatically wanted to live at home and be a companion to her mother, but at the time of the interview had been placed in a residential home for the disabled where she hoped to learn more independence. She found this placement so unsatisfactory (it offered her no daytime occupation whatsoever) that by the end of the year she was prepared to accept anything, at home or away. The other, a boy, had never been away before, was very dependent on his family and simply hadn't been able to deal with the separation. Both he and his parents regretted the decision to leave in retrospect: 'Now I wish I hadn't left . . . it was much better than sitting at home with absolutely nothing to do.' In both cases the careers officers appeared to be annoyed with the young people for not persisting with the original placement, but in each case, with sympathetic support during the first few weeks of college and extra visiting, the difficulties could probably have been overcome.

The third teenager who had originally been placed in a residential college had to leave for medical reasons (he developed a bad pressure sore and urine infection which the college were unable to cope with). He resented this rejection very much, and the fact that, through neglect, his condition eventually required extensive hospital treatment. At the time of the interview he was still in hospital awaiting a skin graft and various urological procedures. He hoped very much to be allowed to return to college when his treatment was completed.

The fourth teenager had hoped to get into a training college on leaving school, and when she failed to do so had tried very hard to get a job. Various agencies had been involved but she'd been unable to obtain a place and had spent the year at home doing the housework. She had parents who were not very supportive and who were, furthermore, immigrants and consequently not well versed in which services to consult. She still preferred the option of further education but felt so desperate that she was prepared to take any kind of job. She was very competent and, though with marked upper limb problems, was acting as housekeeper to her family of seven while her mother went out to work. She had lots of initiative, mixing well with the local able-bodied young people and probably could have managed in an ordinary further education college with support, but no one had suggested this.

The fifth, a boy, had also been at home all year. He was very nervous, very dependent on his family, and had left school rather suddenly because he was depressed having originally intended to stay on an extra year. He'd been assessed by the Spastics Society who suggested a residential course and was waiting for a vacancy, meanwhile doing nothing at home.

Two of these young people had tried local day centres but both left after a very short time because the occupation was so trivial and all the other attenders were elderly. ('Day centres are like glorified play centres to me – useless and boring.') Two others were offered day centres but resisted the placement for the same kind of reason, and because they felt that once they were there, nothing better would be forthcoming.

*Subsequent outcome.* At our most recent contact with this group only one of the young people appeared to be in a satisfactory placement, while one was still in hospital and three were at home and unoccupied. Four of the five were not easy to place, though their difficulties were no greater than (and in many cases less than) other young people in the study who had been successful in getting satisfactory occupation of some kind. However, one was a very competent, very personable girl who was still quite optimistic at the interview about her future, despite very understandable bouts of depression, and she should have been able to get a college place, given informed help – but this help was simply not forthcoming from the agencies she'd explored. As one teenager, who had left school full of enthusiasm to get a job and be independent, said of the agencies she'd consulted, 'They put a barrier up straight away – now I'm defeated.' The very severe stresses suffered by the young people in this group as a consequence of their unemployment are dealt with in more detail in chapter 8, but their plight clearly indicates the failure of statutory and voluntary services to provide adequate post-school services. (This is discussed further in chapter 11.)

### Comparison of handicaps between the placement groups

It seemed worth comparing the handicaps present in the different placement groups in order to demonstrate that placement was not determined by handicap alone, and to show that many in 'special' placements of some kind were no more handicapped than some of those in 'ordinary' placements.

To make this comparison each individual's problems were examined to see how many different handicaps he had, and how seriously each interfered with daily living and might therefore cause problems in a non-specialized setting. A locomotor problem was counted as serious if the individual was entirely or mainly in a wheelchair, or if he were unable to use public transport unaccompanied. Clumsiness or only slight problems with the upper limbs were not counted as serious; however, if both limbs were affected this was counted as two problems. For speech defects any real difficulty in understanding the young person was counted as a serious problem, as was any degree of deafness, epilepsy or incontinence, or if the young person was of very low ability (borderline ESN). This way of categorizing and combining handicaps, therefore, was very pragmatic and based entirely on the young person's current functioning, rather

Table 7.5 *Comparison of handicaps between the placement groups*

| Category of handicap | In employment | Ordinary FE | Special FE | Day centre | At home |
|---|---|---|---|---|---|
| No serious problems | 6 | 2 | 2 | 0 | 0 |
| One serious problem: | | | | | |
| one upper limb impaired | 2 | 1 | 4 | 1 | 0 |
| poor walking | 0 | 1 | 1 | 0 | |
| Two serious problems | 1 | 3 | 6 | 3 | 4 |
| Very serious multiple handicaps | 0 | 1 | 4 | 7 | 1 |

than on any standardized scales like the Pultibec. The results are shown in Table 7.5.

The table clearly shows that those in 'ordinary' placements were less likely to have problems and multiple problems than the others. However, it also shows that there were seven people in special colleges and two in day centres who were less handicapped than many of those in ordinary placements, and who should have been able to manage in an ordinary college of further education. Indeed four had been to an ordinary school. Five young people in ordinary placements had two or more serious handicaps. Despite their difficulties they had managed well in an integrated setting with a little sensible help. In the special further education, day centre and at home groups there were thirteen young people counted as having two serious problems. While clearly some of these young people would not have been able to attend an ordinary college without special facilities and teaching, there is no doubt that some were no more severely impaired than the most handicapped teenagers who were managing in an integrated setting. One must conclude that, considering degree and multiplicity of handicaps alone, about half of those in special college could have managed in ordinary establishments, given goodwill by the staff, without any major special arrangements being required, while the same would be true for one-third to a half of those in day centres, and for two of the five in the at home group.

The problems of those with very serious multiple handicaps were such that it is most unlikely they could have managed in an ordinary college without a special unit of some kind. But with the possible exception of four teenagers, all were capable of benefitting from some of the courses offered at ordinary colleges, especially since the latter are totally familiar with the problems of teaching students of lower ability.

The advantages of integrating as many young handicapped people as possible into ordinary facilities as soon as they leave school are clear; it gives them more self-confidence, broadens their experience and range of interests, and gives them an opportunity to begin making social contacts with the able-bodied. For those who are more competent, it helps bridge the gap between the very protective atmosphere of a special school and the competitive world of work, and must make the handicapped teenager more attractive to potential employers than those who have never had the opportunity to prove that they can compete on equal terms with their able-bodied peers.

There are of course particular advantages that some residential special colleges offer to young people and which could only be provided within ordinary colleges if a special residential unit were provided. First, the experience of living away from home is maturing in itself, particularly if the college treats its students like young adults, giving them considerable freedom and responsibility. Secondly, those colleges which make a special effort to teach ordinary living skills and to encourage their students to become maximally independent are offering something that cannot be provided within most ordinary colleges at present. However, it would not be difficult to provide both these advantages within a college of further education which had a special unit attached and a termly or weekly boarding facility. Such a unit would enable the students to take part more fully in college social activities in the evenings and at weekends, especially if it were combined with some counselling to help deal with this.

Not every college of further education could be expected to provide special facilities to this extent, but it would by no means be unreasonable, and not excessively costly, for each local authority to make provision for handicapped pupils within its FE system, offering varying degrees of extra help or support in different establishments. It should be possible to provide a special unit with residential facilities within one college in each large authority, while smaller education authorities could combine with others to find a residential unit.

# 8

## *Stresses encountered during the transition year*

In this chapter we are concerned with the question of the stresses experienced by disabled teenagers during the first year after they left school. Most of those who write about non-handicapped school leavers assume that this year will often be a difficult one, and we expected that it would be even more difficult for disabled young people. However, since little research evidence was available we wanted to establish, first, what proportion of disabled school leavers found the transition year stressful, and to what extent; and secondly, the nature of the stresses they encountered.

In approaching this question there are three theoretical models of considerable interest and relevance. The first is the model proposed by Lazarus in *Psychological Stress and the Coping Process* (1966). Lazarus suggests that we need to understand what are the conditions and processes that determine when stress reactions will be produced and when they will not. In trying to explain what is or is not stressful Lazarus makes use of what he calls 'the intervening variable of *threat*'. Threat, according to Lazarus, implies a state in which the individual anticipates a confrontation with a harmful condition of some sort. Whether or not a particular stimulus is perceived as threatening will depend on how the stimulus (the potentially threatening situation) is appraised by the individual. This depends upon factors in the situation with which the individual is confronted and include such things as the actual harm that the stimulus could produce and the imminence of the harmful confrontation; factors within the psychological structure of the individual, including what Lazarus calls his 'motive-strength or patterns' (which determine how much *meaning* the situation has for him); his general beliefs about transactions with the environment (for example, his past experience of the amount of control he has over his environment); and finally his intellectual resources, education and knowledge. If a stimulus is appraised as threatening, then coping processes (discussed more fully in chapter 12) are set in motion.

If we accept Lazarus's model, a concrete example would be as follows: A and B are sixteen year old, mildly handicapped hemiplegic boys who have attended ordinary schools and will leave in about a month's time. Both wish to obtain jobs in open employment but both are confronted with a similar situation in so far as jobs are currently hard to obtain, even for non-handicapped leavers. A is a boy who identifies strongly with his able-bodied peers. His mother, who is single, works full-time and becomes rather depressed, and has never been someone he felt he could confide in or look to for help. He has no absorbing interests and has, like most of his peers, been eagerly anticipating the time when he can leave school and start earning. His careers officer has, after a preliminary vaguely optimistic chat some months ago, passed him on to a specialist careers officer who has told him rather bluntly that his prospects of obtaining employment are very poor. A, hitherto a rather happy-go-lucky boy, suddenly finds the whole situation enormously threatening. B, on the other hand, faced with the same potential threat, is not experiencing the same level of stress. His parents have prepared him for the idea that it may take several months to find work, and in the past have been very supportive. He feels they will eventually help him to 'sort out the problem'. He has already faced up to the prospect that it may be more difficult for him than for his able-bodied peers to find a job, and while he feels some resentment about this he is able to discuss the implications of his disability quite openly, as he has been accustomed to doing this with his parents.

A second theoretical model which we have found useful is the one proposed by Adams *et al.* (1976) in *Transition, Understanding and Managing Personal Change*. While Lazarus focused in his model upon threat, Adams *et al.* focus on *transition*. Since in Phase II of the study we were particularly concerned with young people making what is usually described as 'the transition from school to work' (or to adult life) their model is highly relevant. A genuine transition is defined by these authors as 'a discontinuity in a person's life space of which he is aware and which requires new behavioural responses'. The important elements in the transition are first, that the person must actually *experience* it as a discontinuity, and secondly that new behavioural responses are required either because the situation is new, or the required behaviours are new, or both. If these two criteria are taken into account a severely disabled spina bifida teenager, for example, leaving a residential school for the disabled and going with two school friends to a residential further education college for the disabled may not be making a transition at all, whereas a similarly disabled peer, for whom the only available provision is a day centre whose clients are mainly elderly, will be making a major transition. Even among those in our study who did experience a 'transition', their experience of 'stress' varied greatly, some being affected very markedly and others not at all.

The third model we want to refer to is the one proposed by Brown and Harris (1978) in their study of the social origins of depression in women. The psychological problems of the great majority of teenagers in our study were still of a kind more typical of childhood than of adult disorders (a distinction which Rutter *et al.* also noted in their study of psychiatric disorders in the Isle of Wight fourteen year olds). Nor were our young people, with possibly one or two exceptions, clinically depressed. Nevertheless, they showed many symptoms similar to (although less severe than) those described by Brown and Harris as 'borderline' between women having and not having a depression.

Brown and Harris suggest that there are essentially two factors which produce depression: 'provoking agents', which influence *when* the depression occurs, and 'vulnerability factors', which influence *whether* the provoking agents will have an effect. The provoking agents, as identified by Brown and Harris, are 'severe life events involving long-term threat'. The distinctive feature of the great majority of these events is 'the experience of loss or disappointment, if this is defined broadly to include *threat* of *or actual* separation from a key figure, an unpleasant revelation about someone close, a life-threatening illness to a close relative, a major material loss or general disappointment or threat of them, and miscellaneous crises such as being made redundant after a long period of steady employment'. In more general terms the loss or disappointment could concern a person or object, a role or an idea. They also emphasize that they found that feelings of hopelessness could arise 'simply in response to thought about a possible loss', not only to actual events.

Like Lazarus and Adams *et al.*, Brown and Harris note that change is not in itself threatening, rather that 'everything turns on the meaningfulness of events', and that it is only events involving long-term threat that are signficant, since these usually involve loss and disappointment. The authors see an actual or anticipated loss as depriving the individual of sources of value or reward, and as leading to 'an inability to hold good thoughts about ourselves, our lives and those close to us. Particularly important . . . is the loss of faith in one's ability to attain an important and valued goal'. Another relevant point is that it is not simply the loss of a particular 'object' that is important, but the implications of this for his or her ability to find satisfactory alternatives. A sense of hopelessness produced by a particular loss or disappointment can therefore lead to thoughts of hopelessness about life in general, and it is this *generalization* of hopelesness which the authors see as the central core of a depressive disorder.

While the authors give a central role to 'severe life events' as 'provoking agents', they also note that 'ongoing major difficulties' (of at least two years' duration) can also play an important part in the onset of depression. This distinction between 'major ongoing difficulties' and 'severe life events' is a very relevant one where chronically disabled people are concerned. Certainly for most disabled youngsters and their families the disability is considered to be 'a major ongoing difficulty', often giving rise to symptoms such as more frequent worrying, as already noted in this study, and to lack of self-esteem. Despite this, as many teenagers and parents said to us, they had 'learned to live with' disability. The situation may be altered, however, when a disabled teenager is faced by the equivalent of Brown and Harris's 'severe life event', or by a transition involving stress. The likelihood of this confrontation with threat taking place is greatly increased at the time of school leaving, although it may be postponed for several years if the youngster goes straight into a special college of further education.

What sorts of 'severe life events', 'transitions' or 'threats' may a disabled teenager be faced with? One is the realization which often comes on leaving school or college that it may be impossible to get a job. If this is something to which the teenager has aspired throughout school (and he will almost certainly have been encouraged by our whole system of education to hope for this) a large part of his sense of identity and self-esteem will depend on getting a job, and the loss of this hope may be highly threatening. Another severe life event may be placement in a day centre of the kind which many of the young people in our study experienced. It is very easy to see how this could engender a sense of hopelessness. On the personal side, it may not be until late adolescence or early adulthood that a severely handicapped boy or girl is confronted by the recognition that they may never find a partner or marry.

However, while only a minority of teenagers in our study were faced by 'severe life events' of the kind which Brown and Harris describe, a great many were exposed to 'transitions' involving 'stress', as defined by Adams *et al.*, or to 'threats' of the kind described by Lazarus. This chapter discusses the major sources of stress experienced by the young people in the follow-up study, and indicates how many suffered unhappiness as a result of transitional stresses, or threats to their self-esteem.

We were mainly concerned with the stresses imposed by the actual placement, whether this was a job, a college course or attendance at a day centre, and it is these that we have therefore concentrated on. Other sources of stress, however, for instance health problems, or events occurring within the family or in the young people's relationships outside of work or college, were also considered. Accordingly, the chapter is divided into three parts, the first dealing with stresses related to the placement, the second to stresses related to health and disability problems, and the third to stresses engendered by personal and family relationships.

### Overview of the findings

Before looking at each of these three areas in detail, we thought it would be useful to provide readers with the broad pattern of our findings, and to explain briefly why the particular stress items were chosen and the method of rating.

When the interview was completed, the researchers discussed the experiences described by the young people and their parents, and then drew up a list of the stress situations most commonly referred to, or those which, even if they did not occur frequently, were very distressing or had caused a major disruption to the young people's career at any point throughout the post-school year. The list of potential stresses selected is shown in Table 8.1.

The interview material from each of the young people included in the sample was then reviewed to see whether that individual had been subjected to any of the stresses listed during the previous year, and was rated for each potential stress on a scale of 0–2, a rating of 2 indicating a marked stress, a rating of 1 a mild or dubious stress, while a rating of 0 indicated that that individual had not encountered that particular form of stress at any time during the post-school year. In Table 8.1, however, we have shown only the number of young people in each of the placement groups experiencing marked or definite stress on a particular item, that is, we have used the more stringent criteria.

This table shows that of the items selected, by far the most common stress experienced was social isolation, which was a marked problem for nearly 40 per cent of the sample. Problems within the family or the home also affected quite a high proportion of the sample – over 25 per cent. Where social isolation was combined with family difficulties, the young people concerned were often very distressed indeed and this will be discussed more fully later in this chapter.

Anxiety with regard to future placement was also a common experience (for about one-third of the sample). Frustrations because of the feeling that their abilities were not being fully utilized in their current placement, while not so common (affecting only about 20 per cent of the young people), caused much disillusionment and humiliation among those individuals who endured it.

Two other common sources of stress experienced by about one-quarter of the sample, were health problems (either hospitalization, or deterioration in function, or some other serious health problem not warranting hospitalization); and 'time to first placement', involving young people who had to wait for two months or more after leaving school before they were placed; in many cases this involved several months of uncertainty and distress.

About one-quarter of the sample described difficulties they had encountered on first starting their new placement, but although these caused severe stress at the time they rarely persisted, and so this was a temporary situation which cannot in reality be considered a marked problem in the same way as the other items discussed here. In fact the sense of achievement in overcoming the initial difficulties in many cases probably more than compensated for the initial anxieties.

When all the young people considered to have experienced stress in

Table 8.1 *Marked stresses experienced by teenagers in different groups*

| | Employed N = 9 | Ordinary FE N = 8 | Special FE N = 17 | Day centre N = 12 | At home N = 5 | Total N = 51 | (%) |
|---|---|---|---|---|---|---|---|
| *Placement stresses* | | | | | | | |
| Time to first placement | 2 | 0 | 4 | 4[1] | 4[2] | 14 | (27) |
| Problems first starting | 2 | 2 | 2 | 4[1] | 2 | 12 | (23) |
| 1 or 2 changes in placement | 2 | 0 | 0 | 0 | 3[1] | 5[1] | (10) |
| Job/course very demanding | 3[1] | 3[1] | 1 | 0 | 0 | 7 | (13) |
| Frustrated as abilities not utilized | 0 | 0 | 0 | 5[1] | 5[2] | 10 | (20) |
| Anxiety re future placement | 1 | 2 | 5[1] | 4[1] | 5[2] | 17 | (33) |
| Other placement stress | 1 | 0 | 0 | 1 | 0 | 2 | (4) |
| *Personal social stresses* | | | | | | | |
| Social stress related to placement | 0 | 0 | 2 | 4[1] | 0 | 6 | (12) |
| Loss of friends not replaced | 0 | 1 | 2 | 1 | 2 | 6 | (12) |
| Stress with close personal friend | 1 | 0 | 1 | 1 | 0 | 3 | (4) |
| Relations within family difficult | 1 | 2 | 6[1] | 1 | 3 | 13 | (25) |
| Living arrangements | 0 | 1 | 1 | 0 | 4[2] | 6 | (12) |
| Social isolation | 2 | 2 | 6[1] | 5[1] | 4[2] | 19 | (37) |
| *Health/disability stresses* | | | | | | | |
| Hospitalization | 1 | 1 | 2 | 0 | 1 | 5 | (10) |
| Other health problems including deterioration | 1 | 0 | 3 | 2 | 1 | 7 | (13) |
| Management of incontinence | 0 | 0 | 0 | 0 | 0 | 0 | (0) |
| *Other* | | | | | | | |
| Major stress during year | 2 | 0 | 2 | 1 | 0 | 5 | (10) |

[1] Experienced by approximately one-third of young people in that placement group.
[2] Experienced by over one-half of young people in that placement group.

either a marked *or* a mild form are included a very similar pattern occurs, with social isolation still being the most common problem (present for over 60 per cent of the sample), followed by problems on first starting (affecting nearly half of the group), anxiety concerning future placement (44 per cent) and time to first placement (a problem for nearly one-third of the group). Problems within the family, frustrations concerning abilities not utilized, and social stress related to placement also figure prominently.

Looking at the frequency with which the different stresses were encountered within each of the placement groups, it is apparent from Table 8.2 that by far the greatest distress was suffered by the 'at home' group, while the group in day centres also experienced a high level of stress.

Table 8.2 *Distribution of marked stresses by placement group*

|  | Employed N = 9 | Ordinary FE N = 8 | Special FE N = 17 | Day centre N = 12 | At home N = 5 | Total N = 51 |
|---|---|---|---|---|---|---|
| No stresses | 3 | 1 | 2 | 3 | 0 | 9 |
| 1 stress | 1 | 4 | 6 | 0 | 0 | 11 |
| 2 stresses | 1 | 2 | 4 | 3 | 0 | 10 |
| 3 stresses | 1 | 0 | 2 | 3 | 0 | 6 |
| 4 stresses | 2 | 0 | 2 | 0 | 1 | 5 |
| 5 stresses | 1 | 0 | 0 | 1 | 1 | 3 |
| 6 or more stresses | 0 | 1 | 1 | 2 | 3 | 7 |

*Teenagers' own perception of previous year as stressful*

*(a) Teenagers' experience of the post-school year as 'difficult'.* The young people were asked whether the last year had been a difficult one since, as we noted earlier, change or difference in itself may not be experienced as stressful. The actual question was: 'Would you say that you've found the year after leaving school quite a difficult one in some ways or not?' (If necessary the interviewer then added: 'Would you describe it as definitely very difficult or quite difficult or only a few difficulties or not difficult?')

The majority of the young people (almost 60 per cent) were quite positive about the year, because they had enjoyed leaving school and entering adult life, especially those in ordinary further education, despite the fact that some individuals in this group had been subject to quite demanding situations in their attempt to compete on equal terms with the able-bodied. However, the majority of those in the 'at home' group said they had found life difficult, as did over 40 per cent of those in day centres and in employment.

*(b) Comparison between teenagers' experience of difficulty and the number of marked stresses.*   When a comparison is made between the interviewer's assessment of the number of marked stresses experienced, and the teenagers' self-assessment of the year as being 'difficult', although the two sets of data do not fully concord, there was a large measure of agreement (see Table 8.3). Twenty-four of the twenty-nine young people rated as having two or fewer stresses (82 per cent) said that the year was not a difficult one, while of the twenty rated as having three or more marked stresses, fifteen stated that they had experienced the year as being quite or very difficult.

Table 8.3 *Comparison of number of marked stresses with teenagers' experience of difficulty*

|  | Teenagers' experience of the past year as difficult | | | | |
|---|---|---|---|---|---|
| Number of marked stresses (Interviewer's assessment) | Not difficult | A few difficulties | Quite difficult | Very difficult | Total |
| 0 | 4 | 4 | 0 | 0 | 8 |
| 1 | 6 | 2 | 3 | 0 | 11 |
| 2 | 5 | 3 | 1 | 1 | 10 |
| 3 | 0 | 1 | 2 | 3 | 6 |
| 4 | 0 | 1 | 1 | 2 | 4 |
| 5 | 0 | 1 | 0 | 2 | 3 |
| 6 + | 0 | 2 | 1 | 4 | 7 |
| Total | 15 | 14 | 8 | 12 | 49 |

*Stresses related to the placement*

*Time to first placement and resulting stress.*   We assumed that one of the most potentially stressful situations facing the young people would be when the teenager had no definite placement arranged within a few weeks of leaving school, and we asked each one how long a period had elapsed between their leaving school and starting in their first placement. In cases where the waiting period had been more than six weeks (that is, longer than the summer vacation) they were asked what the problem was, whether they had any idea why it had taken so long to obtain a placement, what they had felt like, and who had helped them. The parents were asked a similar question, including whether their son or daughter got 'upset or depressed or worried' if he or she had left school without a definite job or placement to go to. On the basis of the information from the teenagers and the parents, the teenager was then given a stress rating of 0 (no stress) 1 (dubious/mild stress) or 2 (definite and/or marked stress).

Nearly 70 per cent of the young people were placed very quickly (within about six weeks of leaving school) regardless of the type of school attended. Of the three attending ordinary schools who had to wait longer, one had taken only just over six weeks to find her first job. However, she had found this a very distressing experience, since most of her school friends had found jobs much more quickly. In contrast, while 68 per cent of those attending special schools were also placed very quickly, near one-quarter waited over three months before finding some form of occupation (usually a special further education college or day centre), and two individuals had had no occupation of any kind during the year following school.

Looking at time to first placement in relation to severity of handicap, as one might expect the majority of those who had to wait a long time, three months or more, were those who had more serious handicaps. Those who had to wait longest (over 6 months) tended to be cerebral-palsied with multiple handicaps.

There were fourteen young people altogether who had experienced delays of over 6 weeks in time to first placement, and all were considered by the interviewers to have suffered from severe stress as a result. In one case this was a consequence of protracted orthopaedic procedures and the subsequent need for physiotherapy, which made it impossible for the girl to take up her intended employment. Another girl who had a mild hemiplegia took two months to find an employer who would accept her. In neither of these two cases could the careers service or the post-school follow-up services in any way be held responsible for these delays, but this was *not* the case in the remaining twelve cases, and it is worthwhile discussing their problems at some length to illustrate in what way the services are deficient at present.

First, there were four young people for whom a place in a special college of further education had been arranged before leaving school but who had to wait from 3–6 months before a vacancy occurred in the recommended college, and they were very bored at home during this time, and worried about the uncertainty over just when they would start. Although too handicapped to get out of the house easily without support, some kind of activities could have been arranged for them, for example they could have participated in the out of school activities of their own or other local schools or day centres, or perhaps some voluntary work could have been found to help them through this period.

The history of the remaining seven cases demonstrates the very serious deficiencies in services if a young handicapped person leaves school without a pre-arranged placement, because there is no single agency within the community responsible for follow up. For example, one young man, who had confidently expected to enter a training establishment and had stayed on an extra year at school in order to qualify for entry, was turned down on the grounds of his low ability a little before leaving school. Because his careers officer had left the area about this time, no one took up his case, and despite repeated 'phone calls to the careers service nothing was provided for him for twelve months. On the advice of a friend, the mother contacted the Disablement Resettlement Officer (DRO), following which a day centre place was provided very quickly. During this year the boy became very irritable and depressed. He was obviously quite a capable person, since at our most recent contact with him he had found himself a job in open employment.

Another girl had a similar history but a less favourable outcome, perhaps because she did not have supportive parents. She was of average ability with good locomotor function, and ability to use public transport. She had a slight speech impairment, but no difficulty in making herself understood, and although both her upper limbs were mildly spastic, she could manage most manual tasks very competently. She left her special school unplaced, having failed to get into the training college of her choice because her academic attainments were inadequate. No alternative placement was suggested. Again, the careers officer who had been advising her left the service and though the local office said they'd let her know 'if anything came up', they failed to contact her. Day centre places were suggested by the Spastics Society, but there were no immediate vacancies, and they were in any case unacceptable to the girl who wanted, quite reasonably, further education or a job. The DRO suggested Remploy and an application was made but with no result. The girl herself applied for many jobs without success and became increasingly despondent over the year, although she was basically a very competent and outgoing person, with many non-handicapped friends within her own locality.

The support which the teenagers received during this difficult period varied considerably. Most young people had found the most supportive people to be their parents (only three of the fourteen young people said that they got no help from their family). That they badly needed additional support during this period is indicated by the fact that nearly all said they were worried and depressed during the waiting period, eight indicating that the depression was quite serious. Eleven had had contact with the statutory services, but only three found this to be helpful.

*Problems when first starting in initial placement.*   The next area to be explored was whether the teenager had experienced any problem when he or she started in his job or college or other placement. The interviewers rated twelve young people (just over 20 per cent) as having had marked problems with the initial placement, while a further 40 per cent were considered to have had milder problems. Those with milder problems on the whole referred to the same kind of difficulties and worries that any young person is likely to have on making the transition from school to a post-school placement. The most common worries were about how they'd get on with other people and about the work itself presenting a bit of a challenge. Usually these problems were not related to the actual handicap, except of course that those in open employment or ordinary further education felt themselves to be somehow 'on trial' in this situation of competing with the able-bodied on equal terms. A few going to residential college were homesick and found the change from living at home hard at first, but again this is not an uncommon experience for many young people who go away to college. However, some young people did have problems related to the handicap such as 'how to tell the others about my handicap and explain it to them', or difficulty in getting acclimatized to all the walking that was required of them. One teenager worried that the staff at the day centre wouldn't know how to cope with her if she had a fit, and another about a mild pressure sore (with good reason because this subsequently developed into a very serious problem, as described in the next section).

Of those considered to have serious problems on first starting, the majority were placed either in day centres or in special residential colleges. There were four young people attending day centres who found it very hard to adjust to the idea of being placed there. One boy said he felt 'on the scrap heap', especially since he had been turned down for a hoped-for college place. Another boy travelled to his work centre in a bus labelled 'Spastics Society Work Centre', which he said made him feel 'like an animal in a cage'. One teenager described her depression when she first went to the work centre: 'I felt useless . . . I nearly cracked up . . . it took a long time to settle, nearly eight months.' Another boy described how he used to feign illness so as not to go, and persisted with the Centre only because he realized that in going there daily he was relieving the strain of care on his mother.

Four young people were very homesick in their residential colleges, including one boy with a very severe speech difficulty which made it a great effort to communicate with the other students. This college recognized his problem and invited the mother to live in for a few days to help him settle and ensure that care staff knew how to interpret his needs; he was also allowed to go home frequently at weekends. In another case the girl in question was not allowed home visits at all, though her parents had recently separated and she very much wanted to spend more time with her mother, to whom she was very close. After a few weeks, the principal asked the mother to take her home on the grounds that she couldn't cope.

Only three (less than 20 per cent) young people in 'ordinary' placements (employment or ordinary further education) had marked problems at first. For example, one boy had been placed in a college a long distance from home and he found the two-hour journey, which included a change of bus, too tiring. On the advice of the student counsellor, a place was found for him in a college closer to home after a few weeks. Another found the walking and climbing stairs a great strain at first, especially during fire drill, which occurred on a couple of occasions when she first started; she lost a stone in weight which she attributed to the walking.

In fact most of the problems the young people described were relatively short-lived, and all but one of those with mild problems eventually settled down. Of the twelve whose difficulties were rated as marked, three were able to change their placements, while three others gradually overcame their problems within their initial placements. The situation remained very unsatisfactory for five, however – three in day centres, who never really found this acceptable, and two who solved their problems with residential college by leaving for no alternative placement. This result suggests that there are a small number of young people (10 per cent in our sample) who have serious problems with their first placements which remain unresolved, and who definitely need more help and advice than is currently available through this difficult transition period.

*Stress resulting from breakdown of placement or one or two changes in placement.*   There were five young people (10 per cent of the total sample) who experienced such difficulties within their first placement that they had to abandon it. Two were young people who had found themselves jobs on leaving school, but both were found to be too slow and given the sack. Naturally both were very upset, and it was a great blow to their self-confidence; both were unemployed for some months after. Nevertheless both were later successful in getting another job, using the careers service. The other three, however, were unable to solve their difficulties satisfactorily. One was the boy attending a special residential college mentioned in the previous chapter who had to leave because the college couldn't cope with his pressure sore. This had developed just before going to college, but it was not adequately cared for there and progressed to a stage where clearly he needed medical help. Unfortunately, because his mother was unable to provide him with a home, on being sent away from college he was placed in a community care centre where the staff were even less experienced in coping with his medical needs than those at the college. His condition deteriorated until eventually the boy himelf contacted the paediatric hospital under whose care he had been as a child, and he was immediately admitted for major surgery. The last two young people whose residential placement failed have already been referred to. Neither of them found a satisfactory alternative during the rest of that year, and indeed one still had no alternative placement eighteen months after leaving school.

These accounts again demonstrate the need for follow up during the post-school year by someone with a fairly wide knowledge of handicap and of the placement possibilities. If such a person had been available with the responsibility to oversee these young people, these serious problems could have been avoided.

*Demands of course or job very stressful.* Seven young people were assessed as finding their job or college placement very stressful because of the demands made on them, while a further three encountered mild stress in this respect. Three of the ten were in special colleges, and the other seven were in ordinary placements (representing about 40 per cent of those in ordinary placements).

Three experienced severe stress in relation to work placements. The history of two of these was mentioned in the previous section, both had lost their first job and were consequently very nervous in their second in case they would not make the grade, though both eventually were quite successful. The third person with severe stress at work was a young man in a Remploy placement who had found the work very arduous, particularly during his three month probation period, mainly because he also had a journey of two hours each way. He commented: 'When I was at school I didn't think it [work] was as hard as what it is . . . now I know different . . . you can tell you've done a day's work at the end of it, you feel beat.' (Nevertheless he was at pains to insist that it was 'well worth it'.)

Three young people in ordinary higher or further education had found the work very difficult because of problems of hand control, though each managed to find his own solution to this difficulty. The one teenager in special further education rated as having a serious problem was a girl doing an assessment course, which of necessity introduced her to a number of work areas which she found very difficult to manage as she moved from one course to another.

On the whole the problems presented by this group were not very serious viewed objectively, although they were often experienced by the young people themselves to be very stressful indeed. None was radically different from the kinds of problem encountered by many able-bodied young people during their post-school training years, and there is certainly no evidence that, even where this was experienced as very stressful by the young people, they were unable to cope with the problem, and all in some way or other produced their own satisfactory solutions.

*Frustrations because placement does not fully utilize the teenagers' abilities.* This was a common problem, experienced by thirteen of the young people in the sample (25 per cent), and was considered to cause severe stress in ten cases. The majority in this group (N = 8) attended day centres where the work was boring and tedious (see chapter 7). It was considered to cause severe stress in five cases. Because this has been dealt with at considerable length already it is only necessary to quote a few instances here. One girl said, 'We don't do intelligent things here', another felt he was 'wasting his time' because the work was so tedious, and a third said that the necessity of the staff to create work some days made it 'ridiculous – you put paper in envelopes one day and take it out the next'.

Five young people, comprising the at home group, were without any occupation for very long periods and had become very bored and despondent about the apparent lack of interest anyone in authority showed towards their plight. Again, since this has been explained fully in chapter 7 it is not necessary to go into details here, but obviously their situation caused these young people severe stress, and because they had been unoccupied for so long (8–12 months in some cases) they had begun to believe that life held nothing for them.

The last young person in this group was in open employment, having found himself a job as a warehouseman, but both he and his mother felt his talents to be very under-utilized. His mother said, 'He's not stupid' (indeed he was regarded as of normal ability by his school and left there with three CSEs). His discontent was heightened by the fact that he was poorly paid, as will be described later. He felt that his employer was taking advantage of him because of his (mild) handicap and that his prospects for improving his situation were fairly slight.

Again, the implication from the histories of these young people is the need for someone in the post-school period who can supervise their placements to ensure that their talents are fully utilized in some way, by vigorously pursuing the possibilities of alternative placements or, if this is not possible, finding other outlets for the young people's energies through the use of adult education courses or voluntary work of some kind.

*Anxiety about future placement.* Altogether twenty-two people (about 43 per cent of the sample) experienced anxieties about their future, and this was considered to cause severe stress in seventeen cases (over one-third of those interviewed). One was the young man in open employment described in the previous section, and ten who were coming to the end of ordinary (two cases) or special courses without firm prospects. Some were realizing that they might well have no option but a day centre. One teenager said: 'Nobody's interested in me . . . no one will talk to me' about alternatives.

Six of the young people in day centres were considered to have anxieties about the future, while the five young people at home for all or most of the post-school year were clearly worried about their future prospects. The experience and feelings of both groups have already been described.

At our most recent contact with the teenagers, 12–18 months after the

Phase II interview, ten of the twenty-two with anxieties about the future appeared to have solved their problems, at least temporarily, while four had found a partial though somewhat unsatisfactory solution. The remaining eight had not found any means of meeting their needs, nor was there much prospect of this in sight.

*Other stresses related to placement.* There were six young people with problems of varying degrees of severity related to their placement but which did not fall neatly into any of the other categories. Two, who were attending ordinary further education, had found it difficult to get grants; one of these was an Asian being supported by his brother, and the other was a member of a large single-parent family. Neither was clear about what he was entitled to, nor how to apply for a grant. In both cases the problem was rated as mild, since although it was a cause of concern to the young person, it was the brother and the mother who were taking the brunt of the financial strain.

One young man, already mentioned, considered that he was not receiving adequate pay for his work – £28 for a 44-hour week. His work-mates supported his claim for higher pay but with no success. The boy resented greatly what he considered to be exploitation of his situation as a handicapped person with limited job opportunities, and we rated this stress as severe.

The three others in this group had problems with travelling to college, one being considered to have a severe problem because he had a very long journey by public transport each day to reach his day centre, which he disliked intensely, and which cost far more than his IRC allowance of £2 per week.

## Conclusion

In concluding this section we must make the comment that since so many of the young people interviewed were still in higher or further education or training of some kind, we could not really examine the full extent of placement problems, the most severe of which would only come later when the young person left college, or if he failed to improve his employment situation as he grew older. (It is quite acceptable at seventeen or eighteen to start in a fairly menial position, as a junior clerk or warehouseman, but if promotion is too slow this will lead to frustrations.) We attempted to overcome this problem by a limited follow up by 'phone contact at the time of writing, but even at this point twelve young people (23 per cent) were still at college, and of the sixteen at work, none had been in their job for more than 18 months. It will require a later follow up to determine the full extent of the problems discussed in this section.

However, one can say, on the basis of the evidence available to us, that the services were deficient in adequately following up the welfare of those young people with particular problems of occupation, either because of the severity of their handicaps, or because their own or their families' knowledge of what services or opportunities were possible was insufficient to allow them to make the best use of what was potentially available.

### Stresses related to health problems or handicaps

*Stresses related to health or disability.* There were fourteen young people (27 per cent) with health worries during the post-school year, seven involving hospitalization. The stress that the health problems caused was considered to be severe in eight cases, five of whom required hospitalization. These young people missed a great deal of college, or had a long delay to first placement, or were unable to participate fully in college life because of their illnesses. For example, one teenager had needed three shunt operations within five months, missing about eight weeks of college life altogether in consequence. She also suffered from pressure sores and urinary infections during the year which produced further periods away from college. By the end of the year she was seriously worried about her health, especially about whether her shunt problems were likely to continue. Another girl went into hospital for a foot operation soon after leaving school. She was in plaster for three months and then broke her leg during convalescence so that she spent nine months altogether either in plaster or receiving rehabilitation treatment, and this delayed her starting work for eleven months from the time of leaving school. Another teenager suffered from regular occurrences of pressure sores over the whole of the year, which although they never developed into a serious problem, kept her in her wheelchair most of the time and were a constant worry.

Of the five people with less stressful health problems, two needed short periods of hospitalization – a few weeks only – while one teenager, though not seriously ill, was ailing most of the year with various complaints and had a great deal of time off work. This group also included a couple of young people who, though very concerned about their problems, did not objectively appear to have serious reason to do so.

It appears, therefore, that while there were relatively few people with serious health problems in the post-school year, this usually caused serious disruptions to the careers of the teenagers concerned. In at least two cases this might have been avoided if they had had better care when the problems began. It is interesting to note that of the eight young people with severe problems, five suffered from spina bifida, several of whom had had difficulties finding an interested and competent adult doctor – indeed, one had only secured adequate treatment for himself by personally contacting his former paediatric surgeon, who agreed to admit him despite the fact that, procedurally, one is not normally allowed to admit someone over the age of sixteen to a paediatric hospital. This difficulty in finding an adult surgeon or physician who understood their problems exacerbated both the problems and the worry to the teenager and his family. Just at this critical point in their lives they had lost not only the supervision and support of the experienced nurses in their special school, but they had also been obliged to leave the paediatric hospital where they were well known and which had provided medical cover from birth.

*Stress problems related to the management of incontinence.* Very few teenagers reported continuing problems in this area. Only four of the young people with urinary appliances complained of difficulties, and all these were considered to be mild stresses only. Three young people had worries in case the new people they encountered would discover their incontinence because of accidental leaks or by feeling the bag when lifting was required. A fourth young person had become careless about his appliance because he'd got fed up with having to cope with it, especially since he was depressed as a result of a year of severe pressure sore problems. However, on the whole, the year had been a positive one in this respect, several young people finding that since going to college they'd got more confidence about self-care and some having received better advice about appliances which had helped to avoid accidental leaks.

The problem of telling other people, especially boy or girlfriends, even as a hypothetical difficulty, was an ever-present one for these young people, nonetheless, especially for those whose experience of social life had been restricted previously to special school and home, and who had never before had to think about discussing the subject with someone who was not already aware of the problem and what it entailed. This is discussed in more detail in chapter 9.

*Stress due to difficulty with relationship within the family and those in need of alternative accommodation immediately or in the near future*

Thirteen young people were judged to have serious problems in relation to their families, while four had minor problems. There were five teenagers for whom problems were so acute that they were considered to require alternative accommodation rather urgently. A few typical examples are given as illustration.

One has already been referred to – a boy whose mother could not offer him a home because she was unsupported and had five other children living in her small house. She was fond of her handicapped son but simply couldn't manage him at home permanently, and felt it would also be unfair to the others. After leaving his residential school, he spent a few months with a foster family until he went away to a residential college, but when that broke down because of illness he was placed in a community care centre for the lack of any suitable alternative. This he greatly resented, calling it a 'centre for juvenile delinquents', which indeed was probably not far from the truth. This boy, though quite severely handicapped, emphatically did not want to live in a hostel or home for the disabled, but wanted eventually an adapted flat or a mixed hostel with both able-bodied and physically handicapped residents. He was also rated as having severe stress due to family relationships because he resented not being able to live at home, and was upset by the fact that he did not have a close relationship with his mother or feel as happy when in his home as he felt he should.

Another was a girl whose parents divorced just before she entered residential college (her history has already been referred to, see p. 203). She was an only child and very close to her mother who had always been an over-anxious person and suffered from agoraphobia. When her college placement broke down she returned home for a while, but the mother's social worker arranged for her to be admitted to a residential hostel closer to home where the mother could visit frequently, without having to cope alone with the full responsibility for her care. Despite the frequent visits she never became reconciled to the placement, especially since almost a year passed until a suitable daytime occupation was found for her. She said of the hostel, 'It's not Colditz Castle or anything but it's just not home.' She wanted to live at home until she was capable of moving into a shared flat – perhaps an unrealistic ambition within the present context of accommodation available, but not an impossible one given her potential level of independence. This girl was also rated as having severe stress because of family relationships since she was very distressed about the divorce (she had previously been very close to her father also but now had no contact with him) and because she was very concerned about her mother's mental condition.

A third teenager, who had always been at residential school, considered previously that she had had a close relationship with her divorced mother. She was looking forward to living at home and entering the local further education college for secretarial training. However, in her last year at school her mother remarried and was so engrossed in her new relationship that she had little time to spare for the daughter on her return. She tried hard to conceal her feelings from her mother, but simply did not take to her stepfather and felt greatly the loss of her former closeness with her mother. She felt very isolated at college, where she did not make any friends, and very much missed her residential school where she had been very popular and had had a confiding relationship with one of the teaching staff. She said, 'At school they did everything for you, they were always there. Now I feel there's no one to fall back on if I do things wrong.' She was overwhelmed by the sudden transition from the warmth of her school to the relative coldness of her present situation. 'It's thrown on top of you all at once. It takes time to find your balance again.' She saw the solution in the long term as getting a good job which would allow her to move out into a flat on her own, quite a realistic ambition in her case in terms of self-care, although perhaps not in financial terms. Because of her distress about her family situation she was rated as severely stressed on this account also.

*Difficult relationships within the family only.* There were eight other young people who were rated as having severe stress because of family relationships and four whose stress in this respect was considered to be less severe. None was currently thinking of moving out of home, although for some this seemed to be the best solution in the long term, if a suitable alternative could be found. Two young men had very poor relationships with their whole families. In both cases the difficulties were of long standing and had been solved partially during their school years by their attendance at residential schools.

The history of one girl demonstrates the problems. She had previously had a violent temper, but over the years as she matured, she had overcome this and the family situation had somewhat improved. However, the effects of the previous stormy history still lingered, and she was seen by the rest of the family as irritable, sullen and miserable. Apart from her sister, no one in the family appeared to appreciate Sheila's real difficulties arising from her handicap. Her father said, 'She just sits and refuses to meet people.' Though she had had difficulties with relationships at school, at her residential college she was thought to be a pleasant and mature girl, well liked by the staff and other students. She had obviously made great strides in confidence and in skills in personal relationships, but the difficulties at home persisted. While she was prepared to live at home immediately after leaving college, she saw that she would ultimately need to leave. She wanted, if possible, to live in a specially adapted flat which, from the viewpoint of her independence skills, should have been a possibility although in practice such flats are very hard to find.

Two boys had rather bleak home backgrounds because their mothers were themselves very disturbed, one with frequent depression, the other being a very unconfident and isolated lady who was herself slightly spastic. In the latter case the son had, not unnaturally, acquired much of his mother's lack of confidence and was described by his (ordinary day) school as being solitary, not much liked by the other children, and frequently worried and fearful. On leaving school he was successful in gaining a place in an art college, but this was a long way from home and this fact, plus his reticence, meant that he had been unable to participate in college social life, though he seemed to have good, if superficial, relationships with his fellow students.

Another girl had a very disturbed home life, but was rated as only having a mild problem since she had never yet lived permanently at home, and because she had a good relationship with her mother, though not a close, confiding one, since, as she said, 'She [the mother] had enough problems of her own'. This girl was the eldest of three, her brother was mentally handicapped, and her sister was very wild and had recently had an illegitimate child, whom the mother was also caring for. The father had been in a mental hospital previously, and frequently got drunk and became quarrelsome with the family. Added to this there was a serious problem with overcrowding and when she was at home she had to sleep in the living room, with no privacy for dealing with her urinary appliance. Despite all this, she insisted that although her family life did get her down, she never got really depressed about it or felt that life was hopeless. She was accepted at the residential college of her choice, but unfortunately, lost a lot of time during the year due to illness. On our most recent contact with her she was in hospital and awaiting a Remploy assessment course. Because of her loyalty to her mother she did not wish to move away immediately. She hoped eventually to be able to live in an adapted flat, but was prepared to consider a home or a hostel of some kind 'if it came to that'.

In summary there were thirteen people (one-quarter of the sample) suffering from severe stress because of their family relationships, and four in addition who had milder problems. Five of the thirteen were in immediate need of alternative living accommodation, two of whom were capable of caring for themselves independently, while two were very dependent currently, though both hoped, perhaps unrealistically, to be able to live in adapted flats. The fifth young person was quite willing in principal to accept a hostel placement. In addition there were four young people whose family situation was such that one could foresee the need for alternative accommodation at some stage over the next few years, since it seemed unlikely that anything would happen to improve things within the family itself. Two of these might be capable of living independently with special adaptations, though neither had an income which would allow this at present.

However, the prospects of any of these young people finding suitable hostel or adapted accommodation are, at present, fairly slim – there is a great paucity of suitable places available for disabled young people. The only boy whose accommodation situation was so urgent that alternatives simply had to be found had spent time with a foster family and then in a community care centre. In the case of the only girl facing such a problem, she had been placed in a hostel largely for older people and with many restrictions which she had found quite unacceptable.

Again, running through all of this is the general feeling of inadequate follow up for the post-school leavers, of lack of help or advice with family problems and of someone to ensure that a residential college place is found early if staying at home seems likely to exacerbate a family problem. The other obvious deficiency was the lack of suitable alternatives to home where this became necessary. Most young people's preference was for an adapted flat rather than a hostel, but the chances of obtaining one, especially considering their incomes, were fairly slender.

*Stress resulting from the social aspects of placement*

Twelve young people suffered from stress related to the social aspects of placement. For half, all of whom were in day centres or special colleges, this was considered to be severe. None of those in ordinary placements was thought to suffer marked stress in this respect.

Examples of young people in ordinary placements (either ordinary college or at work) included a teenager who had had difficulties with her workmates in her first placement, who initially were over solicitous, but later seemed to resent giving her help. This problem was short-lived, and not repeated in her second job. Another young person was attending an ordinary local college where she found the students not unfriendly, but unwilling to enter into a closer relationship with her. Her current situation contrasted markedly with her school experience where she'd been very popular both with staff and students. Describing the change from school to college, she said, 'It's like having a custard pie thrown in your face, that's it.' She felt that the other students were 'too busy worrying abvout themselves to be friendly'. However, since she had always attended a special residential school and was not used to the company of the non-handicapped, it is likely that she was lacking in the skills necessary to help her to accept rebuffs and to make satisfactory overtures to the other students, who at this age were no doubt too embarrassed by the presence of handicap to know how to relate to her in a natural way, and therefore tended to avoid contact. Some simple counselling would probably have been both effective and welcomed in this case.

Three young people attending special colleges had some social problems (one considered only to be slight). One was a girl who had a long-standing difficulty in controlling her temper, which though much improved with maturity, still caused her difficulties at college with staff but especially with the students, where her over-reaction to teasing was the main problem. Another complained that her special (day) college was so small (only six attenders) that she felt she had no choice of friends, and no possibility for an active social life with such a restricted range of companions.

Four out of the twelve attenders at day centres were considered to have severe problems stemming from the social aspects of the placement, while one had less severe problems. These problems have already been referred to, and need only be mentioned briefly here. One teenager had spent his first eight months after leaving school in a day centre with largely elderly attenders which had made him very depressed. He said, 'It was as if I left school and was retired, all in one week'. Another young man was in a Centre where the other attenders were much more severely handicapped than he, both physically and mentally. He was very upset by this and felt isolated and different from the others. The third young person had no speech and found that she was ignored by most of the other attenders because of this. She used a language board for communicating and was of average ability, but obviously the elderly attenders found the effort to enter into a dialogue with her to be too great.

In summary while about 23 per cent of those in ordinary placements had problems with social relationships at work or college, none was considered to be severe, while about 30 per cent of those in special placements had such difficulties, the majority causing severe stress. In other words, while it would be naïve to suppose that the placement of a handicapped person within an ordinary setting immediately opens the doors of society to him, there is no evidence from this study that social stress for those placed in an ordinary setting was either more common or more severe than for those placed in special environments. Indeed, if anything the reverse is true, especially for those in day centres. Failure to find satisfying social relationships was particularly distressing for the latter, where the work was boring and the pay poor, and so unless the day was at least enjoyable because of the company, it made the whole thing seem like a total waste of life.

### Stress arising from loss of friends not replaced or loss of a close friend

Ten young people were considered to suffer stress because of the loss of school or college friends not replaced with others over the previous year. In six cases this was thought to cause severe problems. All these young people had attended special schools and none had made friends in their own locality with non-handicapped youngsters. Four had been in residential schools, where in many ways they felt closer to the staff and students than they did to their own families, so it was particularly difficult for them, especially as in three cases there were also severe difficulties with family relationships. The loss of a special adult confidant on the school staff was felt very acutely.

It is difficult for any young person to initiate new social contacts without the assistance of another young friend whom they can trust. If there is also a handicap this compounds the problem in many ways, not least the sheer physical difficulty of getting out of the house. One of the main drawbacks to attending a special school, even if it is a day one, is the consequent lack of opportunity to make friends in one's own locality who can act as confidants and give support in initiating new social contacts at clubs, and so on. This is an age where the peer group is very important and without peer support social initiatives seem to be excessively daunting.

Four young people had lost close personal friends over the previous year, and this was considered to cause severe stress in three cases. Two other young women had lost boyfriends, one because she'd met him at her residential college and he lived far away. They 'phoned each other regularly, but she felt her parents didn't understand how deeply she felt and were not sympathetic to her distress. Another girl made friends with a boy at her day centre but when she brought him home her parents greatly disapproved of him and forbade any more contact. Again the parents appeared to underestimate the girl's feelings and how disappointed she was at their reaction.

## Stress due to social isolation

This was the most common form of stress experienced by the young people. Over 60 per cent of the sample were thought to have experienced it in some form, and in nearly 40 per cent of cases the stress was considered to be severe. Because this subject has already been covered to some extent and will be dealt with more fully in chapter 9 it is only necessary to make some brief comments here. Perhaps first should be noted the fact that eight of the thirty young people considered to have stress from social isolation also had severe stress arising from family problems. The situation of these young people was quite desperate in that they were almost totally bereft of support from family or peers.

The second point is that in the majority of cases of social isolation the young person had previously attended special school and had therefore had little opportunity to make friends in his own locality. Once having left school they were too distant from school friends to continue with these contacts, especially if they had attended residential schools or had a severe locomotor handicap.

Seven of the seventeen young people in ordinary placements were considered to be severely isolated partly though not entirely due to the fact that they had made no friends since leaving school. In most cases, the young people would have benefited from counselling to help them acquire the necessary social skills to develop easier relationships with their non-handicapped peers.

Twelve of the seventeen young people who attended special colleges had a very poor social life at home, which contrasted greatly with their excellent social life at college. In six cases the stress caused by social isolation at home was thought to be severe. It seemed surprising that so few efforts were made to keep up contacts made at college, at least by 'phone and letter. Since all the young people had had to travel by public transport to residential college, it should have been possible for them to make an occasional visit out of term-time to one of their friends, but this very rarely happened. In no instance did the college appear to have discussed with the young people how to go about making friends in their own locality, through joining Adult Education (AEI), classes for example*, and either seemed to be unaware of the problems facing the young people in transfer from the richness of college life to their bleak social situation at home, or to feel that there was nothing they could do about it.

Eight of the twelve young people in day centres suffered from social isolation, in four cases thought to be severe, which was the result both of losing friends from school and the impossibility of making new ones in the daily environment they now found themselves in. Only one boy found that he mixed socially with his day centre mates, he attended an Adult Training Centre for the mentally handicapped which seem generally to be more attuned to the issue of improving the attenders' social lives than are day centres for the physically handicapped.

Of those in the 'at home' group, all but one were considered to suffer from severe stress due to social isolation. Two spent most of the year moving between different residential settings, one having been bedridden much of the time. Another had a severe locomotor handicap, and, because the family had no car, hardly went out at all. He went to a school club once a week, and once a week with his father to the local pub, and that was the full extent of his social contacts outside the family. Only one girl in this group did not suffer from severe social isolation. This was the relatively mildly handicapped, very personable young lady (see p. 204) who had a close relationship with her sister, through whom she had made many local friends, and she usually had a regular boyfriend also.

This problem of social isolation among the young handicapped is probably the most serious issue revealed by our studies. It affected a high proportion of the sample, and was so distressing to many young people that they had begun to feel that life was worthless and pointless, and some had had suicidal thoughts.

Although there are real physical problems in helping these young people to make a good social life for themselves, this does not appear to us to be the main issue. The root of the matter lies in the need for true 'education for life' courses at school and at residential college which would discuss the problem generally with the young people and suggest solutions, coupled with concerned follow up by someone with a knowledge of local resources in terms of clubs, AEIs, and transport possibilities, and who could help each individual to enrich his life by making use of whatever local opportunities were on offer. This local person could give individual counselling, initiate discussions between handicapped young people, act as a support when rebuffs occurred, and

* We understand that this is now being included as part of the Beaumont syllabus.

encourage within the young person the confidence he needed to break out of the family circle and initiate contacts with the world around him.

## Summary

Of the areas of stress looked at in relation to placement difficulties, the most common problems that the teenagers described were anxieties caused by long delays to first placement, distress that their abilities were not being fully utilized currently, or concern about their future prospects.

These forms of stress were found most frequently among the teenagers in day centres or those without occupation, though concern about the future was expressed by a number of young people in further education also. The teenagers' worries in these respects were quite firmly founded in fact, of course, in that employment for the more severely handicapped is not easy to find and the facilities available for alternatives to work are not adequate at present, although it is certainly true that more interesting opportunities do exist if the personnel were available to help each teenager find his own solution within the opportunities existing in his area.

A breakdown of placement, while not such a common stress, caused much anxiety to the teenager and to his parents when it occurred. Perhaps in some cases these could not have been avoided no matter how good the services, but in some cases it was likely that professional help at the appropriate point could well have avoided the crisis.

Problems of some kind as the young person settled into his placement were also very common, but although sometimes posing quite serious difficulties, these were usually resolved satisfactorily. However, there were a few instances where the right help was not forthcoming and the problems persisted, the majority of these being young people in unsatisfactory day centres. Relatively few young people described stress due to demands made on them by their placement and where they occurred a satisfactory solution to the difficulties had been found in all cases.

Stresses arising directly from poor health or the effects of the disability itself were, fortunately, relatively uncommon. In terms of incontinence management things seemed to have improved during the year following school, although the social problem of how to explain their disability to others remained. However, a small number of young people, mainly those with spina bifida, had quite severe health problems, some involving prolonged hospitalization, which caused them to miss a good deal of time from their placement, in addition to the stress arising from the condition itself. In a few cases the medical problems of the teenagers were exacerbated by the lack of adequate medical cover, in part because of unfamiliarity with their problems in special colleges, and in part because there are as yet few centres which can give proper medical cover for spina bifida young people once they have passed through the care of the specialist paediatric hospitals.

Many young people were undergoing strain because of disturbed family relationships, in some cases resulting in general family strife or continuous tension, and in others in the silent misery of the handicapped young person. Some family problems were probably no greater than those to be found in many families with a teenage member, although where the teenager is dependent on his family the effect of any family tension is experienced more acutely. However, there were a number of instances where the difficulties were quite severe and likely to be resolved only by the young person moving away from home and into a satisfactory substitute. In five cases the need for an alternative to home was considered to be quite urgent, and in several others, although there was no immediate crisis, a need was likely to arise in the near future.

Social isolation was by far the most common source of stress among the teenagers, affecting over 60 per cent of the sample to some degree and judged to be severe for 40 per cent. Most of those with severe difficulties were moderately or severely handicapped and had been to special schools, so that they had the dual difficulty of not being socially mobile as well as not having had the opportunity to make friends during their school days within their own locality.

Young people in ordinary placements, who were usually rather less handicapped, did not so commonly have such severe problems with relationships as those in special placements, but there were some difficulties in relating to non-handicapped peers and some form of counselling would have been beneficial. On the other hand all but one of those in the 'at home' group had very little contact with anyone at all outside the family, while most of those in day centres could derive little social benefit because few or no other young people were attending. Many of those in special colleges, while having a rich social life at college, were entirely dependent on their families at home.

Many young people missed their friends from school, especially those who had been to residential school who sometimes felt closer to the staff and friends there than they did to their own families. Once having left school or college it is exceedingly difficult for young handicapped people to make new social contacts, unless they are in a placement which provides opportunities for social outlets outside work-time as well as within it.

What is a cause for even greater concern is the fact that nearly one-third of the young people suffering from social isolation also suffer from stress due to family relationships. These young people were bereft either of adequate family support or the support and comradeship of their peers, and the plight of some in this group was very distressing indeed.

# 9
## *Change and development in the post-school year*

## Introduction

The follow-up study had three main aims. One was to look at the placements of the young people, the processes by which they were placed, and their satisfaction and that of their parents with placements. The second was to try to identify some of the factors causing stress during the post-school year. The third aim was to take advantage of the longitudinal aspect of the study by looking at changes in the young people during the year after leaving school. We did not expect to see marked changes in the majority of the group, first because a year is a comparatively short period and secondly because, unlike non-handicapped school leavers, many young people did not have a very marked change of environment during this time, since they moved on the whole from one type of segregated institution (a special school) to another (a college or day centre for the disabled).

The first area to be considered was the development of personal independence and maturity. Although we were not able to collect very detailed information on this we were able to assess changes with regard to basic self-help skills (including driving) and to get some idea what changes occurred both in the teenagers' and the parents' attitudes to independence and self-help. Another general area of potential change was in the social lives of the young people, including their peer relationships, and the use they made of their leisure time. Here the crucial question was whether the quality of their social lives, particularly away from work or college, had improved since leaving school. The third area to be considered was whether or not there were detectable changes in the young people's present situation and aspirations with respect to relationships with the opposite sex and their hopes and expectations about marriage and children.

Another important area was the young people's emotional adjustment, including their relationships with their families. Were there changes in overall psychological adjustment ratings, and if so how could these be accounted for? Could changes be identified in specific areas found to be important in Phase I of the study, in particular in fearfulness, worrying and depression? Had the mother's mental health changed at all over this year? Did they worry more or less now? Had the relationship between parents and their children changed at all over this period? To end this chapter we discuss the responses of the parents and the young people to questions about the way in which they viewed the long-term future.

## The development of personal independence after leaving school

### Attitudes to independence

This was an area where the parents were definitely pleased with the progress made by their sons and daughters over the year. Over 45 per cent (N = 22) said that they thought the young person was definitely striving for more independence now. As one mother put it, 'There's no stopping her now. She really thinks for herself'.

About 20 per cent of mothers felt that their own attitude had changed over the year; many blamed themselves for having been too protective in the past and, in the case of those at residential college (a third of the sample), saw the advantage to the child of having lived away from home in an environment where he was expected to take care of himself. One said, 'I've had to change a lot of my ways. He's grown up a lot since he left college and he says I must let him do things now'. Another said, 'It was a good thing him being away at college . . . At home . . . I was running round after him all the time'. However, some mothers, quite understandably after years of anxiety and total responsibility for care, obviously found it difficult to 'let go'. One mother of a seventeen year old boy who was managing very well at his residential college said, in a tone of some surprise, 'He doesn't want his hand held now, so I just walk behind him in case he falls'. Another said, 'I've still got at the back of my mind she's my little girl. I blame myself a lot'.

### Self-help skills

In terms of improvements in the basic self-help skills such as hair washing and dressing there had been some real progress (see Table 9.1) as well as in being able to stay unattended at home and in making a snack. However, over half were still unable to make themselves a meal while even on such basic tasks as washing, dressing and taking a bath or shower between 13 per cent and 24 per cent of the teenagers still needed help.

Parents were also asked about the management of incontinence and epilepsy, and again progress had been made – eight out of the ten with urinary appliances were now fully able to care for and change these, and only one mother reported any major problem (she had a very depressed son who was going through a phase of not caring). All seven teenagers who had epilepsy were fully responsible for taking their medication, three of them reordering their prescriptions when necessary without

Table 9.1 *Self-help skills*

|  | Total | Could do previously | | Could not do previously, can do now | | Can't yet do | |
|---|---|---|---|---|---|---|---|
|  |  | N | (%) | N | (%) | N | (%) |
| Dressing | 49 | 34 | (70) | 7 | (14) | 8 | (16) |
| Washing | 49 | 39 | (79) | 4 | (8) | 5 | (13) |
| Washing hair | 50 | 30 | (60) | 8 | (16) | 12 | (24) |
| Bath/shower | 50 | 37 | (79) | 2 | (4) | 11 | (17) |
| Making a snack | 50 | 34 | (68) | 4 | (8) | 12 | (24) |
| Making a meal | 49 | 20 | (40) | 3 | (6) | 26 | (54) |
| Alone in day up to four hours | 49 | 37 | (75) | 6 | (12) | 6 | (13) |
| Alone in evening up to four hours | 47 | 25 | (53) | 11 | (23) | 11 | (24) |

assistance, three others informing their parents when more drugs were needed.

## Mobility

All the teenagers were asked about use of public transport over the last year. As previously there was a marked difference between the spina bifida and the cerebral-palsied teenagers in this, less than 30 per cent of the former having used a bus regularly over the past year, compared with over 60 per cent of the cerebral-palsied group. Some who didn't use public transport regularly, especially trains or the underground, thought that they could have used it more frequently, though again this was more true for the cerebral-palsied group. Only just over half of the total group could use buses without assistance, and about one-quarter were unable to use a bus at all.

In terms of car use, although only three teenagers had passed their driving test (two of them could in any case use public transport), a further nine had provisional licences. All these nine definitely thought that they would be able to drive, however about one-quarter of the whole group thought they definitely would be unable to do so. Rather more parents than teenagers were doubtful about the possibility of driving, but on the whole agreement between the teenagers and the parents over this issue was greater than in Phase I of the study, suggesting that there had been more discussion about this within the family over the previous year. However, about half the teenagers and the parents were still unclear about whether driving would be possible.

*Friendships*

Friendships at work, day centre or college have already been considered in chapters 7 and 8. Briefly, all but four of the young people had at least one friend in their placement, the majority being friends whom they hadn't known previously. However, very few (only 12 per cent) said that they saw their friends regularly outside work or college although nearly half said that they definitely wanted to have more contact. Indeed 40 per cent of the young people had no friends at all whom they saw outside work, college or day centre, and of those who did see friends, the majority were ones whom they had known from school days rather than new ones. The proportion who didn't see friends in evenings, weekends or holidays was very similar to that reported in Phase I of the study. Over half the teenagers could name a special friend, but again most of these were long-standing friends rather than ones newly met. Nearly one-quarter could never meet the friend at the weekends, evenings or in the holidays, and only half met as often as once a week.

Despite the new friends made at work or college, the majority of teenagers (over 70 per cent) felt that they did not have enough opportunity to make new friends, and one-quarter of the teenagers felt that they had fewer friends overall this year than when they were at school. Those who felt this most commonly were the ones without occupation or in day centres. Nearly three-quarters of the young people felt themselves to be alone too much and this was related, as one might expect, to severity of handicaps, since nearly twice as many of those who were moderately or severely handicapped said this, compared with those with a mild handicap. Again, a higher proportion of the young people felt themselves to be 'too much alone' this year compared with Phase I of the study.

When the young people were asked about loneliness nearly half said that this was a definite problem, compared with only a third who did not feel lonely. While some young people (under 20 per cent) felt less lonely than they had previously, twice that number appeared to be feeling more lonely. One boy said, 'We were protected at school', another 'I used to have loads of friends at school, but not now'. One boy who had had no placement throughout the year, and whose family had also moved house said, 'I'm a hermit. I don't see anyone here to even say hellow to in the street'. Many said they were particularly bored and lonely when the other members of the family were out and they had only the television for company. This didn't happen all that frequently, except in the case of those without a placement during the day, but subjectively it was felt quite strongly. It is one thing to have solitude from choice but quite another if one has to accept it without any option. It was the weekends particularly which dragged. As one girl said, 'I see nobody my own age. Even though Mum and Dad take me out when they can, it's not the same as being with someone your own age'.

Questions to parents suggested that while over one-third felt that their son's or daughter's social life was definitely unsatisfactory outside of work or college, they tended on the whole to overestimate the extent to which their children accepted the poor quality of social life available to them; perhaps because the teenagers appreciated the outings provided by the family, and the parents did not realize their need for more peer contact. As one girl said, 'I've got my family around, but I still feel lonely – I just wish there were more people my own age'.

*Opposite-sex relationships*

In Phase I of the study, the majority of the young people expressed an interest in the opposite sex, and by the time of the second interview all but four young people said that they were interested in having a boy- or girlfriend. The percentage who had a boy- or girlfriend had increased only slightly from the Phase I of the study, and only fifteen young people (one-third of those who wished for it) actually had a boy- or girlfriend currently. Nearly half had never experienced such a relationship. Where such a relationship existed, the boy- or girlfriend was usually handicapped and most had met at college or day centre, while a few had met at a club. Only half saw their friends as often as once a month, and many could only keep in touch by 'phone. One-third had never met at all outside college.

Again, as in the previous interview, a major worry for the teenagers was whether they would ever be found attractive to the opposite sex. One boy said, 'I've tried hard. Everyone else has a girlfriend, but not me'. One girl in a wheelchair said, 'I'm just not attractive from the neck down', and another boy, 'I'm very popular with the girls at college but not as a boyfriend or husband. When I ask them, they say they don't want to go out with me'. A few were worried about sexual relationships, the boys in particular, whether they'd be capable of this. As before, nearly all said they were hoping to marry and have children, but most who had worries about this still had no opportunity to talk things over either with a friend or with anyone who might have given them sensible advice. About 60 per cent of both parents and teenagers found the idea of a disabled partner acceptable, provided that they were 'right in other ways'.

*Clubs*

Only about 40 per cent of the teenagers were in a club of some sort (usually a PHAB-type club or one for the handicapped) when they were at home, a rather lower percentage than was found in Phase I, when, it will be remembered, many of the teenagers were in clubs attached to their schools. Some of these school-based clubs do allow former members to attend after leaving school, but since they tend to be run only in term-time, this virtually excludes the young people who leave school for residential college. In fact nearly all those attending residential colleges were not members of a club at home, although about half were in clubs at college. This lack of continuity with social contacts built up while at school is a cause for great concern, since once lost they may be quite difficult to revive, and when the student returns from residential college, his social life contracts abruptly.

## Contact with able-bodied teenagers

The young people were questioned about contact with able-bodied teenagers, how the able-bodied responded to them, and what their own feelings were when they met able-bodied young people. While they clearly wanted to have more contact with the able-bodied, most admitted to having difficulties in relating. Over one-quarter said that they definitely felt more comfortable in the company of the handicapped, making remarks like, 'I feel more at ease with those that are handicapped, same as me', and nearly half felt some kind of nervousness or anxiety when meeting able-bodied teenagers. It was noticeable that those with restricted social lives commonly expressed anxiety about meeting the able-bodied, and although this group included the most severely disabled, it also included many with relatively mild handicaps. One good looking boy with a right hemiplegia, who was not noticeably handicapped despite his awkward gait and partially paralysed right arm, said that in his home area he hadn't any friends at all. 'It must be because I'm disabled, I can't think of any other reason.' When he met able-bodied teenagers he always felt that they were feeling, 'What's the good of having him for a friend'. Many teenagers made comments such as, 'I get a bit apprehensive', 'I'd like to feel more at ease with the able-bodied but I just can't', 'I worry about how they're going to take to me, about my speech and whether they'll understand me – I reckon that's why I'm a bit shy', 'I feel a bit uneasy because I think how are they going to take to me?'.

Many found the embarrassment and curiosity of the non-disabled to be off-putting. 'I get the feeling that they stare at me – as though you're not human.' 'They mainly have quiet glances at my behaviour, looking a bit put off.' Several said they'd had the experience of being ignored. As one said, 'Some behave as if you had a disease.' However, over half the teenagers either felt that non-handicapped young people had a neutral or a positive attitude ('They want to help'), or that it all depended on the individual ('There are some . . . they'll call you names and you've just got to accept it'; 'Those at PHAB react very well, they want to help'). Some young people were so insecure that they distrusted even friendly reactions: 'I've always got a doubt in my mind – they're only taking me for a ride – they're being nice out of pity.' Saddest of all, however, were the many young people who, in response to these questions about the able-bodied, simply said, 'I don't really meet any' or 'No one has ever introduced me except at youth clubs.'

There were, of course, some young people who didn't worry about contacts with the able-bodied. One said, 'I forget I'm disabled.' But on the whole the findings suggest that handicapped teenagers do need support in mixing with the able-bodied, and advice on how to overcome the embarrassment and unease which both sides are likely to feel initially. As one boy said, 'I would like to mix with able-bodied people, but I haven't got the nerve to go up to them – I think it's because I'm handicapped – they won't come up to me and I won't go up to them.'

### Quality of social life

In respect of our global ratings of quality of social life, over 40 per cent were considered to have a very restricted social life compared with less than one-quarter whose social life was judged to be 'satisfactory'. These ratings were made on the social life of the young people while *at home*, not while in any residential establishment. The findings indicate no overall improvement in the quality of the young people's social life since leaving school, and the majority of those who previously were thought to have a very restricted social life still had very few social outlets (see Table 9.2).

Table 9.2 *Comparison of current social life ratings with social life ratings from Phase I*

| Current social life rating | Previous social life rating | | | | | | | |
|---|---|---|---|---|---|---|---|---|
| | Very restricted | | Limited | | Satisfactory | | Total | |
| | N | (%) | N | (%) | N | (%) | N | (%) |
| Very restricted | 14 | | 9 | | 0 | | 23 | (45) |
| Limited | 5 | | 9 | | 3 | | 17 | (33) |
| Satisfactory | 0 | | 7 | | 4 | | 11 | (21) |
| Total | 19 | (37) | 25 | (49) | 7 | (14) | | |

The eleven young people whose social lives were thought to be satisfactory were all either mildly or moderately handicapped, and over half were in ordinary placements. Of the twenty-three whose social lives were felt to be very restricted, 60 per cent were severely handicapped, while only two were mildly handicapped and only three were in ordinary placements. Clearly, severity of handicap was an important variable, as it had been previously, as well as type of placement.

Table 9.3 *Quality of social life in relation to placement*

|  | Total | Satisfactory | Somewhat restricted | Very restricted |
|---|---|---|---|---|
| Employment | 9 | 5 | 3 | 1 |
| Ordinary further education | 8 | 1 | 5 | 2 |
| Special further education | 17 | 2 | 4 | 11 |
| Day centre | 12 | 2 | 5 | 5 |
| At home | 5 | 1 | – | 4 |
| Total | 51 | 11 (21%) | 17 (33%) | 23 (45%) |

In contrast to the relatively good social life for those in ordinary placements, (all but one of whom were living at home) over two-thirds of the
young people in special colleges (most of whom were residential) were
judged to have very restricted social lives, as were nearly half of those in
day centres and four of the five young people without any placement at
all (see Table 9.3). It should be noted that none of the young people in
the at home group had been given a social life rating of 'very restricted'
in the previous year, but their outlets had then been closely linked to
school, and they had not had the opportunity to find alternative social
contacts during the post-school year.

Ability to use public transport unaccompanied was looked at in relation to the overall quality of social life, since one of the problems
frequently mentioned was difficulty in going out because of transport
problems. The results are shown in Table 9.4, quoting those who could
use buses. A rather higher proportion could use a train unaccompanied,
but this was not included here since, for most local journeys, bus travel
would be a more relevant skill. It suggests that ability to travel by bus
unaccompanied was a *necessary* condition for having a satisfactory social
life, in that all those who had a satisfactory social life had this skill.
However, it was not a *sufficient* condition in that almost as many as those

Table 9.4 *Use of bus in relation to quality of social life*

|  | Quality of social life | | | | |
|---|---|---|---|---|---|
|  | Very restricted | Somewhat limited | Satisfactory | Total N | (%) |
| Uses bus alone | 8 | 8 | 11 | 27 | (56) |
| Thinks could use alone | 2 | 2 | – | 4 | (8) |
| Must be accompanied | 1 | 1 | – | 2 | (4) |
| Can't use bus/no car | 11 | 4 | – | 15 | (31) |
| Total | 22 | 15 | 11 | 48 | (100) |

who could use a bus were rated as 'very restricted' as were considered to have an adequate social life. The other factors which seemed to be important were type of placement, the distance of the placement from home, and the diffidence and reserve of the teenager himself.

These findings suggest that every possible effort should be made to ensure that all who are capable of doing so are taught to use a bus unaccompanied and encouraged to do so regularly while they are still at school. Over and above this, however, many young handicapped people need support in finding satisfactory social outlets, especially those who are timid or shy of making contact with the able-bodied. Those whose disabilities are such that they cannot use a bus unaccompanied need to have volunteer transport and to be taught how to use a mini-bus or taxi with the minimum of assistance, as well as support to help them find and maintain their own social outlets independent of their families.

## Parental perception of changes in psychological adjustment

Before asking about changes in relation to specific behaviour, we asked the mother this general question about psychological adjustment, early on in the interview: 'I wonder whether you have noticed any changes in X's behaviour since he/she left school, either changes you are worried about, or changes you are pleased with.'

As might be expected, because the time interval between the first and second interviews was so short, many mothers (nearly one-third) felt that there had been no noticeable changes in their child's behaviour. However, nearly half the mothers reported improvements in the young people – they were, 'more mature', 'more adult and grown up', '[has] come out of herself more', 'gained in confidence, does things on her own more'. One or two referred specifically to the young person's attitude to his handicap – 'He's beginning to accept things more now that he's older.' As one might expect, there were a few parents who said that while in some ways the young person had matured, this had brought some problems also. ('She rejects me as a normal process of growing up, but she's definitely matured.' 'He's more aggressive now, but also more self-confident and sensible.')

Only five parents (10 per cent) reported changes for the worse. In one instance it was simply that the daughter was becoming more argumentative and assertive, from being formerly very timid and docile, and the mother recognized this to be part of the growing-up process. Another teenager had been miserable and depressed all year because he was unplaced, but his family were very sympathetic to this. The behaviour of the other three young people had become very difficult to tolerate, however. They had always been rather aggressive and resentful towards their parents, but this had become much more pronounced over the last year and they were now very difficult to live with.

Overall, eighteen parents (36 per cent) reported some difficulties in the teenagers' behaviour, usually because their son or daughter was unhappy or depressed much of the time (with good reason in some cases, owing to placement difficulties or constant illness), while others described general timidity and lack of self-confidence. One or two were worried because their teenager was 'a loner, doesn't mix at all' or because it was difficult to get them to do anything. ('She just sits doing nothing.' 'He won't do anything unless you tell him.') A few reported irritability due to boredom and frustration, and one or two that the young person was resenting the disability and becoming truculent in consequence.

## Worry and anxiety

Both the parents and the teenagers agreed that the teenagers had been more inclined to worry over the previous year than in the past – 25 per cent of parents said this and 43 per cent of teenagers, compared with only 12 per cent who said that they now worried less. The parents of the 'at home' group thought they were more worried, now, 'about the future', and this was confirmed by the teenagers themselves.

The teenagers usually described worries about getting a job or getting married. One said, 'It keeps me awake at night', another 'I'm bored . . . I've got so much time on my hands because I haven't got a job. I don't see myself breaking down but if this carries on I suppose I will'. One or two contrasted their carefree state at school with the present reality. 'At school you're always there, going there tomorrow . . . it's all planned . . . Now I don't know what to do.' 'I used to put things out of my head, now I face up to them – my disabilities. I realize now I have to come to terms with it.' Several teenagers expressed concern about their handicap, either in relation to specific problems ('In case I have a convulsion') or more generally ('Being with people who think I'm different', 'Why I can't go out on my own . . . like my brother does', 'Things I can't do').

## Fearfulness and lack of self-confidence

This seemed to be an area of general improvement. No teenager was thought to have a severe problem with fearfulness (compared with 5 per cent in Phase I) and none was thought to be more fearful now, compared with over one-third who were thought by their parents to be less timid now. The parents made comments such as, 'He's come out of himself a bit', 'She's getting more independent now', 'She's more confident in meeting people' and 'She's more self-confident because she knows now she can make friends'.

Nonetheless, on the Malaise Scale twelve young people (23 per cent) described themselves as fearful, and nearly 40 per cent of parents still felt there were some problems with this, despite the fact that there had been improvements. Many instances were cited. 'He's always been with people and he fears to go out alone.' 'She's fearful about travelling.' 'He gets scared stiff about things sometimes and won't sleep.' 'She's nervous about trying new things. I have to talk to her.' However, this did seem to be an area of improvement and it was encouraging to find that even in such a short space of time the young people were gradually gaining in confidence provided that they were in supportive situations where they had opportunities to make new friends and learn new skills.

*Misery and depression*

As in Phase I, more teenagers than parents reported that depression was a problem (60 per cent of the teenagers, 35 per cent parents). In fact, one-third of the teenagers said that they'd felt life to be hopeless at some time during the previous year, and 10 per cent had thought of suicide. The same sorts of issue were discussed by the parents in relation to worrying ('He gets unhappy about not being able to do things', 'He's got no job to go to') but other problems were raised ('She found it difficult having to be independent at college', 'She didn't want to leave school . . . she misses her friends'). The teenagers themselves, in describing their unhappiness, commonly referred to feelings of lack of worth because of not having a job or other suitable placement. One said, 'All the people I know have got things to do. I haven't got anything'. Another said, 'I felt terrible . . . when I went to the DRO and he said he'd help and then nothing came of it', and yet another, 'I just don't enjoy life any more. People think I'm not capable of anything'. In describing her feelings on leaving school and having no placement one girl said, 'I thought, is it all worth it? – I thought I wanted to die'. Another girl (who was doing an FE course) said, 'Most of the misery at the moment is caused by being unemployed and stupid. I feel I should be working but I can't.' Those who had been ill a lot during the year because of their condition said how depressed this had made them. Others said that they were unhappy because of leaving school – they missed their friends, teachers and care staff. 'You have no social life at all . . . I think, how long am I going to be like this? I need someone to talk to about it.'

The sixteen young people who had felt life to be hopeless at some time during the year also frequently mentioned despondency about their placement: 'I've thought this many times when I haven't wanted to go back to my day centre', 'I think I'll never get a job. I'll be like this all my life'. Indeed, nearly 60 per cent of those with suicidal thoughts were either in the day centre or the 'at home' groups (comprising over half of the young people in these two groups), compared with only two in employment or ordinary colleges (less than 12 per cent of all those in ordinary placements) and only five (30 per cent) of those in special colleges. Teenagers in ordinary placements or special colleges who felt like this were very often those who had poor or deteriorating relationships with their parents.

Conversely, those who were thought by their parents to be happier since leaving school (about half of total group) were usually those who had placements they enjoyed. 'He's happy to be working and earning money', 'He's been much happer this year – he really liked [his special training college]', and 'He's much more contented now he's at college.' Greater independence was also seen to contribute to happiness: 'He can do his own thing more now in a different environment' and 'He's more independent and therefore happier.'

### Irritability

Although irritability was not felt to be a serious problem, there was a slight increase according to the parents in the amount of irritation and aggression now shown. According to the parents 14 per cent of the teenagers had a severe problem with this, and 40 per cent a mild problem. (As previously, the teenagers themselves gave lower figures, only 4 per cent stating that they had a severe problem.)

Sometimes irritability was seen as a response to boredom: 'He's got very moody but only through boredom' and 'If he gets frustrated or wants to go out and can't.' In other cases it was seen as a sign that the young person was trying to establish his independence. Only a few obviously reacted with anger and irritation as a reflection of a generally poor relationship either with their parents or with other members of the family. The teenagers themselves usually referred to feelings of frustration when asked to describe the situations which made them irritable 'When I can't do something other people can', 'If I think too much about how I am', 'When I feel sorry for myself' and 'When I think about the future'. Few teenagers openly admitted feelings of aggression towards their family even when this was reported by the parents, and when, in other parts of the teenager's interview, it had been clear that problems did exist.

### Changes overall in psychological adjustment

In making our overall ratings of psychological adjustment we followed the same procedures described for Phase I (p. 118). Most of the questions put to the teenagers and their parents were identical, or very similar, the main difference being that we probed in some detail to find out whether changes in behaviour had taken place. Taking into account all the data available, the overall ratings of psychological adjustment in the follow-up group are shown in Table 9.5. They are compared with the findings for the same group of teenagers in Phase I of the study.

Table 9.5 *Overall psychological adjustment before leaving school and one year after leaving school*

| Current rating | Previous rating | | | | | | | |
| | Marked problems | | Some problems | | No overt problems | | Total | |
| | N | (%) | N | (%) | N | (%) | N | (%) |
|---|---|---|---|---|---|---|---|---|
| Marked problems | 8 | | 3 | | 2 | | 13 | (25) |
| Some problems | 4 | | 3 | | 6 | | 13 | (25) |
| No overt problems | 4 | | 5 | | 16 | | 25 | (50) |
| Total | 16 | (31) | 11 | (21) | 24 | (48) | 51 | |

Overall about half the young people were judged in exactly the same terms as they were on the previous occasion and only six teenagers (less than 12 per cent) had changed their status radically. The majority of those young people judged to be without overt problems in their last year at school were still seen as having no major problems at the time of the second interview, and only two were thought to have major problems at the time of the second interview. Both of these were teenagers showing severe anxiety and depression as a consequence of a disappointing year of inactivity with little hope for improvement.

Of the sixteen young people previously rated as having marked problems, half were judged still to have severe difficulties, but four were thought to have no problems currently, all young people for whom the year following school had gone well and who had gained much in confidence and stability as a result. Another four had considerably reduced problems in consequence of their better circumstances and opportunities to enhance their self-esteem.

Of the eleven young people previously rated as having mild difficulties, most were judged to be the same or rather better, and only three were thought to have more serious problems at this stage. In one case this was the result of an unsatisfactory placement with no prospect of improvement which had increased all the anxiety and fearfulness the young person had previously shown. In the other two cases, this was because of deteriorating relationships with their families. Both were young people with long-standing personality problems which had become more marked over this period.

## Factors associated with a change in psychological adjustment

As already indicated, whether the year had been satisfactory in terms of placement seemed to be a major factor in psychological adjustment in that a very distressing year in terms of placement was commonly associated with a deterioration in adjustment, while a good year, offering opportunities for enhancing self-esteem and improving confidence, frequently resulted in a lessening of difficulties. The prospect of improvement in placement, such as the promise of a place on a training course, helped to make a poor situation tolerable, and conversely the lack of any hope for improvement caused unhappiness which was close to despair.

Relationships with parents appeared to be another important factor associated with psychological adjustment, although of course it was often difficult to say whether poor relationships were the cause or the result of psychological problems in the teenagers. However, all but one of those teenagers whose mothers claimed to have a poor relationship with them (N = 6) were judged to have marked psychological problems, and all but four of those judged to have marked problems appeared to have considerable difficulty in relating to their parents.

Although on the whole relationships between parents and teenagers were fairly harmonious, in this respect things were not as good as they had been in the previous year. On the teenagers' own assessment only one-third thought that they got on 'better than other teenagers' with their parents (compared with 50 per cent in Phase I), while 13 per cent (six teenagers) thought that they did not get on as well as others (and in our judgement this was something of an underestimate) compared with 10 per cent in Phase I. Surprisingly, the parents' perception of family relationships did not always coincide with that of their son or daughter, except in the most extreme cases of family disharmony. A few teenagers definitely felt more distanced from and more out of tune with their parents than previously, which their parents appeared to be quite unaware of, and similarly in a couple of cases the parents viewed a relationship as poor or deteriorating when the teenager apparently did not feel this.

Where relationships were strained this caused a severe problem for the teenager, however, especially if this handicap was more than fairly mild. It is difficult to adjust to the idea of long-term dependence on one's family at a point in time when one's non-handicapped peer group is becoming increasingly independent. If the dependence is on family with whom one is out of sympathy, the distress involved is difficult to contemplate, especially since the prospects of an alternative congenial living situation are so poor.

## And what of the future?

### Mothers' feelings about dependence

Surprisingly, when asked about the amount of physical care needed by the teenager, over half the mothers said that their teenager needed no extra help (N = 26) compared with their other children. Of those who admitted that their son or daughter needed considerable help (40 per cent) most said that this did not really worry or depress them; only one said that this worried her greatly. This was the elderly mother of a very severely handicapped girl who had already made enquiries about a residential placement for her daughter and was fully aware of the difficulty of finding anything suitable.

When asked about the future, however, the picture was somewhat different, and over 20 per cent said that they worried about what arrangements could be made to ensure that their child got adequate care, while a further 20 per cent said that this was a major source of worry to them. Some of those who were not depressed were optimistic about the degree of independence that might eventually be achieved, partly because so much progress had been made in the past year. One said, 'I think it'll slowly come to him. He'll probably learn to live independently.' Another said of her daughter, well settled on a three-year residential course, 'She's made the break now'. And another, 'I'm not worried because I can see she's still developing.' However, many were fending off anxiety simply by just not thinking about the future, for example, 'I say when the time comes we'll see', or 'I'll just have to live forever'. Others declared that they were employing the same tactics that they had always done with regard to their handicapped child – 'We just live for today'.

Apart from the physical care needed, many parents felt that their teenager still needed help with such things as handling money and decision taking. A few said that this was changing – 'He takes more decisions now' – but others saw this as a permanent problem – 'She'll always need help in making decisions', or 'She needs to be more aggressive, she's too sweet, doesn't answer back enough, I don't think she ever will'.

*Teenagers' accommodation preferences*

Quite early on in the interview, the teenagers were asked about their accommodation preferences for the future. First of all they were asked, If they had a choice in a year or two's time of living away from home, would they prefer this? Quite a large number (20 per cent) were quite definite about preferring to live at home. Although the others did not on the whole have very clear ideas about what kind of accommodation they would prefer, most spontaneously suggested flats rather than hostels. However, when we asked them to consider a list of different types of accommodation that might, in theory, be available to them, they were much more definite. The choices included adapted and serviced flats, lodgings and mixed hostels, as well as hostels specially for the handicapped, or fully-staffed homes. When given these choices the majority of teenagers liked the idea of adapted or serviced flats or lodgings as opposed to special hostels or homes. The results suggest that in order to meet their preferences, a much wider range of provision is required, with a lot more emphasis on adapted or serviced housing, although hostels and homes were an acceptable option for some young people, especially those who were more severely disabled. Although some young people's ambitions in terms of independence may have been unrealistic, many who wanted this should have been able to manage in adapted or serviced accommodation. These, of course, would need to be provided at subsidized rents.

*How the parents and teenagers viewed the future*

At the end of the interview both parents and teenagers were asked to imagine the future. The parents were asked, 'What sort of life do you think X will be leading in about ten years from now?', while the teenagers were asked, 'What do you really hope to be doing by the time you're in your mid-twenties?'

Those parents who expressed a definite view about their child's future usually gave suggestions which were quite realistic in terms of their child's capacity, even if over-optimistic in terms of what services can at present be provided. Fourteen parents (28 per cent) thought that their son or daughter would be living independently in some way, though perhaps needing adapted accommodation, while a further ten (20 per cent) spoke of marriage and a job – in most cases quite a reasonable ambition. 'She'll be looking after herself, I hope, leading an ordinary life and being independent' (the mother of a hemiplegic girl who was at a special college when interviewed, but who subsequently found herself a factory job). 'Working and leading an ordinary life like anybody' (the mother of a bright hemiplegic boy with a speech defect, in a day centre at the time of interview and hoping for a place in a special training college). 'I hope he's met a nice girl, is planning to get married and have his own car. I'd like him to live with us' (the mother of a cerebral-palsied boy with an awkward gait and slight speech defect who was working as a messenger boy in the City and saving up to buy a motor bike).

Nine parents (18 per cent) thought that their child would either be in an institution of some kind or still fully dependent on them. 'I'm not sure. She'll probably be away from home somewhere – she'll always need help, but I hope she'll be working' (the mother of a severely handicapped spina bifida girl of average ability, who was at a special college). However, nearly one-third of the parents (N = 16) could give no answer to this question. These were mainly mothers with a moderately or severely handicapped teenager, who were clearly very confused and anxious about what the possibilities might be, and one suspected many feared that the future was likely to be fairly bleak. Some openly admitted this: 'I dread to think. There are so many people out of work with qualifications and he hasn't any' (the mother of a cerebral-palsied boy with an awkward gait and little use of one arm who was in a special college).

When the teenagers were asked what they were hoping for themselves by their mid-twenties, the most common thing mentioned was a job (referred to by over two-thirds of the group, although this was quite unrealistic for at least half of those who hoped for it, given the current employment situation). 'I hope to have a job, like gardening, and earning good money' (a boy with a marked right hemiplegia, of borderline ESN ability who was also epileptic, and currently in a day centre). 'Have a secure job' (a severely handicapped spina bifida girl of low average ability at a special college).

Being married or having a boyfriend was mentioned by sixteen young people (over one-third), while a further eight spoke of their hope of living independently. 'I hope to marry, have a child, a house and a car' (a moderately handicapped cerebral-palsied girl of low ability, currently in a day centre). 'I hope to get married, to get a lot of money and to be a better person' (a severely handicapped quadriplegic boy with a marked speech defect and lowish ability). 'To settle down in a place of my own and I'd like to be quite near home' (a severely handicapped spina bifida girl). Nine young people also mentioned having a better social life ('Go out more often', 'Going out when I want to'), while several others said, 'Enjoying myself generally'. A few young people expressed a wish to help others, one very specifically wanting 'to help other people with the difficulties I've had – to go to clubs and give people advice'.

In many cases it seemed likely that, given the present level of services and opportunities for work and social interactions, the hopes expressed by the teenagers were unlikely to be fulfilled. This was particularly so in the case of those who hoped for a job, and it seems unfortunate that so many had not been helped to realize that open employment would not be feasible for them, nor to discover alternative ways of feeling useful and wanted, or of achieving the far more reasonable ambition of getting about more and making more friends. In terms of independent living we found again this desire for one's own home, although given the amount of suitable accommodation available at present this was another ambition unlikely to be achieved.

## Summary

In many respects both parents and teenagers saw the post-school year as a constructive time during which the young person made progress towards greater independence both in attitude of mind and in actual self-help skills. Although timidity was still a problem for many, the parents noted a general growth in confidence and a greater willingness by the young people to attempt new things. The experience of living away from home for those who had the opportunity appeared to be beneficial both for the teenagers and the parents, and contributed to the growth of independence and to building up self-confidence.

One important area of independence where there was little change from the previous year was in the ability to get about outside the home unaccompanied, although this is so crucial a skill particularly in establishing an independent social life. Only half the group were able to use a bus unaccompanied, and less than one-quarter had a full or provisional driving licence (and most of this group were also able to use public transport). About half the young people were not sure whether or not they would ever be able to drive, and clearly had not had the opportunity to discuss this with anyone outside the family. It is quite remarkable that a skill which is so important if a disabled person is to achieve an independent adult life had not been thoroughly explored by this age so that the teenager would know whether or not this was a realistic ambition.

While most of the young people had made new friends at work, college or day centre over the previous year, there had been no improvement in the proportion able to see friends regularly in the evenings or weekends or in the holidays (in the case of those at college). Forty per cent never saw friends in their leisure time, while of those who were able to do so, one-fifth met less than monthly, or could make contact only by 'phone or letter. At the same time, rather fewer young people were members of clubs compared with their last year at school. Three-quarters of the teenagers felt themselves to be too much alone, a rather higher proportion than had said this in the previous year. With regard to the able-bodied, most of the disabled teenagers wanted to have more contact, but did not have much opportunity to do so, unless they were in an ordinary placement. Many young people said that they felt anxious and uncomfortable in the presence of able-bodied peers and clearly needed help and support if they were to overcome their anxieties.

In general we did not find substantial differences in the overall quality of social life between Phase I and Phase II of the study, in that at both interviews about the same proportion of this group of young people were rated as having a 'very restricted' or a 'satisfactory' social life. In other words, their situation was still very poor; less than one-fifth were thought to have a 'satisfactory' social life compared with nearly half rated as 'very restricted'. Where individuals had changed their status, the most important variable seemed to be the placement situation (although of course this is closely related to severity of handicap). We found that a poor social life when at home was common among those in special residential college, those in day centres and those without any occupation. The fact that the proportion of young people in these last two categories is likely to increase as the young people pass through special colleges (see chapter 7) does not give one much hope that social isolation will decrease as the young people move into adult life unless more help is offered so that they can overcome the very real difficulties they have in making better social contacts.

By the time of the Phase II interview, nearly all the young people were expressing an interest in the opposite sex, though only half of those interested had had any experience of this. About two-thirds of the teenagers wished to marry and most of these believed that this would be possible, although their parents were a great deal more pessimistic about their chances. Most of those who hoped to marry wanted children, although they expressed many anxieties about this, such as whether or not they were capable of parenthood, what effect the presence of a urinary diversion would have on pregnancy, and how they would physically manage to have intercourse. The most common worry expressed was that their child might be handicapped. The spina bifida teenagers were more likely to worry about this, with good reason, but they had had little opportunity to discuss this, and a few seemed quite unaware of the potential risk. Some cerebral-palsied teenagers were also worried about this, quite needlessly, and again had not had the opportunity to voice their fears to anyone who could reassure them. Their parents were often quite unaware that the teenagers were worrying about parenthood or the genetic risk of child bearing, but in any case they were in no position to help because they did not themselves have enough information to do so.

In terms of psychological adjustment, the parents were inclined to see an improvement because they were aware of the increased maturity and greater independence, although nearly 40 per cent thought that their child still had a definite problem, usually described as depression or as lack of confidence. In fact, apart from some improvement in confidence, the teenagers did not show a decrease in psychological problems. Nearly two-thirds said that they suffered from depression and one-third had felt life to be hopeless at some point during the previous year. Misery was particularly a problem for whose who did not have a satisfactory placement, and conversely those who were content with their placement were less likely to have been depressed. Many teenagers said that they worried more this year than previously – usually about their future, whether and how they would get a job or get married – and those without occupation or in an inadequate day centre with no prospects for improvement were, very understandably, the ones showing most concern. The other major factor contributing to adjustment in Phase II was whether or not family problems were present.

When considering what the future might hold for their children, many parents felt encouraged by the progress made in the last year and were hoping that their son or daughter would eventually be able to lead some kind of an independent life. However, one-fifth said that they were very worried about the future while another fifth admitted to some anxieties. Getting on for 20 per cent thought that the teenager would either be in an institution or fully dependent at home, compared with almost one-third who thought that their son or daughter would be independent to some extent.

When the teenagers were asked to say what they hoped for themselves their wish to live as independently as possible came across very clearly, as did the extent to which their self-esteem was bound up with achieving this. Although some could not conceive of living away from home, when asked to consider possible accommodation options, about twice as many young people said they'd prefer adapted or serviced flats to hostels or homes. To 'get a job' was the most universally expressed wish even by many whose chances of doing so were minimal or non-existent, and this again emphasizes that no one appeared to have helped the teenager appreciate this fact or to consider alternative ways of feeling useful and fulfilled.

It is a cause for great concern that both the psychological well-being of the disabled teenagers and the degree of social isolation are related so closely to achieving a satisfactory placement, when the long-term prospects for many are so poor in this respect. At the time of the second interview, most of the teenagers saw themselves in a transition stage, and if not satisfactorily settled, many clearly hoped that their situation would change for the better. Consequently, although the distress caused by uncertainty about the future and the lack of social outlets was high, many were protected from its worst effects by their expectation for progress. In addition those in residential colleges were better able to tolerate the boredom and social isolation while at home in the holidays because for most of the year they were busy and active at college. However, once their furthur education course was complete, many young people were likely to be greatly disappointed with the lack of opportunities available to them at home and disillusionment and despair were likely to result.

One would be naïve to deny the difficulty in ensuring that the more disabled teenagers develop their skills and talents in some way which will give them contentment and a feeling of self-worth, or the problems involved in helping them extend their social contacts. Nevertheless, it is apparent that they are being offered a very poor service in this respect at present, and that at school and at college we are seriously failing to prepare them adequately for adult life.

# III
# Support from society and the family

# 10

## *Provision made in schools to facilitate the transition to adult life*

Adolescence is generally recognized as a time of particular stress. The 'symptoms' of adolescent turmoil, and those of the handicapped teenagers in particular, have been discussed in chapters 5, 6 and 8. The years around the age of leaving school are of crucial importance for all young people in gaining personal independence and confidence, but even more so for handicapped teenagers. Moving from the secure and sheltered environment of school to the unknown, outside world can be extremely traumatic and, apart from the search for employment, coping with daily living and getting out and meeting new people requires social skills and confidence which may not develop unaided at school.

Anderson and Spain (1977) suggested that spina bifida school leavers have three main kinds of problems to deal with. These include the physical factors of impaired mobility (and possibly incontinence), problems related to general or specific learning difficulties, and finally personality or social factors. These are essentially the same kinds of problems which cerebral-palsied teenagers also have to face, although of course the physical problems for any particular cerebral-palsied young person often include other faculties, such as speech, which are not usually affected for teenagers with spina bifida.

In the opinion of Mary Greaves (1972), it is the level of social maturity and personal adjustment which are important when considering employment prospects, rather than the severity of the handicap; and while this may be true, nonetheless the handicap itself will limit the young person in many ways. It will obviously influence the extent to which he can engage in particular activities, but over and above this it will influence the extent of his experience and depth of understanding. There may be many gaps in the experience of very common things which able-bodied peers take for granted – for example walking in the countryside, going to clubs or discos, or shopping in a busy shopping centre. In addition limitations in social contact are inevitable where the handicapped young person cannot use public transport and does not have a car.

Schools, whether ordinary or special, can do much in preparing school leavers for the world of work and making the transition to adult life as trouble-free as possible by helping the handicapped pupils to learn ways of coping with some of these problems and come to terms with them before leaving school. Projects, discussions, visits and assignments can help to substitute for 'lost' experiences. The handicapped teenager must be prepared for citizenship in a complex and highly literate society which will make few allowances for his disabilities.

As early as 1963 the Newsom Report considered the education of 13–16 year olds of average or less than average ability. It was pointed out that 'the school programme in the final year should be deliberately out-going, an initiation into the adult world of work and leisure'. This same emphasis for handicapped pupils was recommended by Younghusband *et al.* in *Living with Handicap* (1970): 'The school curriculum, especially in the last year, should give due consideration to the need for prepar-ation for life after school, particularly personal independence, social relationships and pre-work experience.'

The Warnock Report has more recently drawn attention to the gaps in services for young people with special educational needs in the transition from school to adult life. It emphasizes that skilled support must be available to teenagers and their parents at this time and that this should be provided according to each individual's requirements. The Report recommends that 'a pupil's special needs should be reassessed with future prospects in mind at least two years before he is due to leave school . . . [and also] that both ordinary and special schools should give pupils with special education needs more help to acquire the basic skills and to develop social competence and vocational interests' in order to prepare them at school for the demands of adult life.

The fact that the handicapped teenagers do have special needs that are not being catered for is exemplified by the fact that most of the young people in the follow-up study who had either no occupation or quite un-satisfactory occupation appeared to be completely unprepared for dealing with this situation, and also by the high level of social isolation found particularly, but not exclusively, among those who had attended special schools. In general, the teenagers were poorly prepared for life as an adult handicapped person on leaving school, and in most cases were still unprepared at the end of a year in further education.

Preparation in school for adult life must embrace two important areas. The most obvious is helping in the transition to work which must include all the things that can be done to maximize the teenager's chances of finding a satisfactory placement after school – whether this be employ-ment, further education or some alternative to work. (The subject of careers guidance, education and advice will be considered in more detail in chapter 11.) However, preparing school leavers for work and helping them to find placements is not the only problem area. It is just as im-portant to foster skills needed for general social competence, such as making friends, use of leisure time and dealing with bureaucracy, and it is here that schools can play a crucial role. A recent study for the OECD of the 'preparation for life after school' programmes in nine local authorities in Great Britain (Rowan, 1980) noted that courses of this kind have become more numerous recently, and will be increasingly important for both handicapped and non-handicapped secondary age pupils given the diminishing employment prospects generally.

In fact, in all schools some form of 'social education' or 'education for living' takes place whether or not it is on the curriculum. Certain standards of behaviour are established by school rules and others may be learned unconsciously by the response of peers and staff to different behaviours. However, certain aspects of this kind of learning may need to be made more explicit, and this is especially true for handicapped pupils who have not had the same opportunities to build up social confidence and experience in the daily routines of independent living. Teenagers may need specific guidance about the appropriate behaviour in social settings which they may have never encountered while at school. A most important element of this, for special schools, is to find ways of establishing contact between their pupils and able-bodied young people in both formal and informal settings, so that leavers are not inhibited in their social relationships with the able-bodied in adult life. The importance of a well prepared programme of 'education for living' was pointed out in the Scottish Report (1975) but it does not minimize the difficulties involved: 'The achievement of personal identity and satisfactory relationships in the adult world and with the opposite sex poses problems to which there are no simple answers.'

Social education programmes in special schools will be particularly important for pupils who, although theoretically employable, may be unable to find employment at the present time, or for the more severely handicapped who will never be able to work. Whether pupils are to enter open employment, further education or some alternative to work they must be prepared to cope with their future place in the outside world. At the very least, they need to achieve maximum independence and develop social skills so that a more fulfilling life without work can be enjoyed.

In recent years these kinds of programme have been developed in schools for the educationally subnormal (ESN) but not in those for the physically handicapped (Tizard and Anderson, 1979). The changing nature of handicap, due to the decline of conditions like polio, together with the move towards the integration of the more able into ordinary schools means that most of the children in PH schools are now very severely or multiply handicapped and a high proportion have marked learning difficulties. Spina bifida and cerebral palsy together now account for about two-thirds of the population in special schools. It would seem that there has been a time lag in developing a curriculum more suited to the fact that less able and more handicapped children now predominate in the special schools.

The OECD Report notes that although many of the transition programmes in the ESN(M) schools are new and have had their difficulties, the curricula are constantly being improved and the valuable experience gained in the process could be passed on. The courses reviewed for the Report, covered 'such aspects as personal life, health, hygiene, shopping, home management and getting on with other people, to bring public services like the post office, library, telephone and transport into familiar use, and to introduce the routines of work – from job applications and time-keeping to travel and canteens. Visits to local firms and public offices are arranged and nearly everywhere there is work experience for one day a week in the final year' (Rowan, 1980).

A survey of the provision for 'social education' for special school leavers, and the facilities available to them while still at school to make contacts and relationships with their peers in ordinary schools, was recently carried out by PHAB (1979). Replies to a postal questionnaire were analysed for the 128 schools that replied out of 146 contacted. The survey looked at out-of-school activities, youth clubs, other groups, contact with other schools and formal links between schools as well as families' and teachers' views on the need for social education. It found that the kind of provision most often seen as desirable in these special schools was for greater links with ordinary schools. It concludes: 'It was evident that many head teachers were extremely well aware that their school leavers needed help with the difficult transition between the special school environment and the outside world. Many were trying hard to prepare their pupils for this while they were still at school.' But it also adds the important proviso: 'The impression gained from this study is that there is still a long way to go in enabling special school pupils to widen their horizons.'

It is apparent that schools play an important part in the social development of teenagers. The type of school attended and the scope of the curriculum will either create opportunities for developing confidence in different social settings or will greatly inhibit this possibility. For this reason, the staff of the sixty schools attended by the teenagers in the study (including class teachers, year heads, pastoral care staff, careers guidance staff and social education staff) were questioned about the services they offered and their suggestions for improvements. In addition the teenagers and parents in both phases of the study were also asked about their personal experiences in receiving advice and help and for any ideas they had on the improvements needed to be made.

This chapter examines the services offered by the different schools, including any special arrangements made by ordinary schools to cater for handicapped pupils, as well as the pastoral care arrangements in all schools. The social education ('education for living') programmes will also be discussed, and the views of the parents and the teenagers are then considered to compare the schools' and the families' perception of the effectiveness of these programmes. We shall also consider education for use of leisure, and how much the schools promoted integration with the able-bodied outside school hours. Sex education and preparation for parenthood programmes are next examined and compared with the teenagers' knowledge and opinions about which areas need to be developed further. In the final section, the schools' suggestions for improvements will be described, together with the teenagers' and the parents' complaints and feelings looking back at their schooling a year after they have left.

## Services provided by schools

Handicapped pupils in both ordinary and special schools are likely to need extra help and support in the transition to adult life although they may face different problems and the solutions will, of necessity, differ according to the school setting. While it may seem obvious that attending a special school will make it much less likely that a teenager will have friends who live nearby, attending an ordinary school does not automatically solve the problem of friendship, as shown in chapter 3. The attitudes of the handicapped teenagers to themselves, and the attitudes of others to them, will greatly determine their social competence and sociability in general. Both ordinary and special schools can provide a supportive framework and make imaginative attempts to help a teenager overcome these physical, social and emotional difficulties which determine whether satisfactory social relationships developed at school and in adult life.

The Spastics Society has been concerned with this very subject, setting up a working party on 'The Special Needs of Handicapped Adolescents' which reported in 1978. This points out that in special schools it should be easier to identify the needs of handicapped teenagers than in ordinary schools. It considered that coming to terms with one's situation may be considerably more difficult in a large comprehensive school where a handicapped youngster is the only handicapped pupil than in a small special class with other handicapped peers and staff who are aware of their problems. Also in ordinary schools at present, there are few teachers or counsellors who understand the wide and varied range of individual needs which many handicapped adolescents and their parents are likely to have.

In our study, we looked first, therefore, at what special arrangements had been made by any of the ordinary schools we visited to accommodate handicapped pupils or to make their participation in the normal school activities as full as possible.

### Special arrangements in ordinary schools

The level of the physical adaptations and back-up services required in ordinary schools will obviously depend on the number of handicapped pupils in attendance, the severity of their handicaps, as well as the size, physical layout and general organization of the school concerned. The characteristics of the ordinary schools involved in this study have already been outlined in chapter 1. The number of physically handicapped pupils on the school registers varied greatly according to the completeness of the records and the school's own definition of physical handicap. One school said that fifty pupils out of a total school population of 1000 were physically handicapped, but this included very minor deafness or eyesight problems, as well as epileptics and cerebral-palsied pupils. On closer examination, and with stricter definitions, no school had more than ten handicapped pupils, and most (thirty-one schools out of thirty-four) had between one and five.

Only three schools said that they had made some physical adaptations in the school for handicapped pupils. One had built a ramp in the hall so that the spina bifida girl in the study could wheel her wheelchair in and out, and they were also planning to make a ramp in front of the school so that she could get herself in by this. Another school had also built a ramp into one of the classrooms (not for the survey pupil but for a girl severely handicapped with muscular dystrophy). Another school, which had two thalidomide pupils and one muscular dystrophy pupil as well as the spina bifida boy we interviewed, had arranged for a lift to be installed. A fourth school had specially arranged the timetable of one of the survey pupils to minimize the amount she had to move about the school because they could not provide a lift.

Few schools had arranged special medical supervision of their handicapped pupils, although five said that the school doctor would have extra involvement with the handicapped pupils. Only five said that the school doctor systematically saw handicapped pupils and had extra responsibility for them, although in only three schools had the doctor actually seen the survey pupil during the last year. (Two boys had been seen for medical check ups, and one so that a medical report could be sent to the careers officer.) Some schools had a school nurse, but only three of these had special responsibilities for the handicapped pupils, and in only two was there systematic involvement. Three of the survey pupils had seen the school nurse in the last year. One was trying to arrange hydrotherapy at a local special school for a cerebral-palsied girl, and one saw a cerebral-palsied girl about personal problems. The third saw a spina bifida boy on the occasions when his bag leaked, but since she had received no instruction on how to change a bag, she merely arranged for the boy to be sent home when accidents occurred. However, she had arranged on her own initiative for this boy's mother to have a telephone installed through the Rowntree Fund. In another school, which did not have a school nurse as such, the spina bifida girl in a wheelchair had a part-time welfare assistant who was employed by the LEA for this girl's benefit and who, in fact, acted as an unofficial matron to the entire school. She assisted the spina bifida teenager by helping her with toileting and in getting around the school in general, had taught her to type while the other pupils had physical education lessons, and also worked with this girl in the lunch hour helping her with independence training. This woman had been given no information at all when she started this work, but by chance met the Advisory Teacher for the handicapped in Hertfordshire who was very helpful and arranged for her to spend a few days at the local special school and to attend a course for school matrons.

None of the ordinary secondary schools which the handicapped pupils in our study attended had designated a member of the teaching staff to have special responsibility for handicapped pupils. There were also no individual teaching arrangements. All the schools, except three, said that the handicapped pupils attended ordinary classes and no special arrangements were made for them. However, all but four of the schools (three of these being grammar schools) had a teacher who was mainly responsible for the slow learners. This was usually the head of the remedial department or a teacher with a graded post responsible for slow learners. The majority of schools (N = 20) had a remedial department while others had 'remedial sessions', 'special classes' or a remedial advisor who gave help in ordinary classes. Two schools said that the handicapped pupils were in full-time remedial classes, and two used the remedial facilities regularly. In another school there was a special unit, 'The Communications Unit', for pupils with learning difficulties which the survey pupil concerned was due to enter the following term. This unit comprised twenty children from the fourth and fifth years with special learning difficulties. Each pupil spent eight 1 hour 10 minute sessions a week in this 'workshop' getting extra individual help and social skills training. For example, they were taught how to use the telephone, go shopping and other such activities. In addition, fifteen schools said that the physically handicapped pupils occasionally used the facilities for slow learners. Examples quoted were a boy with spastic quadriplegia who was learning to type as he could hardly write; a boy who had always been given extra tuition in English, maths and science; a girl taking the 'Right to Read' course; and a boy getting extra individual help with reading.

On further questioning, eleven of the schools said they had other special arrangements or facilities for handicapped pupils or other pupils with special needs. Four of these had recognized the need to cater for pupils with behaviour problems separately in special withdrawal units of some kind. One was planning to take all the maladjusted pupils in North Hertfordshire into a newly opened unit for twenty children. Two schools had peripatetic teachers for the partially hearing, and one of these had, in addition, a remedial specialist who also acted as a counsellor and teacher of social education. She gave extra support to pupils with emotional as well as learning problems. One large comprehensive school with a very large Asian population had appointed a special teacher to help these immigrant children learn English with the use of the language centre at another school.

## Pastoral care in both types of school

We have already pointed out the emotional and behavioural problems that the group of teenagers in this study are likely to have (see Chapter 5). In the light of this, and the general probability that adolescence will be a particularly stressful period for handicapped teenagers, the pastoral care organization in school would seem to be of prime importance in providing support at this time.

This is very important in both special and ordinary schools but for rather different reasons. The special school will need to stimulate the confidence of their pupils to mix in the wider community and to face the prospect of leaving the protective atmosphere of the special school. In the ordinary school the special emotional problems faced by the handicapped pupil may well be overlooked, but the evidence from this study suggests that these pupils did appear to need special help, particularly for girls in their relationship with the opposite sex. A counsellor who understands the handicapped teenagers' situation and empathizes with the teenagers' special worries can help in their transition to adult life and in coming to terms with their position in life. The Spastics Society's Working Party (1978) has recognized this, and has called for personal counselling services to be readily available to handicapped adolescents in all types of schools as one of the major priorities for this age group. They further point out that as fewer people in mainstream education are likely to be aware of the needs of handicapped adolescents this should receive priority consideration, although of course they state that it is equally important to recognize the needs of those in special schools.

With this in mind, it is interesting to look in detail at the pastoral care and counselling arrangements in both the special and ordinary schools that we visited. When asked generally about pastoral care in the school, the staff in ordinary and special schools demonstrated a distinct difference of opinion about how such matters should be conducted.

The ordinary schools tended to outline a formal system of pastoral care, describing a hierarchical system of responsibility starting with the form teacher, the child being referred on, if necessary, to the year head and sometimes to the head of the lower, middle, or upper schools. A number of schools also said that the deputy head was an important person in the pastoral system. Alternatively, the house system was the pastoral unit, and the house tutor or head of house was the key pastoral figure. Four schools also mentioned a school counsellor who played a part in individual guidance in addition to the more formal structure of care. Most of the ordinary schools (N = 25) said the person likely to have the most knowledge of a particular pupil's personal and emotional development was the form tutor or class teacher, while a number (N = 8) said this would be the year head, and a few (N = 4) that this would be the head of house, the head of middle school or the head teacher. Only one school said the school counsellor knew pupils best.

The picture given by the special schools was quite different. They were generally in favour of an informal, personal approach made possible by their small size compared with the ordinary schools. Most said that personal problems were dealt with on an informal basis by a variety of staff members – the class teacher, the head teacher, medical staff, welfare assistants or house parents. It may seem surprising that only two special schools mentioned formal arrangements in the form of a regular counsellor, although two said that structured case conferences were held regularly about pupils. In no school was there a member of staff with specific responsibility for the pastoral care of pupils.

Like the ordinary schools, the form teacher was the person named most often (by fourteen of the twenty-six special schools) as the person who knew pupils most intimately, yet in only one school was time assigned for form teachers to discuss personal and social relationships with the pupils in their classes. Some mentioned other members of staff in conjunction with the form teacher. Four of the residential schools mentioned the matron, and three others mentioned either the houseparent or the form tutor. Two schools thought the welfare assistants or child care staff would know the children best, and one school said that the head or deputy head would have most knowledge of each pupil. It was difficult to see how most of the systems described could adequately identify any but the most severe and obvious problems, and this would appear to be an area in which great improvements could be made to help the handicapped teenager cope with this particularly stressful time of life.

## Counselling

Chapters 5 and 6 describe how the physically handicapped teenagers suffered from a higher rate of psychological problems – especially the so-called 'neurotic' disorders – than their able-bodied peers. The specific problems described include depression, anxiety, loneliness and lack of self-confidence. Over half the handicapped teenagers had problems in adjustment, and one-quarter had marked problems which indicated the need for counselling by someone experienced in the field of handicap. The Spastics Society Working Party (1978) named 'the need for personal counselling services to be readily available to handicapped adolescents in all types of school . . . as one of the major priorities for this age group'. Warnock also recommended 'that better counselling on personal relationships should be available to young people with special needs and their parents from a variety of sources, including the health and social services and voluntary groups' (para. 10.96).

First, let us look at what is meant by 'counselling'. The Spastics Society define it by its aim: 'The ultimate aim of counselling is to help people to come to terms with their difficulties and solve their own problems.' They note the problem in defining counselling by method because of the wide range of counselling techniques currently used, which include group or individual counselling, while the role of counsellors may be seen as giving advice or guidance or, to follow Carl Rogers' philosophy, simply to listen, understand and accept (Rogers, 1942). There is also a blurred distinction between social work and counselling. Counsellors can include trained, partly trained or untrained personnel appointed by statutory or voluntary agencies, or friends, teachers and parents. As far as trained counsellors for adolescents are concerned, there is a lack of information about the number throughout the country and how many are currently working with handicapped teenagers.

The Warnock Report concluded that 'young people with special needs may require advice on a range of personal matters including health, and personal and sexual relationships'. Counselling on sexual relationships is discussed separately, pp. 281–2, and we shall deal here with counselling in schools on other personal matters.

*Ordinary schools.* Most of the ordinary schools had no special counselling service as such, but two had full-time counsellors, and seven had part-time school counsellors. These counsellors mainly gave help with personal and social problems, either in group sessions or individually, but a few said that they gave some educational and vocational guidance as well. Two schools also had informal arrangements for counselling, which were very interesting. In one the two heads of the upper school – a married couple – took charge of the pastoral care of the boys and the girls separately. Every six weeks pupils who were considered not to be working for one reason or another were seen by them and this often generated counselling for personal problems. Pupils would often approach them to talk about personal matters. In the other school a well organized system of 'communities' was set up with the specific purpose of pastoral care. The communities were like houses in structure, but had no competitive element. The head of the community kept files on all the pupils and would deal with any individual problems. The form tutor would get to know pupils in tutorial periods but refer any pupils who needed extra help to the respective community head.

As far as their teachers were aware, only three of the thirty-seven survey pupils in ordinary schools and one of the control teenagers had been to see the school counsellor in the past year. One girl had been

referred to the senior mistress by her form teacher because she
isolated, nervous and depressed; another had sought help of her
accord because of headaches and feeling the pressure of impending
O level exams. A third survey pupil had been seen by the counsellor on
casual basis because of complaints from the staff about her laziness and
untidiness, and she also saw this pupil in connection with funding her
travelling expenses to a Spastics Society's assessment course. One control
teenager had been to see the school counsellor on several occasions about
feeling upset and inadequate in comparison to her sister who was
brighter and doing much better at school.

The majority of the ordinary schools said that they had no contact with
social workers. Only three had social workers attached to the school (all
on a part-time basis) while ten said that they could contact a social worker
if necessary. One school said that they used the health visitor (who visited
weekly) to contact families if there were problems, while another said
that the educational welfare officer (EWO) acted as a 'special sort of
social worker'. In fact, most of the schools mentioned the EWO's as
sources of help to deal with general family problems as well as with
truancy. The social workers who were used in ordinary schools usually
dealt with particular families and not with the teenager personally unless
referred by the school because of discipline problems. Only one of the
survey pupils in an ordinary school had been in contact with a social
worker in the last year as far as the school knew. This was a hemiplegic
boy whose family were quite notorious with the police in the neighbourhood, and he received no personal support from home. He had mixed at
school and outside with 'criminal types' according to the school counsellor and had recently been put on probation.

When the school staff were asked what sort of problems adolescents
with spina bifida or cerebral palsy generally wanted guidance about,
most of them said they did not know, or could not generalize from their
limited experience of individual cases. Two said that handicapped pupils
usually had very similar problems to their peers, and only three thought
that they were also likely to have problems specifically related to the
handicap. Indeed it seemed unlikely, with the counselling systems
described by the schools, that many handicapped pupils' needs would
have been identified, or that any extra help they required would have
been recognized.

*Special schools.* Since special schools are dealing with handicapped
pupils who are known to have more problems to cope with than able-
bodied adolescents it might be expected that individual counselling
would be an integral part of the special school structure. However, only
eight of the twenty-six special schools visited (four residential and four
day schools) said that either members of staff (N = 2) or visiting professionals (N = 6) were given time specifically for individual counselling.

Two of these were visiting educational psychologists, one who came weekly and the other fortnightly; two were attached social workers who visited at least once a week and would deal with pupils' problems or act as a link between the school and the pupils' home, offering help and assistance to the parents as well. In another school the social worker had started to hold group sessions where teenagers could talk about their personal problems. Only one school had a formal arrangement with a visiting counsellor for the sole purpose of in-depth counselling of pupils. This scheme seemed so successful that it will be described in detail later in this section (p. 267).

Of the two schools which had staff members who acted as counsellors neither had had any special training. In one the matron was always available to both parents or pupils, and in the other the deputy head's post was seen to be primarily of a pastoral nature, while the head of the upper school was also free every afternoon to deal with the pupils' personal problems. Three other schools mentioned *ad hoc* arrangements. Two said that their social workers did counsel pupils on request and if necessary referred them on to an educational psychologist or some other professional. In another the matron was always available to the pupils, and an educational psychologist visited if consulted over disturbed pupils.

Few schools, therefore, could offer a special counselling service, but it might be expected that where local authority social workers were attached to special schools they would be available to give advice to individual teenagers or their families if necessary, as well as dealing with such things as aids and benefits or other special services. Only five of the twenty-six special schools visited had a full-time social worker attached, while six had a part-time social worker. In addition, ten schools said that they would contact someone to give advice when help was needed, usually the educational welfare officer or a local authority social worker, while one school used a health visitor to liaise with parents and to refer any problems to the appropriate authorities or local family doctor.

In fact, only nine of the eighty-two survey pupils in special schools were reported to have seen their teacher or counsellor for help or advice with personal or emotional problems over the past year. We also asked what proportion of the secondary age pupils in the special schools (not just the survey pupils) had received some personal counselling over the last year. Seven of the schools said they had no idea, while five said that no pupil had received personal counselling. However, in eleven schools counselling was commonly provided for children of secondary age, but this included four residential schools which provided regular counselling for families although the pupils themselves could not approach anyone for help or were not seen for counselling individually.

Most of the special schools maintained that there did not appear to be particular problems associated with teenagers with cerebral palsy or spina bifida. Most schools thought that the majority of problems the teenagers were concerned about were the same ones that any teenagers face or worry about at this age. Many schools mentioned problems at home, marital discord or family breakdown, worries about leaving school and what they would do when they left. Some schools also mentioned sexual worries, going out with friends independently and meeting the opposite sex as being a concern of pupils of this age. However, while these are subjects that may concern all teenagers, they are certainly much more difficult for handicapped adolescents to overcome without assistance. Only one school mentioned loneliness as being the biggest problem for handicapped teenagers and thought this was especially apparent in the teenage years.

Given that our study revealed that the handicapped teenagers had many problems and worries specifically connected with handicap, such as incontinence, epilepsy, and worries about sexual relationships and relationships generally with their able-bodied peers, it seems extraordinary that the special schools were unaware of their pupils' anxieties and of their great need for counselling during the adolescent years.

One residential school (for cerebral-palsied pupils of secondary age) did provide a service which seemed far and away the best of any described to us and it seems worthwhile explaining this in some detail as an example of good practice. The head teacher, while stressing the importance of encouraging young people to raise problems with school staff, felt strongly that pupils should have the right to discuss their personal problems on a strictly confidential basis with someone who was not connected with their day-to-day life at school. For more important worries the head felt that skilled counselling was much more appropriate from an outside expert, and consequently a counsellor with considerable experience in marriage guidance has been visiting the school for some years. This counsellor worked with pupils in a variety of ways. She visited the school three evenings a week to work with groups and was also available to do individual counselling if any teenager wished this. At about 13 or 14 years, groups of about eight pupils were taken for a period of at least three weeks (and sometimes much longer depending on the interest shown) to discuss their sexual development and personal problems. Attendance at these sessions was not compulsory and any teenager could opt out if he or she felt uncomfortable, but all pupils were encouraged to go. These groups might be mixed or single sex according to the pupils' own preference; no member of staff was present. These sessions were entirely confidential and pupils knew that they could go to the counsellor on an individual basis at any time. The head arranged the appointment but would not ask about the problem. The head thought that this arrangement was a great success and that there had been a definite decrease in general tensions since formal counselling had been available. Also during the past few months the school had been trying out counselling for those with no speech, since the needs and problems of this group of young people is considerable. They felt that some success had been achieved by involving the speech therapist on the same basis of confidentiality as the counsellor. The therapist discussed with the child what he or she wanted to talk about and the counsellor dealt with that subject. The head pointed out that this was very time-consuming but was showing positive results as tensions were being reduced. From his experience, he thought that counsellors must be prepared for the fact that more problems will arise as young people are taught to examine themselves, and emphasized that parents must be involved at an early stage to help them face their own problems and understand more about their child's development and adjustment to adult life.

*Schools' perception of the adequacy of counselling and pastoral services.* Given the paucity of counselling services available, it is interesting to note that a large proportion of both the special (48 per cent) and the ordinary (42 per cent) schools thought that the counselling or personal guidance services available within the school were meeting the needs of the handicapped teenagers quite adequately. However, almost equal numbers thought that while services were fairly good they could be improved in some way, while about 10 per cent of special and ordinary schools felt that they were definitely inadequate.

Of the three special schools which felt their counselling services and pastoral care organization was definitely inadequate, one had only been opened for two years so had not fully established any arrangements yet; another said that the teenagers did not approach the staff with their problems and felt that perhaps a person from outside the school could be more helpful in counselling; while the third, a residential school, felt that the teachers suffered from a lack of contact with the teenagers' home background which limited the kind of help they could offer. The three ordinary schools which thought that their services were inadequate applied this judgement as far as all pupils were concerned, and not just for the handicapped pupils. Two of the schools felt that their pastoral staff did not have enough time to devote to personal counselling and hence only crisis cases or behaviour problems were seen, and that no self-referrals were possible. The other school felt that their school pastoral team (the educational psychologist and social worker) was inadequate to deal with all the problems since the children came from a very deprived neighbourhood with many social problems: they felt they needed a full-time counsellor.

Some of the ordinary schools (N = 74) and special schools (N = 8) thought that their counselling services were fairly adequate but could be improved. Some of the special schools felt that they would benefit from having a social worker or another visiting professional attached to the school to help with counselling, for example with genetic and sexual counselling. Most of the ordinary schools complained that the staff did not have enough time to deal with pupils' personal problems as they were so busy teaching, though this was seen as a general problem for all pupils and not the handicapped pupils in particular.

These figures again indicate that schools simply did not appear to appreciate the extent of problems or anxieties experienced by the handicapped teenagers in their care, or that the amount of counselling being offered was insufficient to meet the teenagers' needs. In our judgement only five of the special schools were providing anything like an adequate service in this respect. It was a little more difficult to make a similar judgement for the ordinary schools in respect of their non-handicapped pupils, but certainly no ordinary school appeared to provide a service at all tailored to the needs of the handicapped.

## Social education

As already mentioned at the beginning of this chapter, a school's responsibilities towards its handicapped pupils do not consist solely of academic teaching but also include preparing the pupils for life after school, which should include a comprehensive 'education for living' programme and should, where possible, also act as a mediator in finding a satisfactory post-school placement. PHAB concluded in their survey (1979) that most special schools now recognize the need for social education programmes to foster social competence and personal independence as an important preparation for the transition from school to the outside world. In the nine local authorities surveyed by the OECD (Rowan, 1980), all the ESN(M) schools looked at had begun to develop programmes for preparing handicapped teenagers for the world outside before they left school, and nearly all of those were geared to building up social competence as much as helping the transition to work.

Since nowadays far more children in schools for the physically handicapped suffer from central nervous system damage they are often of low ability, while a high proportion have complex and multiple handicaps; this means that such programmes must now become a more central part of the special school curriculum as they have been for some time in the ESN schools. For the most severely handicapped youngsters such social education programmes will be a question of nurturing the most basic independence skills, but for others they should include the encouragement of attributes of a general nature, such as a willingness to accept responsibility and make decisions, as well as more specific skills, such as coping with money and the transport system or various household activities (buying and cooking food, washing up, cleaning, bed-making and budgeting). All activities must be aimed at encouraging maximum physical and also personal independence. Other aspects of 'education for living', that will affect a special school leavers' social independence, are general hygiene and self-care, while health education should be a regular feature of the curriculum in all schools. Handicapped pupils will have to face special problems in this area; in the case of spina bifida teenagers, for example, incontinence management is crucial, while all paraplegics are prone to pressure sores so that self-care of skin must also be learnt.

The Scottish Report (1975) indicates another function of the special schools when it recommends that 'each PH child should leave school with a sound knowledge of the aids and equipment which are available to him as an adult and also exactly how to obtain these, so that he will be able to assess in a realistic way the extent to which he can achieve domestic independence and travel to work'. Teenagers also need to be taught while still at school about the services available to them and about how to claim for benefits for themselves.

Education for leisure is another important area, especially for the majority of special school leavers who are unlikely to get paid employment. Learning how to make use of adult education facilities, developing hobbies, and considering the possibility of voluntary work are all important since they suggest to the school leaver ways of making his life more interesting and satisfactory, and of helping him to meet non-handicapped peers on equal terms. This is most important for handicapped teenagers both in ordinary and in special schools since, as we have shown, social isolation was a great problem for the majority of teenagers in the study.

However, it is not only in the special schools that education for adult life is important. Ordinary schools have also started covering this area, often combined with careers education, and no doubt it will become increasingly important if unemployment continues to rise and alternative arrangements to active work have to be considered. If this happens the amount of leisure time for all school leavers will increase, but especially for the handicapped whose employment prospects are poor, and who are likely to have long periods of unemployment. The constructive use of leisure is a major area in which all schools can prepare its leavers for life after school.

It is often assumed that these different aspects of education for living will be part of the curriculum of a special school. This is not usually the case as our results will show, and the Scottish Committee in their visits to schools for the handicapped found only *one* school in which education for living was an established part of the curriculum and recommended that much more be done in this area. One example of such a course, offered by a college of further education rather than a school, is provided at Beaumont College opened by the Spastics Society in 1977. It aims specifically to provide a social learning curriculum for slow learners or pupils in the ESN(M) ability range. The college sees its main task as 'preparing physically handicapped and intellectually retarded young people for an adult life which is to be lived, where possible, within the wider community; our main concerns are with developing attitudes and skills associated with a person living a life as independently as would be possible. A preparation for life in the wider community would for most of our students involve obtaining optimum independence from the various effects of physical handicap and acquiring a satisfactory and satisfying degree of personal growth and social independence.'

*The schools' attitudes towards preparation for adult life.* When asked about things that the school was doing to prepare its PH pupils for life after school, the ordinary schools unanimously felt that special arrangements for their PH pupils were not appropriate because each school had so few. This does present a problem since these one or two pupils in a school will often need extra support and help in adjusting to adult life although it is very difficult to know how to provide this without stigmatizing the pupil as 'different'. Any extra help offered would have to be given discreetly, although this should be possible with a good pastoral care system.

Many of the special schools, however, were able to describe ways in which they were attempting to facilitate the broadening horizons and social competence of their pupils. Most schools had not specifically developed an organized leavers' programme, but involved the pupils in shopping expeditions, visits to supermarkets and local facilities like the library, and encouraged them to attempt washing and cooking in school. Four of the residential schools had 'independence flats' or bungalows which they used for leavers. Pupils were usually placed in this flat in a small group for a week or two and had to look after themselves entirely – shopping, budgeting, cooking, washing and cleaning; their attempts were usually monitored.

Four of the special schools had developed special 'leavers' courses' and these will be described briefly since they are quite rare at present, but offer useful models to show what it is possible to do within schools in this respect. In one this involved the occupational therapist and domestic science teacher and emphasized independence training both in the school and on a week's intensive course by the sea in an ASBAH bungalow. Some of the leavers went on a one-week residential course for handicapped school leavers, originally designed for ESN leavers. Another school (for the ESN(M)), was aiming to make its pupils 'socially acceptable' during their last year at school through a special programme. They took pupils out to introduce them to local facilities like the sports complex and youth centre, and also actively made use of certain public facilities like the library, telephone box, careers office and social services offices. On one day each week pupils were given work experience in the school, including clocking in and out, 'working' at packing boxes on a simulated conveyer belt system, learning about work routines and wage slips, and how to fill in various forms. The third school leavers' programme formed part of an overall social studies programme which was provided both for younger pupils and for those in their last two years at four levels, according to ability. The course for older pupils included topics such as contraception, alcoholism, smoking, marriage and family relationships, as well as subjects related particularly to handicap, such as the hereditary risks of spina bifida and the management of incontinence in relation to marriage. The teacher of the leavers' class, who also dealt with careers, emphasized that she was trying very hard to make pupils think about how, as adults, they would use their leisure time. She felt very strongly that not enough time was available to spend on this subject which she saw as a priority for handicapped school leavers. By far the most extensive leavers' programme was in a residential secondary school, only in its infancy at the time of the survey but laying great emphasis on social education, especially in the last two years of schooling, that is, for 14–16 year old pupils. There were five main components to this programme – personal self-reliance, functional mobility in the community (e.g., shopping, using buses, etc.), classroom/practical knowledge (e.g., social security and benefits, use of money, using the telephone, etc.), citizenship 'training' (e.g., discussions on topical issues) and the use of leisure. Each term teachers rated pupils in these areas so that shortcomings could be identified and gaps in the programme could be overcome. This school was also doing some questionnaire research in the school with the view to improving the programme.

*Information on handicap.* A central problem faced by physically handicapped teenagers, which has been discussed already in earlier chapters, is how to achieve the normal adolescent desire to become independent of their parents and form relationships with other adults, peers and members of the opposite sex. Achievement of personal identity and of satisfactory relationships will be hindered by the severity of handicap itself, but could be further hindered if the young person and his family do not have a clear idea about the extent of independence it is possible for him to achieve. A sound knowledge of the nature and extent of his ability, the modern aids and equipment, and the special services (for example health and social services) and benefits that are available to disabled adults are needed to prepare each school leaver for the problems of adult independence. The first thing that is needed, however, is a good knowledge about his own condition so that the young person can have a better understanding of his needs, limitations and potential and thus acquire a greater feeling of autonomy over his own future.

According to Philp (1978) there is little documentation about how much handicapped children know about their condition, but what there is suggests that knowledge about the nature of handicap or treatment given is poor. Scott, Roberts and Tew (1975) in a small study of twenty adolescents with spina bifida looked at knowledge about the need for penile and urinary appliances. They found that very few knew much about the nature of their handicap or the reasons for surgery and that only two adolescents 'felt that they had a good understanding of their condition'. This is also a clear finding in Dorner's study (1976) where only four of the forty-six adolescents interviewed had a good understanding of the nature of spina bifida, eight an adequate understanding, while twenty-four had only a limited understanding, and the other ten were unable to give any description of the condition. Studies of children handicapped in other ways (e.g., Feinberg *et al.*, 1974; Burton, 1975), show that this lack of information on the part of young people about their handicaps is the rule rather than the exception.

Questions to teenagers in our own study (see chapter 2, pp. 41–7) showed that only about one-third had a good or even fair knowledge of the nature of their disabilities. It is significant that the majority of teenagers said that they would like to know more about their handicaps. Some of the other studies mentioned (e.g., Scott *et al.*, 1975; Dorner, 1976) also make it clear that teenagers wanted to know more.

This unfulfilled desire to be informed about one's condition is often seen as resulting from 'ignorance among parents'. It seems to be assumed that parents should and will inform children about their handicap and the reason for any medical intervention, but Philp's review of the relevant research concludes that the information received by the parents of handicapped children is itself quite inadequate. He quotes numerous studies of parents of children with spina bifida, cerebral palsy, diabetes and cystic fibrosis which show that they have had insufficient explanation of their child's condition. Pless and Pinkerton (1975) show that this lack of understanding and information is true for parents with children handicapped in many different ways. If parents themselves are poorly informed they obviously cannot inform their own children adequately. However, the majority of teenagers in this study said that it was from their parents that they had derived most of their information, although some also mentioned medical staff, especially the hospital consultant. Very few mentioned the school as a source of information.

Surprisingly few, only six of the special schools, did attempt to ensure that their pupils left school well-informed about the nature of their own handicaps. Three schools said that this was done on an informal basis, usually by the form teacher, and in only three schools (all residential) was a *systematic* attempt made by school staff to inform pupils about their condition. All the special schools felt that it was important that their pupils should have acquired a good understanding of their own handicaps by the time they left school, but varied greatly in who they thought should be responsible for this. It is interesting that only two of the special schools saw the parents as being responsible. Most thought of it as something requiring special knowledge and coming most appro-priately from a doctor, nurse or other trained expert, although few ensured that these specialists were available and actually did undertake this responsibility.

It was of course much more difficult for ordinary schools to arrange that their handicapped pupils be given knowledge about their conditions. Anderson (1975), Halliwell and Spain (1977) and Cope and Anderson (1977) all report that there is a dearth of information about handicap available to teachers who are expected to integrate a handicapped child into a normal classroom. Apparently the major source of information to ordinary school teachers is the parent, and direct contact with medical personnel is rare since school doctors do not appear to see it as part of their role to inform the teacher about the medical problems of their pupils. With information coming largely from the parents, who are themselves not well informed, little accurate knowledge can be expected of teachers in ordinary schools, and it was hardly surprising to find that only one of the ordinary schools made any attempt to inform handicapped pupils about the nature of their handicap, although all of the schools, except two, felt that it was important that handicapped pupils should have acquired a good understanding of their own handicaps by the time they leave school. However, they did not feel that this was the school's responsibility. Ten said it was the job of the pupils' parents, two schools thought it should be a social worker, and only two mentioned the school doctor. Eleven said that they didn't know who should be responsible for this.

*Services and benefits.* The Scottish Report suggests that the school should allow time in the curriculum to make sure that each pupil leaves school with a sound knowledge of the aids and equipment which are available to him as an adult and also exactly how to obtain these. This means the teenager will need to be given information about organizations such as the Disabled Living Foundation, the Disablement Income Group and others (see Appendix B). Teenagers also need to be taught at school about services available under the Chronically Sick and Disabled Persons Act, about the Attendance Allowance and Mobility Allowance and about how to claim for benefits themselves. The Warnock Report repeated the importance of covering these topics within the school curriculum.

Anderson and Spain (1977) have suggested that the close co-operation of a social worker might be needed as teachers may not know in detail exactly what is available to disabled adults. They also point out that the reasons for teaching teenagers about benefits and facilities should be explained to parents so that they too can take part in encouraging the young people to assume as much responsibility as possible for themselves in claiming and using them.

It might be thought that most special schools' curricula would nowadays cover the many services and benefits available to disabled people.

However, in chapter 2 when we looked at the teenagers' knowledge of benefits and how to obtain information about them we concluded that the majority of teenagers were very badly informed indeed. We commented that the findings suggest that there is still great scope for more to be done about these matters in the social education programmes in school. Our findings from our examination of the schools themselves confirm this conclusion. Most of the schools agreed that it was important that handicapped pupils know about the services and benefits available to them, although one special school felt that there was not enough time to cover this as part of the curriculum. However, in only nine of the twenty-six special schools was a systematic attempt made to teach older pupils about what is available, or how to contact local authority services on their own behalf. The nearest the ordinary schools came to this was as part of general civic studies programme designed for all students and not for handicapped pupils in particular, though only seven of the thirty-four ordinary schools said that they provided general civic studies lessons.

Again, the ordinary schools generally thought that providing handicapped pupils with this kind of information was not their domain, and tended to name parents, social workers or other experts from outside the school. The special schools also named these people but they did see members of the school staff, including house parents or occupational therapists, as being appropriate sources of information in this respect, despite the fact that so few actually taught this.

*Mobility and driving.* Adequate transport to work and to social facilities is absolutely vital for adults with limited mobility. The mobility allowance is a step in the direction of providing this even if the level is not yet a realistic alternative to the provision of a special vehicle. The Warnock Committee has recommended that 'further consideration should be given urgently to the needs of young people with disabilities for help with mobility, particularly those aged sixteen to seventeen and those who need special help to travel to and from work'.

Getting about is much easier for the handicapped teenager if he or she can drive. Schools should therefore offer constructive help in this respect, such as helping pupils to decide if driving would be feasible for them and organizing driving lessons for pupils who should be able to drive. This is particularly important in special schools where the pupils are more severely handicapped, but it can be advantageous for many in ordinary schools as well.

Only six of the special schools had any organized schemes for teaching pupils to drive. For example, one school had a link with the local driving school to teach any suitable pupils. Another school (also residential) had arranged for someone from the Ministry of Transport to come in to inform pupils about transport and cars and to arrange for driving lessons. The situation in ordinary schools was similar – only three schools had a scheme for learning to drive (for all pupils not just for the handicapped). No survey pupils at all were learning to drive through their schools.

Those who will never drive, and those who might do so at some future date but have no immediate prospect of a car, need the opportunity to find out about alternative forms of transport, such as the possibilities of travelling by train, to discover whether they can use taxis or minicabs unassisted, and to find out the best way of getting themselves and their wheelchairs in and out of cars. Sometimes very simple aids which can be home-made (such as a sliding board to help transfer from a wheelchair to a car seat) can make all the difference in terms of making use of non-family transport.

Teenagers should also appreciate the fact that the mobility allowance is given specifically to help them with transport, and discussions begun with the parents to see what portion of the allowance is needed to help run the family car and how much could be given to the teenager so that he himself could be responsible for paying for mini-cabs, etc. Volunteer transport should also be discussed – whether there are any organizations in the teenagers' local area, such as the Red Cross or a Rotary Club, which might be able to offer transport provided that petrol costs were covered. It is most important that before he leaves school the teenager knows that there are some other sources of transport available to him, so that he doesn't feel he has to rely solely on his family, and that he has some practice in telephoning and arranging for transport by himself, so that he feels competent to care for himself in this respect. As far as we could ascertain no consideration was given by any of the special schools to raising this important issue with their pupils.

*Leisure.* Another problem that has to be overcome by handicapped adolescents is that of social isolation. In chapter 3 we examined the peer relationships and leisure-time interests of the teenagers in our study and concluded that one-third of those who attended ordinary schools and two-thirds of those who attended special schools were completely isolated once outside school, and many had few leisure-time interests.

Several factors play a part in the social isolation of these teenagers. On the physical side access to buildings and transport are important but there are also social and emotional factors. Placement in special schools can lead to feelings of strangeness and anxiety in social relationships with non-handicapped peers and it also makes it less likely that a handicapped teenager will have close neighbourhood friends, or meet non-handicapped peers. Also the handicapped person may feel anxious or shameful about being handicapped which may itself interfere with the forming of friendship. Kathleen Evans (1974) found that the spina bifida adults she interviewed had many such anxieties. Both ordinary and special schools could do much to ameliorate these problems which play a contributory role in the teenager's social isolation at school and in the post-school years.

Special schools especially could organize their pupils, with help from non-handicapped peers, to carry out surveys of local facilities from the point of view of access and then use this to put pressure on local authorities for modification. This would encourage pupils to become accustomed to speaking out for themselves, as well as introducing them to local recreational facilities. As far as transport is concerned, as already suggested there should be someone in each school responsible for discussing with handicapped pupils and their family the problem of mobility at home and in the neighbourhood, with the aim of ensuring that each pupil knows how to get about his own locality and to visit friends.

In many recent reports (e.g., Scottish Education Department Report, 1975) it has been recommended that contact between children in ordinary and special schools should increase. School staff could do more to help pupils in this way by encouraging them to attend youth clubs in their area. As far as leisure pursuits are concerned more attention could be paid to the sort of leisure activities that any child is likely to enjoy and continue in adult life: music, gardening, reading, collecting, photography, theatre and film going, and sport (either actively involved or as a spectator) being some examples. These will not only encourage the constructive use of leisure, but equip handicapped pupils with skills similar to the non-handicapped and make social contact on an equal basis easier to achieve.

Since the fostering of social development and the constructive use of leisure are important both as ways of avoiding boredom and making friendships, we were particularly interested in the ways the schools we visited attempted this. Most of the special schools said that they would like to see more mixing with non-handicapped peers. This supports the findings of the PHAB study (1978) mentioned earlier which concluded that teachers in special schools recognized the need for social education programmes to enable their pupils to have greater links with ordinary teenagers in order to broaden their experience. Seventeen of the twenty-six special schools named some way in which they were attempting such contacts, but most of these were very minimal (though important) such as having mixed Scout or Guide troops or holding a PHAB club or other 'mixed' youth club on the school premises. Some also had volunteer helpers from local secondary schools who visited the school for one or two afternoons a week, often as part of a community service option in their timetables.

Only three of the schools mentioned linked courses with ordinary schools although this is the most obvious way in which the schools could encourage contact. In one school this included junior pupils who went swimming with the local school, in another pupils from the special school joined remedial groups from a nearby comprehensive for games lessons, while some of the able-bodied boys attended the special school for the CSE cookery course. One of the residential special schools had developed this exchange more fully so that junior pupils were spending one morning each fortnight in the local ordinary school, while on the alternate week the children from the ordinary school came to the special school for one morning to do joint project work. Also some of the senior pupils at this school attended the ordinary school for typing lessons.

It is not only special school pupils who suffer social isolation however since, as we showed in chapter 3, even handicapped pupils in ordinary schools may lead very lonely lives outside school. None of the ordinary schools was doing anything specifically to help handicapped pupils take advantage of clubs or other organizations for young people in their area. One school, however, did think that these pupils would be catered for in their active social activities scheme for all pupils. This school was arranged in 'communities' like vertical house-groups, and time was allocated on the curriculum for a social education programme which was described as 'getting to know themselves, their family, the school and the resources in the town'.

*Sex education.* During adolescence physically handicapped teenagers will experience the same physiological and emotional changes as all teenagers. The achievement of personal identity and satisfactory relationships in the adult world and with the opposite sex poses problems to which there are no simple answers. Particularly where their sexual development is concerned, handicapped adolescents will face doubts about their attractiveness, about the technical problems involved in achieving a sexual relationship, or about the possible hereditary nature of their disability.

Handicapped teenagers, even if they know about normal sexual development, often know very little about their own particular situation. Very little research into the knowledge and attitudes to sex of physically handicapped teenagers has been carried out in this country. In Sweden, however, Bergstrom-Walan (1978) reported a survey carried out with seventy-five adolescents in special schools. Among these teenagers there was a marked demand for more sex education especially about the ethics, values and norms of sexual relationships, as well as technical information and aids including, in particular, information about contraceptives. Anderson and Spain (1977) point out that 'the restricted social contacts of handicapped teenagers mean that they have less chance to "pick up" such information than do many of their non-handicapped peers'.

For the non-handicapped, while in the past it was assumed that parents would inform their children about the facts of life, it is now usual for sex education to be taught in school. However, the Warnock Committee found that sex education and counselling for the handicapped

Table 10.1 *Subjects on which the teenagers felt they needed more information*

| | Don't want any more information | | How babies are conceived | | How babies are born | | How children grow and develop | | Practical problems of family life | | Total |
| | N | (%) | N | (%) | N | (%) | N | (%) | N | (%) | N |
|---|---|---|---|---|---|---|---|---|---|---|---|
| *Girls* | | | | | | | | | | | |
| Controls | 8 | (44.4) | 4 | (22.2) | 2 | (11.1) | 8 | (44.4) | 9 | (50) | 18 |
| Handicapped | 9 | (18) | 28 | (56) | 28 | (56) | 36 | (72) | 41 | (82) | 50 |
| *Boys* | | | | | | | | | | | |
| Controls | 6 | (38) | 2 | (13) | 2 | (13) | 6 | (38) | 8 | (50) | 16 |
| Handicapped | 21 | (38) | 14 | (25) | 16 | (29) | 21 | (38) | 22 | (33) | 56 |

tended in general to be handled very badly in schools. This is particularly unfortunate for handicapped adolescents since their opportunities for learning about such matters through self-education are limited compared to their able-bodied peers.

The problem of sexual relationships and adolescence will also be confounded by the attitude of society, which tends not to recognize that handicapped young people undergo normal biological and psychological changes and have normal sexual needs. Until recently, the discussion of the sexual needs of handicapped adults and young people was very neglected. The situation is slowly changing, and recent developments include a survey carried out by the National Fund for Research into Crippling Diseases of the sexual problems of the disabled (Stewart, 1975), and the establishment of SPOD (the Committee on Sexual Problems of the Disabled) which provides information, advice and counselling services to individuals, schools and groups. This means that information about sexual development and opportunities for counselling on sexual and related problems can be provided for the handicapped in both ordinary and special schools.

We asked the teenagers if they had been taught about the facts of life in school and if they found this helpful. Nearly 60 per cent of the handicapped pupils in ordinary schools had been taught in general about how babies were conceived and born and had found this helpful. However, between 20–25 per cent claimed that they had not even been given this basic information. Similar results were found in relation to a question about whether they had been taught at school how babies are conceived, although here an even smaller proportion felt satisfied with the information given.

Most of the teenagers in this study, both handicapped and controls but especially the handicapped girls, wanted more information about sex and child development (see Table 10.1). Overall only about 60 per cent of teenagers and an even higher proportion of handicapped girls wanted more information about these subjects.

Let us now compare the teenagers' reports of what they were taught at school and which subjects they felt they need more information about, with the schools' perception of what they cover and their attitudes about this subject in relation to the physically handicapped adolescents.

It appeared that most of the ordinary schools we visited covered sex education; twenty-two of the thirty-four ordinary schools provided sex education to all pupils, six for some pupils only, and only three had no sex education at all. All included contraception in their courses. However, sex education was not so commonplace in the special schools: only thirteen schools (a half of those visited) taught sex education to all pupils and in another seven schools this was provided for some pupils only, while five schools did not cover this at all. Only eight schools taught contraception. The way the schools provided sex education varied considerably. Twenty-two of the ordinary schools and ten of the special schools said that their sex education courses also included the emotional and personal aspects of sexual relationships. In three of the special schools, sex education was covered in biology classes, and in two others as part of social studies, which sometimes also included BBC programmes. Four other schools ran courses that included sex education; one covered personal hygiene and was called 'Good Grooming', another 'Human Relationships' in which family planning representatives gave talks; one school's human biology course covered the subject, while another had a human biology class for 12–14 year olds and then specific counselling for 14–15 year olds from a marriage guidance counsellor. In other schools sex education was not part of a formal course but was left to individual teachers to cover in their preferred manner; while three schools said that the subject was covered on an individual basis.

The ordinary schools also varied in how they taught this subject. Six schools covered it in biology classes, five as part of social studies, seven in biology lessons coupled with some other part of the curriculum (social studies, health education or housecraft). Six schools incorporated sex education within courses which were basically on health education, with various titles – 'Learning to Live', 'Social and Moral Education', 'Health Education'. In one a specialist marriage guidance counsellor talked to small groups and ran discussion groups, while in another group discussions were run by a biology teacher. One school covered sex and more general health education in specific tutorial groups as part of the pastoral care system.

In none of the ordinary schools were any special arrangements made for handicapped pupils to talk over private anxieties about their own sexual functioning or sexual relationships. Only four schools thought that there was a need for this and three of these felt that a doctor or consultant was the best person to do this, while two felt that it should be the school counsellor.

None of the special schools raised with the pupils the specific problems which certain physically handicapped people may have, for example the problems of lack of sensation, incontinence, or difficulty in controlling movement. Most felt that a sex education programme should not cover such problems on a group basis but only on an individual counselling basis, although in fact only four schools said that such problems were ever discussed informally or on an individual basis. However, in one school a SPOD representative had held a discussion with pupils on this subject, while Wendy Greengross's book (1976) was recommended to pupils as informative reading. Most of the special schools did not know what the pupils or their parents felt about the sex education programmes, although nine thought the pupils were satisfied and only one that there was some dissatisfaction. Two of the schools had held parents' meetings, one on adolescence and the other two on sex education (one involving a SPOD representative), both of which were very well attended. Another school broached this subject at a parents' meeting but were told that the parents were pleased with the way the school was covering the subject.

Nine of the schools suggested ways in which their sex education programmes could be improved, including such things as starting at a younger age, making sure that boys are as well informed as girls and more expansion on potential problems that handicapped people might have, including genetic advice. Some schools said that they'd like their own staff to be better informed about sex and the handicapped so that they could advise parents and help them to be more aware of the problems that might concern their child. Others thought they should invite more 'experts' into the school from bodies like the Family Planning Association (FPA), Marriage Guidance Council and SPOD.

Of the five special schools which did not teach sex education, only one felt that this should not be covered in school at all. Most thought it should be discussed on an individual basis because of the difficulty of introducing the subject to pupils of widely differing levels, and felt that group discussion could cause embarrassment and confusion in children who did not understand. However, they had no clear suggestions about how to do this and, as one said, 'No one really has the courage to do this, especially with the boys'. If staff are themselves embarrassed and diffident about approaching this subject, then they are unlikely to be able to allay the fears and anxieties of their pupils.

*Sexual and genetic counselling.*   Anderson and Spain (1976) say that sex education for those with spina bifida 'must encompass not simply the facts of sexual development as related to a particular individual's condition but also the opportunity to discuss the implications of these facts for relationships with the opposite sex and also for marriage and procreation'. Dorner (1976) has also pointed out that the spina bifida teenage boys in his study were very concerned about their potency, and the girls with the question of marriage and whether they could have children. Our own research suggests that many cerebral-palsied teenagers were also worried quite needlessly about genetic risks if they had children while many worried about how their handicap might affect a sexual relationship (see chapter 4).

The Warnock Report has called for more research to be carried out into how sexual counselling can best be provided for young people with special needs, including the training of counsellors and other staff. They suggest courses of training for all professionals working with disabled adolescents so that as many people as possible will be equipped to give support in this area. They also suggest that in this, as in other areas of counselling, handicapped people can often best be helped by others who are also handicapped.

Who the best person is to provide counselling on sexual matters will depend partly upon how services are organized in a particular area and on the confiding relationships a teenager may already have established. There are now a number of psychiatrists with expertise in counselling non-handicapped people on sexual matters and it may be possible to contact them or SPOD.

Genetic counselling also needs to be readily available to handicapped people and their families. This requires expert knowledge of the risks of transmitting different disabilities. Philp (1978) has concluded that there is room for the extension of genetic counselling facilities and for more information to be provided about whom teenagers and parents should contact if they require such advice. We found that in only nine of the twenty-six special schools had arrangements been made for pupils to talk over privately any worries about sexual matters. In five of these schools, survey pupils had in fact made use of this opportunity in the past year. Of the schools which did not provide for individual discussion of worries about sexual matters, nine thought that there was no need, but six felt this should be provided, usually suggesting that the school doctor, the GP, or hospital doctor would be the most appropriate person. Only one of the special schools systematically provided genetic counselling for older handicapped pupils who might require this, for example those with spina bifida. Eight other special schools said that this was done only if the pupil sought advice, and two other schools could not say if genetic counselling was covered or not; one of these was the school where the marriage guidance counsellor handled the sex education, as described earlier in this chapter, while the other said this subject would be dealt with, if at all, by the school doctor.

*Preparation for parenthood.*    Apart from basic sex education, twenty-one of the ordinary schools (nearly 70 per cent) but only ten of the special schools (40 per cent) provided 'preparation for parenthood' lessons. However, these lessons were attended by all pupils in only nine of the ordinary schools and three of the special schools. In the other schools only about half the pupils were involved. Only five of the survey pupils in special schools and nine of those in ordinary schools had actually attended these lessons, and the vast majority therefore had had no instruction on this subject.

The content of this part of the curriculum varied – eighteen of the ordinary schools and eight of the special schools included the care of babies, and about the same number covered child development and the practical problems of family life. In many of the ordinary schools these subjects were covered as part of the CSE course in child development, or in tutorials and social studies programmes. Two schools also taught general household tasks and personal hygiene (including cooking, laundry, first aid, budgeting, diet and skin care) in their social education lessons, and one residential school was experimenting with pupils helping to cook their own lunch, and introducing books about living in a family setting.

*Personal relationships.* Apart from individual counselling or preparation for parenthood lessons, some schools ran discussion groups in which teenagers had the chance to discuss their personal relationships with peers, parents or others. Eleven of the special schools and nine of the ordinary schools reported that they did this, although the organization, structure and depth of discussion varied greatly. Four of the special and four of the ordinary schools said that they had such discussions at least once a week, while the rest held them less than weekly, and two special schools reported that only *ad hoc* discussions were held. In both ordinary and special schools these discussions were usually chaired by a member of staff, though outsiders were sometimes used. Six of the thirty-seven handicapped pupils in ordinary schools had taken part in these discussion groups over the past year, whereas only four of the eighty-two pupils in special schools had participated in such a discussion group.

The four special schools which held discussions about personal relationships regularly (at least weekly) provided this as part of their general social education or school leavers' programme. In one school, as already described, weekly discussions were held by a marriage guidance counsellor from outside the school which covered the facts of life and sexual relationships, as well as general counselling. Another encompassed this as part of the overall social studies programme taught by the form tutors throughout the school, covering topics in varying depth according to age. The third school called one section of its leavers' programme 'The Home' where such topics as living at home and leaving home introduced discussions about relationships with parents, family and friends. In the fourth – a residential school – the general studies curriculum covered personal relationships in great depth.

In contrast, the four ordinary schools which held regular discussions on this topic did not include them within a wider framework of a social education programme for leavers. Three of the schools said that such discussions arose during the periods that were set aside for pastoral activities of tutors but that these were not structured components of the curriculum. The other school had recently started a 'Pastoral Relations' course, run by the head of the upper school, which she described as having the objective of instilling self-analysis and decision making. Only two of the special schools ever held discussion groups of this kind jointly with non-handicapped pupils from neighbouring schools. In one school, which was on the same campus as an ordinary comprehensive, some pupils attended the comprehensive for a course in moral/social studies and so would be involved in discussions in these classes. In the other school three girls attended the local girls' comprehensive to attend the child care course for one day per week and the arrangement was reciprocated by four pupils from the comprehensive joining in the leavers' programme in the special school.

## Section B. Suggestions for improvements

### Schools' suggestions

Some of the special schools were aware of their deficiencies in the field of social education and made some suggestions. These included paying more attention to helping the teenagers develop constructive uses for their leisure time, and by providing more opportunities for teenagers to mix with their able-bodied peers to develop confidences in interaction with the able-bodied. Another suggestion was that schools should aim to make teenagers as independent and socially responsible as possible in matters like coping with money and health problems, and generally to foster a mature self-reliant outlook, and not 'protect' pupils from the outside world. This, they felt, would help in easing adjustment to adult life and avoid the acute shock often experienced by handicapped pupils when leaving school and being forced to face the community and world of work. Other suggestions focused on giving teenagers more vocational training or work experience so that they could leave school with a more realistic opinion of their own capabilities and what would be expected from them at work.

### Parents' and teenagers' suggestions for improvements

In the Phase II interviews, we asked the handicapped teenagers and their parents for their views on ways in which young physically handicapped people could be better helped before and after leaving school. In particular we asked if there was anything they thought their school could have done which would have made it easier for the teenager to cope with life after school.

This question provided a wide range of suggestions. The teenagers mainly spoke about educational matters – being allowed or encouraged to take exams, getting more advice about leaving school, or having more basic maths and English teaching to improve their ability generally. Others specifically mentioned careers guidance and preparation for an independent life-style. For example, one teenager said, 'They could have given you some work to do at school, taught you what it was like to be at work so that you knew what to expect when you left'. One boy in an ordinary school felt he could have gained more confidence if the teachers had supported him and stopped other boys teasing him. It is interesting that three of the teenagers in special schools said that they would have preferred more freedom and challenge in school. One girl said, 'When I was at . . . school I felt closed in, I didn't do much there, it was too protected'.

The parents' comments also consisted mainly of criticisms of the academic curriculum or various aspects of social education. A number of the parents thought that their son or daughter had wasted much of their time at school; some felt that the school lacked discipline in following an academic programme with distinct goals in mind, or felt that more individual attention would have helped their child to achieve his potential. Others felt that the teaching did not concentrate enough on the basic skills of writing and arithmetic, or handling money. One parent felt that her severely handicapped daughter had suffered academically by being in a special school because classes were constantly disrupted by toileting assistance and physiotherapy visits.

The parents, like the teenagers, also felt that not enough time, if any, had been spent on social education. Typical comments were: 'They are all so sheltered there', 'they should have spent more time on outside activities like clubs and discos', 'she was not encouraged to be independent', and 'it was sadly lacking instruction in things like filling up forms and claiming social security.' Some parents mentioned that their child had not mixed with able-bodied teenagers at all and felt that more joint activities could have been held with ordinary schools.

In addition to asking generally about suggestions for school curriculum improvements, we asked the teenagers to rate some ideas provided by us about ways in which schools could help, including some concerning social education. When we asked if schools should spend more time on activities which they could do in their leisure time nearly two-thirds of the special school pupils thought that this was a very good or a fairly good idea, compared with about 40 per cent of those in ordinary schools. On counselling facilities, we asked whether they would have liked someone on the staff or someone from outside with whom to talk over their problems. Nearly 70 per cent of those in special schools thought this a good or fairly good idea, compared with over 40 per cent of those in ordinary schools, indicating that students in both types of school wanted more help, but especially those in special schools.

The teenagers generally were not so enthusiastic about the idea of discussion groups to talk about their problems, just under half of those in special schools and about 40 per cent in ordinary schools believing this to be useful – but quite a sufficient number to suggest such arrangements would be welcomed (on a voluntary basis) by many. However nearly two-thirds of those in special schools and 60 per cent in ordinary schools liked the idea of some *disabled* adults coming to school to talk about their experiences and how they'd got on in life. It is particularly interesting that such a high proportion of students in ordinary schools would have liked this.

### Summary and recommendations

Possibly the most stressful and problematic time of personal development is in adolescence, and the transition to adult life is even more difficult for handicapped teenagers than for their more fortunate contemporaries. The Warnock Report has singled out this age group as having particularly inadequate services and support, and has made several valuable comments and recommendations on how to rectify this. A school's responsibility towards its pupils are not only in academic instruction but in developing social skills and helping in the transition to adult life. The OECD Survey (Rowan, 1980) shows that social education is much more developed in ESN schools than in schools for the physically handicapped. The Warnock Report specifically recommended that pupils with special needs, whether in ordinary or special schools, should be given more help in acquiring basic independence skills and in developing social competence and vocational interests. It also stressed the importance of training teachers to be aware of special needs, and to be equipped to cope with them.

When considering the services offered by the ordinary schools, we noted that there was a distinct lack of supportive help available for handicapped pupils. While it is true to say that some teenagers did not need special help, whether medical or social, some certainly did. *None* of the schools had designated a member of staff to have special responsibility for its handicapped pupils to monitor any problems, nor did they provide individualized teaching arrangements. This is an important omission, given the Warnock Report's emphasis on supporting teenagers with special needs in this way.

Given that fears and anxieties are very common amongst handicapped adolescents then special counselling is a service required by many of these individuals. The young people need help to develop their self-confidence and to take active steps to overcome their feelings of being different. We would also endorse the Warnock Report's suggestion (para. 10.95) that handicapped adults could be used in counselling programmes, and our findings suggest that the majority of young people in both ordinary and special schools would welcome this. A counsellor who understands the handicapped teenager's situation can help him come to terms with his position, whether within a special or an ordinary school. The Spastics Society's Working Party has recognized this and called for personal counselling services to be readily available to handicapped adolescents in all types of schools as a priority.

We found that provision for counselling of the handicapped in ordinary and special schools was not common. Only seven of the twenty-six special schools said that members of staff or visiting professionals provided time for the individual counselling of pupils. In only one special school was there a formal arrangement with a visiting counsellor for the sole intention of in-depth counselling of pupils. As the head reported that this arrangement was a great success and had shown positive results in terms of reducing tensions, we would wish to see this extended *at least* to all special schools and to be available to ordinary schools pupils if required.

It would also be beneficial if social services were more involved with these teenagers and their families. Only five of the special schools had a full-time social worker and six a part-time social worker attached to the school. Warnock (para. 10.96) has suggested that health and social services personnel as well as voluntary groups could all be appropriate sources for counselling.

One way in which schools could help their pupils very easily is in ensuring that they are fully informed about their condition and aware of its implications. We found a high level of ignorance among the teenagers in this matter, and the majority said that they would like to know more about their handicaps. However, only three special schools in our study made a systematic attempt to inform pupils about their condition, and although in some others the form teachers were said to cover this on an informal basis, six schools said that they made no attempt to teach this whatsoever. It is essential that a teenager should have this knowledge and that the schools should ensure that this is so, even if they only act as a referring agency to medical staff with specialized knowledge.

We have also indicated that handicapped teenagers are often not aware of the aids and allowances that are available to them to facilitate personal independence in transport or self-care. Schools are certainly in a position to take the responsibility upon themselves or to call in the advice of professional social workers to enable maximum independence for the teenager in adult life. These topics can be easily covered, especially in special schools, in a civic studies course, but few of the schools in our study covered this systematically. Service needs in this respect have recently been reassessed by the Warnock Committee and we reiterate its recommendation that there is still great scope for more to be done about these matters in the social education programmes in schools. Social workers could be much more closely involved with the social education of handicapped teenagers while they are at school, and schools could do more in using the resources of the social services department for organizing social education programmes.

Mobility is also an important component of physical independence in adult life, especially transport to and from work. If possible, disabled teenagers should be taught to drive before they leave school and the school could make the arrangements necessary or provide their pupils with the information regarding this. Only two of the schools we visited had organized driving lesson schemes and we were asked by many parents or teenagers where and how they could learn to drive, especially by those who took part in the follow-up study. In addition handicapped young people need to know how to order mini-cabs or taxis, how best to get in and out of them with minimal assistance, and what volunteer transport might be available in their area. None of the special schools appeared to give instruction on these topics.

Although most of the schools claimed to teach the basic facts of life, this was certainly far from adequately covered in the majority of cases, and none systematically provided discussion of the special problems which certain physically handicapped people may have. This was an area in which the schools themselves expressed a desire for someone with expertise, whether from inside or outside the school, to handle this topic. Also, within the schools we visited there was a dearth of genetic advice, whether given on a group or individual basis. Very few schools provided 'preparation for parenthood' lessons in addition to basic sex education. A few schools ran discussion groups in which teenagers had the chance to discuss personal relationships. In general, however, this whole area of sex education, preparation for parenthood, and genetic counselling were not covered well in the majority of schools, with the result that many young people were needlessly preoccupied with fears which simple instruction could have allayed.

One important finding is the high incidence of social isolation among the teenagers in this study, indicating that another major area in which schools could do more to prepare teenagers for life after school is in the use of leisure. Unemployment is likely to increase in the 1980s, especially for the more severely handicapped persons whose employment prospects are always poor. The OECD Report has shown that alternatives to work and constructive use of leisure time should be a priority for handicapped school leavers. Much more needs to be done by schools to encourage outside school activities as well as developing pursuits and interests within school that can be continued by individuals later, for example, musical activities, various kinds of sports, reading and craftwork. Pupils should be encouraged to find out about these and other activities in their local area and given support in following up their enquiries.

We have also shown that a child's parents are an important influence on physical and emotional independence (see chapters 2 and 3). For this reason any effort on the school's behalf to foster an independent life for the teenager will be hampered if parents are not made aware of the school's efforts and kept in close contact with the school's work. It is essential, therefore, to involve parents at an early stage and help them to face their own problems and to understand more about their child's development and adjustment to adult life.

Perhaps the most important omission our survey showed is the lack of follow up and supportive services available to school leavers. This is often a period of great uncertainty for all school leavers, but especially for the handicapped. There may be no immediate job, college placement or placement of any description, and even those lucky enough to have employment may experience great difficulty in adapting to working life, especially if they have spent most of their life in the sheltered and supportive environment of a special school. They may easily become isolated at home with no friends in the neighbourhood with whom they can share anxieties. A major problem when handicapped young people leave school is that it is often impossible to identify exactly who has responsibility for them after leaving school as it may be the LEA, social services department, employment services agency or a voluntary agency. The advantage of having a member of the school staff responsible for the follow up of leavers is that there would be a continuing link for the teenager and family, and this would be someone whom they could approach if difficulties arose and if no one else seemed to help. This would also result in valuable feedback for the school about what happened to each leaver and could be instrumental in curriculum design for the future.

# 11

## *Satisfaction with vocational and other services for school leavers*

### Introduction

In the previous chapter we examined how far the teenager was prepared for adult life after school. Now we examine what is done to maximize his chances of finding a satisfactory placement – whether in employment, further education or some alternative to work – when he leaves school.

There is a distinction to be made here between adequate provision for leavers in terms of the actual placements available and adequate provision of careers education, guidance and support from the services. It is very difficult to assess the current provision for disabled or even able-bodied school leavers as this can change quite rapidly according to the general economic situation in the country, and in periods of recession everyone is vulnerable, but the disabled even more so. The current provision for disabled leavers was briefly covered in chapter 7. Our findings, and those of the other studies quoted (Scottish Education Department Survey, 1975; Tuckey *et al.*, 1973; Spastics Society, 1975; Training Services Agency, 1975) show that in practice the facilities for vocational training as well as opportunities and alternatives to work are extremely inadequate.

Given that there is generally inadequate provision of satisfactory placements for school leavers, it is even more disturbing that good guidance and advice about these somewhat limited possibilities are often not available. In Warnock's words 'our strong impression is that existing arrangements for the provision of careers guidance for young people with special needs generally falls far short of what is required' (para. 10.11). They conclude from their own evidence that 'fixed ideas are usually entertained about occupations suitable or unsuitable for young people with particular disabilities' and that 'specialist advice on the problems associated with different disabilities or disorders is often not available'. The Report makes two important recommendations for the improvement of careers education and advice. It emphasizes that careers guidance of a high standard needs to be available for pupils with special educational needs both in ordinary and special schools and makes a specific recommendation about teachers with responsibility for careers and specialist careers officers.

For the handicapped school leaver a continuing link with counselling services is crucial, and it is in recognition of this that Warnock recommended that a 'named person' should be appointed providing a single point of contact for those with special needs during the transition to adult life. Often there is an administrative gap through which the school leaver falls, since those who have responsibilities for school-age children – whether teachers, paediatricians, social workers or careers officers – see their role as finished once the teenager leaves school. Even if they are handed over to other people, without a strong school link the advice and support they receive will at best be disjointed, if not completely conflicting or non-existent.

Obtaining a satisfactory placement depends very much on what is done *before* the teenager leaves school. The key people in shaping a teenager's decision will be his parents, teachers and careers officer. Many ordinary schools now offer specific careers education programmes, and some actual work experience. We shall examine exactly what was provided in the schools we visited shortly. While innovations are being made in this area there is still a long way to go. For example, in a DES survey (1974) of ordinary schools for pupils aged fourteen and over, less than half the schools provided careers education for all pupils, and 28 per cent did not provide it at all.

Other studies (ASBAH, 1975; Anderson and Spain, 1977; Rodgers, 1979) have recommended that it is essential that preparations for school leaving should begin as soon as possible, preferably at the beginning of the third year of secondary school life, as it will take the careers officer time to get to know each pupil, to assess his strengths and weaknesses and to gain his confidence. It is rather disturbing that a recent enquiry by Queen Elizabeth's Foundation for the Disabled suggested that many problems arise with their trainees because of inadequate (or non-existent) assessment of their potential. For many pupils the decisions made about placement need to be very flexible to allow for further assessment and change.

Surveys of handicapped school leavers suggest that the time immediately after leaving school constitutes a period of great uncertainty, although this is becoming increasingly true for non-handicapped young people experiencing great difficulty in finding employment. For the handicapped leaver this situation will probably be harder to cope with as he is also unlikely to have friends he sees regularly with whom he can share his experiences. It is therefore important that adequate support is provided for handicapped teenagers after they have left school. It has previously been suggested (Anderson and Spain, 1977) that follow-up services should cover three main areas: (i) helping with the practicalities of finding and settling into a suitable placement whatever this might be; (ii) continuing help for welfare needs such as accommodation and transport, and also counselling for emotional needs; and (iii) continuing medical supervision.

At present, it is often impossible to identify who exactly has responsibility for a particular pupil after leaving school as this may be the local education authority, social services department, the employment services agency, or some voluntary agency, depending upon the placement. There are now specialist careers officers with responsibility for the handicapped in most districts, who have been trained in giving vocational guidance for the handicapped and should also know what is available in further education and employment. The careers officer can act as a consultant to careers teachers or the school staff who are in everyday contact with a handicapped pupil, whether in a special or ordinary school. Problems may arise, however, when a specialist careers officer is not available or is found unhelpful by a particular school, as many special schools may not be equipped with a teacher trained in careers guidance, and ordinary schools may not be geared to advising handicapped pupils.

In Section A, we shall look at the careers guidance and information on placements provided by the schools in our survey, then at the teenagers' and parents' satisfaction with these services. In Section B we shall examine the services provided after leaving school, mainly from the experience of our follow-up group. Finally, in Section C, we shall examine their views on the general areas where improvements are required, and make recommendations for changes.

## Section A

### Services provided while still at school

As we have already stated, for a handicapped teenager to find a satisfactory placement and adapt successfully to adult life he needs adequate information and guidance about the possibilities open to him, and also some understanding of what life at work will be like. Successful adjustment and adaptation will not be facilitated by giving teenagers false hopes and ambitions for their future employment. The handicapped pupil needs careful guidance and advice, and he must be encouraged to make decisions on his own, realistically facing up to the alternatives open to him. It is *very* important that the teenager is fully aware of his likely prospects and has recognized the problems *before* leaving school. Finding a suitable placement can, and must, be assisted by certain key people in the handicapped pupil's life – his parents, certain members of the school staff, and the local authority careers officer – before he leaves school. Even a disabled pupil who has successfully integrated into an ordinary school may still need special help with guidance about further education, training or employment, and this is not always recognized.

Let us now examine the preparation for work provided by the schools in our survey. The general characteristics of the schools are described in chapter 1 (see pp. 21–5). It will be recalled that of the total sample, just under one-third (N = 37) of the teenagers were attending the thirty-four ordinary schools and just over two-thirds (N = 82) were attending the twenty-six special schools. Three of the thirty-four ordinary schools were private schools, and one of these was a boarding school, while fourteen of the special schools were boarding schools.

We were able to ask detailed questions about the careers education and vocational guidance arrangements in thirty-three of the ordinary schools and twenty-two of the special schools. It was impossible to cover all of the schools as sometimes the teachers who dealt with these matters were absent or unobtainable, and for this reason it was not always possible to get our questions answered. Consequently, the totals quoted in the rest of this section vary between different tables.

Most of the pupils attending ordinary schools in our study were only offered the same careers education and vocational guidance arrangements that were generally available in the school. Three schools said that they gave 'some extra help' to handicapped pupils in addition to their usual programmes, but none of the schools offered a different system or appointed a teacher to be responsible for the guidance of handicapped pupils to give them earlier preparation or the special support for school leaving which, as we mentioned earlier, has been generally recommended as essential.

*Careers teachers.* Whether or not the leaver finds a suitable placement depends very much on what is done before he leaves school. The careers teacher, if there is one, the head, or the class teacher can play an important role by giving pupils information about the possibilities and by developing close links with the careers service. Teachers must ensure that the careers officer is supplied with information about a particular pupil and his needs at an early stage to allow time to consider future placement carefully. The Warnock Committee has gone as far as to recommend 'that a teacher with special responsibility for careers guidance should be appointed in every special school which caters for older pupils and that in every ordinary secondary school there should be at least one careers teacher with additional training or expertise in understanding the careers implications of different types of disability or disorder' (para. 10.14).

Most of the ordinary schools in our study did have a member of staff designated as a careers teacher. Sixteen of the thirty-three schools had one careers teacher, twelve had two or more, and only five had no careers teacher at all. In addition, five of the schools also had teachers who were designated as counsellors who had some special responsibility for careers as well as for personal and social guidance. Two of the designated careers teachers had full-time posts, while in five others the total time given for careers teaching and other careers work (administration, writing reports and references) was up to a total of one half-time post, and in four schools this was more than one half-time post. The other twenty schools said they could not estimate the time they spent as it was not calculated separately from other responsibilities. Most of the ordinary school staff with responsibility for careers had some training in careers education, though this was rarely extensive, it included having attended careers or counselling courses of at least 1–5 days, while seven had attended a course of over one week, and nine of one term or longer. Over half of the teachers (fifteen) in the ordinary schools felt that placement in employment was not part of their duties, while eleven felt it was only a minor or occasional part; but three considered this a major part of their task. They tended to see their role as confined to providing information.

The special schools in our study fell far short of the Warnock Report's recommendations as only five of the twenty-two questioned had designated teachers with special responsibility for careers. These were usually the leavers' class teacher, although in one school there was a careers teacher who did not teach full-time who was responsible both for the careers advice and for liaising with personal problems. Three teachers said they spent up to a total of half of their time on careers teaching and writing reports, while two said they could not estimate this time separately from other responsibilities. Only three teachers had attended a careers or counselling course, and these were all for only one or two days.

In the other special schools a variety of people shared the responsibility for careers in the school. These included the teacher of the leavers' class or the head and sometimes the deputy head, though in only three schools had any of these members of staff attended any formal course. In most instances, the staff could not estimate how much time they spent on careers work separately from their other duties, and in some schools the arrangements were practically non-existent, the issue being left almost entirely to the careers services.

Eight of the nineteen schools who were questioned on this point thought that post-school placement was not part of their duties at all, while only three felt that this was a major consideration for a teacher with responsibility for careers in a special school. This implies that the special schools generally do not see themselves as acting as a continuing source of support for a teenager once he has left school. This makes leaving school even more traumatic for teenagers who have been used to the very supportive environment of a special school, especially if they somehow fall between the mandate of the various agencies that could be involved in their care. We shall discuss this further when considering the follow up of leavers in general.

*Careers service.* Because teachers know the pupils well, they are important as a link with the careers officer, on whom ultimate responsibility for vocational guidance falls, who should provide a bridge for young people between school and work. The careers service in the UK is in the anomalous position of being directed at national level by the

Secretary of State for Employment, but run locally by education authorities. There is, however, some logic in the dual connection since, for the handicapped school leaver especially, the link between school and life after school that a specialist careers officer can offer could be crucial to satisfactory placement. This is why the specialist careers officer was identified by the Warnock Report as the 'named person' to provide the single point of contact for those with special needs during the transition to adult life.

There is some overlap between careers officers and careers teachers in the provision of information and instruction, in giving vocational guidance, in acting as links with further education and industry, and in the follow up of leavers. In relation to finding jobs, there is also an overlap with the Disablement Resettlement Officer (DRO). The careers service may keep its clients until they are nineteen years old (or into their twenties in the case of specialist officers) while the Manpower Services Commission (MSC) Resettlement Service (which employs the DRO) deals with young people of any age once they have left school.

The careers officer for the handicapped is a comparatively new specialism which has developed in the last ten years, and the service was given its first real boost after the 1974 local government reorganization when the number of local authorities which could afford to make a full-time specialist appointment increased. Virtually all authorities now have a specialist careers officer – there were ninety-six full-time and thirty-five part-time according to the careers service staffing return for 1978.

The Secretary of State for Employment's advice to authorities is that they should appoint one specialist officer for every 200 handicapped fifteen year olds (according to Rowan (1980) this is about half the normal case load), but since the method of organization varies widely it is sometimes difficult to calculate how far this advice is followed. The Warnock Report's recommendation that the careers service be 'considerably strengthened' (para. 10.5) to provide at least one specialist careers officer for every 50,000 of the school population has caused some confusion. It is not clear how this would marry up with the currently recommended case-load advice, nor what definition of special need Warnock had in mind in arriving at this figure. The DE calculation is that an additional ninety full-time specialist posts would have to be created to provide one for every 50,000 of the school population.

At present, according to Rodgers (1979), few specialist careers officers will deal with more than 150 leavers per year. However he has estimated that in a school population of 50,000 there will be approximately sixty leavers from special schools alone every year, in addition to which the careers officer will have to deal with handicapped leavers from ordinary schools. He or she will have to cope with at least four year groups at any one time, since Warnock (para. 10.7) recommends that every pupil's needs should be assessed at least two years before he is due to leave school, and that ex-pupils should be in contact with the careers service at least until their eighteenth birthday. It is immediately apparent that with this case-load, the careers officer will not be able to get to know every individual personally.

Warnock (para. 10.16) also considers the problem of liaison where the careers officer in the locality of the school and the careers officer in the child's home area are not the same, and suggests a possible liaison through an appointed home–school liaison teacher. This is particularly important for pupils attending residential special schools who intend returning home when they leave school.

Given the importance attached to the post of careers officer by Warnock it is interesting to examine how far careers officers were involved in vocational guidance in the schools in our study.

*Careers service in ordinary schools.* Careers officers visited all of the thirty-three ordinary schools in our study. Seventeen were visited by the careers officer more than twenty-five times a year, usually to see pupils in the leavers' year individually. We asked in which ways the careers officers assisted the schools; in some they helped in the planning of careers programmes, in the planning of work visits and work experience, and in planning talks to parents or parents' evenings, but by far the most common task (in twenty-nine of the schools questioned) was giving talks and holding discussions with pupils and, in twenty-one schools, giving talks and holding discussions with parents. Only nine of the ordinary schools had ever been visited by a specialist careers officer, and in only one school had he been more than twice. This was mainly for the pupils in the survey, eight of whom had been interviewed by the specialist careers officer. Needless to say, this rate of referral for specialist advice does not match up to the recommendations made by Warnock.

The careers officer's main function is to act as a link between the school and placement after school, and before he can give any vocational guidance he will need to meet the school staff and find out as much as possible about a particular pupil. For handicapped pupils in ordinary schools he may also need more detailed medical and psychological reports. It has previously been recommended that the careers officer's attention should be drawn to the handicapped pupil's needs early on, preferably at the beginning of the third year of secondary school. The ASBAH Report (1975) explained that contact should begin about one year earlier than for other teenagers since 'it takes a careers officer some considerable time to get to know a handicapped pupil, to assess his abilities and personality, as well as the practical effects of his disabilities, and to win his confidence and that of his parents'. In our study, however, only five of the schools said that handicapped pupils were likely to meet the careers officer earlier than other pupils. This does not allow enough time for careful consideration of the problems to be faced in any placements and is clearly an area to which ordinary schools need to attend.

*Careers service in special schools.* It might be expected that special schools would be much more geared to the needs of the individual pupil and so would have well-established contacts with the careers service. In fact the number of times that careers officers visited the school varied greatly, but was generally less often than for the ordinary schools (though this may be merely a result of the smaller size of special schools). Usually it was the specialist careers officer for the handicapped who visited. Only one school was not visited systematically by a careers officer. This was a residential school where the responsibility for post-school placement was designated to the careers officer in the area where the pupils lived, who usually saw clients when they were at home during vacations.

From our results it would appear that the careers officers in special schools were not very much involved in the planning of the careers programmes, work experience or planning talks to parents. As in the ordinary schools, their main role was in talking to the pupils (in eighteen of the twenty schools for whom we have information) and to a lesser extent in talking to and holding discussions with the parents. Most of the schools (fifteen) said that leavers were usually interviewed individually more than once by the careers officer. In only one of the special schools in our study was it usual for the careers officer to meet pupils for the first time in the third year (as recommended by Warnock), while seven schools said it was generally in the fourth year, and eleven said not until the fifth year when the pupils were already fifteen years or older. This is particularly important in the light of the Queen Elizabeth's Foundation for the Disabled enquiry, where it was suggested that many problems arose for disabled leavers because the assessment of their potential at school had been inadequate. This might be understandable for leavers in ordinary schools, but certainly not for special school leavers.

The special schools themselves were very restrained in their complaints about the careers service, and most were favourably disposed towards them. Few named problems that they had encountered in establishing a close working partnership with careers officers. One residential school which had a very large catchment area said that the distance that specialist careers officers had to travel caused problems in communication and in visiting their pupils, while three other residential schools said that it was difficult for their local careers officer to liaise with the careers officer in the children's home area. Only one school felt that their careers officer had insufficient specialized knowledge of handicap. This school had experienced problems in the past with the careers officer failing to judge sensibly what particular pupils were capable of, and in raising their expectations unrealistically.

*Other agencies.* We also asked schools which other special services or voluntary organizations they called on to help in giving advice on careers to individual pupils. Only one ordinary school and four special schools said that they regularly used the schools' psychological service, while eleven ordinary schools and seven special schools said they occasionally used this service. This means that about half the special schools were not using this service at all to assess their leavers. The DRO or Employment Rehabilitation Centre staff were also rarely used – only one special school used them regularly.

More common advisors were the voluntary societies – mainly the Spastics Society – used for assessments of cerebral-palsied leavers regularly by six of the special schools and occasionally by eight special and seven ordinary schools. It is worth noting here that while the Spastics Society assessment courses may have defects (that some teenagers and their parents in our study complained of), at least they are generally available and most useful for cerebral-palsied leavers. No similar assessment procedures are available to the spina bifida teenagers at all as yet. At the time of writing the Spastics Society assessment service appears to be under threat from severe cuts, and since they cannot be replaced by statutory services their loss is likely to have very damaging effects.

Various other people were also called on for careers advice (but not on a regular basis) by the special schools. These included physiotherapists, occupational therapists, social workers, school nurses and, in residential schools, the house parents. Most of the special schools also used the school doctor at least occasionally. In general, however, it would seem that more use could be made of the advice of professional services already in existence when assessing a handicapped teenager's future potential.

*Parents' meetings and case conferences.*   One interesting difference between the ordinary and special schools is that most of the ordinary schools (twenty) regularly held parents' meetings where careers education was discussed, whereas only five of the special schools did this. Special schools tended to favour an individual approach and called case conferences in which parents were included, only four saying this was not the rule. In theory, the conference should have produced a clear plan of action for each student, in practice, as our results in chapter 7 show, the conferences (or at least the follow up from them) were not always very effective. The normal procedure was for the school to hold a case con-ference to discuss the pupil and his future career, usually in the year before he was due to leave school. The format varied, but the conference generally took place after the careers officer had met the pupil, and in two-thirds of the schools the careers officer was present. Various members of the school staff were involved, usually the head and the pupil's teacher, and perhaps also the physiotherapist, doctor, social worker, or any other people who had been involved in the pupil's care. (It was rare for these meetings to occur in ordinary schools – only four of the thirty-four schools reporting that they had case conferences on particular pupils.)

It is worth pointing out here that case conferences and parents' meetings are both valuable and are not mutually exclusive as they serve different functions. It is important for parents to be informed about what, in principle, is available for their child and to discuss the advantages and disadvantages of these in individual case conferences. It is also important that parents have the opportunity of learning from each other and sharing their feelings so meetings are a good idea *in addition* to individual consultations, although of course these are more difficult to organize at residential schools.

*Careers education.* Careers education in schools can include group discussions, outside speakers and films, while some schools also arrange visits to colleges of further education and places of work, or participation in work observation courses, work experience courses or linked courses. These are all important preparations for life after school. On work experience courses the pupil actually gets some experience of work while still at school – for example, helping out in a nursery one day a week – while for work observation a pupil only visits a place of employment with the specific purpose of familiarization with the nature of the work.

Linked courses, on the other hand, can exist between ordinary or special schools and further education establishments, or with adult literacy centres. They enable pupils to spend some time mixing with other students outside school and so can help ease the transition from school to work both socially and occupationally. Linked courses can also serve as useful trial periods enabling teenagers to try out their abilities at different courses before they leave school, introducing them (and the school staff) to the range of courses that are available in further education. The Scottish Report (1975) indicated the importance of this point when it stated 'that some potential students are not aware of the opportunities that are open to them. It may be that they or their advisors feel that the challenge would be too great. We recommend, therefore, that all physically handicapped pupils in special schools should have their attention drawn to the types of courses which their abilities would enable them to pursue in further education. We would also recommend that the special schools should take steps towards more formal liaison with further education colleges'. Judging by the special schools we visited, this is also true in England. As we pointed out in chapter 7, there were certainly some teenagers in our follow-up study who had been at home or in day centres since they left school and could have benefited from further education.

In all but four of the ordinary schools we visited, there was someone on the staff who liaised with establishments of further education, and in about two-thirds of the schools linked courses of some sort were available.

The person who formed this liaison was usually the head, deputy head or careers teacher. A great variety of linked courses were available, including shorthand, typing and commercial courses, nursery nursing, engineering, agricultural studies, catering, art, motor vehicle maintenance, plumbing, transition to work course, practical electronics, indoor maintenance, building and CSE courses. Only two of the survey pupils had been on these linked courses, but half of the ordinary schools had organized visits to further education colleges for pupils to see what these were like and what they had to offer.

The picture given by the special schools was very different. While fourteen of the twenty-two special schools said that they had a member of staff who liaised with further education establishments (this was nearly always the head but in a few cases it was the careers teacher), unlike the ordinary schools only eight had actually arranged linked courses – three with local ordinary schools and five with local further education colleges. Only three of the survey pupils had attended these courses. The courses on which they participated were not very varied or stimulating, and included the Duke of Edinburgh Award course, art, home economics and typing. The lack of participation was not because schools had experienced difficulties in the past. Only one school reported that a local college had been reluctant to take a pupil (who was only mildly handicapped) and this had been solved by the careers officer taking the pupil along to the college concerned.

The fact that so few teenagers had the opportunity of participating in courses outside their special school either in ordinary schools or further education colleges is disappointing, both because mixing with non-handicapped teenagers would be a useful social experience and because it would give them a broader insight into the range of options open to them when they leave school. In fact it was rare for special school pupils even to have the opportunity to visit further education establishments before they left school. Only seven of the special schools said that they organized visits to further education colleges, and only three survey pupils had taken part in this. None had experienced major problems on such visits – apart from those of mobility and access – but in any case, this is good training for the teenagers as they will have to cope with these matters when they leave school.

Twenty-one ordinary schools also made organized visits to firms to familiarize pupils with industry and commerce. This was not common practice in the special schools, however: only two schools said this was done on any scale (for about 20 per cent of pupils) while a few others did this on an *ad hoc* basis only. However, four of the special schools complained that they had found it difficult to do this as firms were not keen to take handicapped employees. No survey pupils in ordinary schools or special schools had been on such visits. It is important that, wherever possible, handicapped teenagers should make as wide-ranging visits as possible. This will inevitably mean that they meet situations which will be discouraging, but the problems encountered can then be discussed, ways to get round them can be suggested, and the sort of work that is possible can be more realistically assessed. While it may be difficult for special schools to take a large group of handicapped teenagers round firms offering open employment with different mobility problems, it might be expected that staff in special schools could cope with the problems of individual pupils or small groups, and it should certainly be possible to provide information about and visits to sheltered workshops, employment rehabilitation units and day centres. Unfortunately, this rarely occurred in the special schools that we visited and is clearly an area needing urgent development. It is important that these visits are not so carefully selected that the teenagers get a distorted view of working life, but should cover the widest variety of places possible, and not only the type of place where particular pupils might eventually be placed. This will at least give leavers a realistic view of the employment world so that they know what other people do at work.

Another invaluable method of preparing teenagers for work while still at school, is work experience. Two-thirds of the ordinary schools (twenty-two) said that work experience was available for at least some pupils, although some schools complained that firms were not currently interested in offering work experience since, with high unemployment, there was plenty of labour available. In fact, none of the handicapped pupils in ordinary schools had been on a work experience placement. Some of these placements were organized by the schools themselves and others by the careers service which operated a scheme for schools in their area. There is also in existence, a national scheme – 'TRIDENT' – which some schools participated in.

Of the special schools we interviewed, eight said they had no work experience available at all, ten said it was arranged for less than 20 per cent of pupils, and only two said it was arranged for over half of the pupils. Surprisingly, only two schools reported that they had encountered problems in placing pupils – one said that transport was a general problem, and the other had found that they had tried one boy with three firms which were very co-operative, but the child himself could not cope. Three of the survey pupils had had work experience. One girl had tried helping in a nursery one morning a week, but the school said she could not manage this very well; she was then transferred to a work centre twice a week with a view to moving there full-time when she left school. Another girl had spent a week working in a local factory and the third had been to a day centre. This girl however was not at all happy there and, since she was given no extra help to find an alternative placement, ended up without any placement on leaving school.

Another method that special schools could employ to give pupils a realistic idea of work before they leave school could take a variety of forms ranging from the setting up of a mock workplace in the school – for example, modifying a woodwork lesson to more structured arrangements – through to attempts to simulate all aspects of working life in a special unit.

*Careers education lessons.* We have discussed two aspects of any careers education programme for handicapped teenagers – vocational guidance by careers teachers and careers officers, and methods of introducing pupils to a working environment by visits or work experience – but we also need to consider the information-giving aspects of the curriculum. This can take a variety of forms including group discussions, outside speakers and films. Vocational elements can of course be introduced into all lessons, for example, the explanation of pay-slips can be brought into mathematics lessons, with the calculation of net pay forming a useful arithmetic exercise. Books describing occupations can be used for those who are receiving reading instruction. Specific lessons can also be devoted to the world of work with discussions on particular jobs, social security and allowances and benefits. The qualifications and social skills that are needed for certain occupations, and for life after school in general, can also be examined and encouraged. This will include general aspects such as accepting responsibility, as well as coping with money and transport (which will overlap with the social education programmes described in chapter 10).

Twenty-two of the ordinary schools in our survey said they allocated periods specifically for careers education, and only nine said they did not. In contrast, only five of the special schools had specific careers education lessons and thirteen did not. (The proportion allocating time for careers education in ordinary schools is in keeping with the DES survey (1973) already mentioned.) It was thus much more common for the ordinary schools to provide careers lessons; special schools were obviously not giving this topic priority, although their pupils need more information about the availability and expectations of different jobs than do those in ordinary schools.

Most of the schools providing careers education started this in the fourth year, when the pupils were 14–15 years old, although some ordinary schools started this in the third year and others not until the fifth year. This might mean that the special needs of handicapped and less able pupils were being overlooked in most cases, and pupils may feel very discouraged and frustrated if most of the jobs discussed are out of their reach in terms of qualification or ability. The careers lessons in the ordinary schools were fairly wide ranging, most including the personal and educational qualifications required for specific occupations and opportunities in industrial training and further education. Slightly fewer provided information about local industry or discussed the various aspects of working life. Only two special schools covered any of the above subjects. (Rather surprisingly only six of the ordinary schools and two of the special schools provided careers programmes for pupils of different abilities.)

The results suggest that, while careers education is becoming the norm within ordinary secondary schools, special schools still tend to favour an individual approach, which is facilitated by their smaller size and may indeed be necessary because of the very different and individual problems to be considered for each pupil when discussing post-school placement. However, pupils also need to know about the world of work in general in order to appraise their own potential realistically and to learn how to cope with the various problems they will undoubtedly experience when they leave school. These aspects can best be discussed in groups, and much can be done by the special schools to prepare their pupils in this way.

*Teenagers' perception of school-based career services*

We shall now look at what the teenagers themselves thought about the vocational advice and guidance they were given while they were still at school. While most of the controls (90 per cent) and the handicapped teenagers in ordinary schools (81 per cent) said that they had spoken to their parents about what they wanted to do when they left school, this was true for only two-thirds (68 per cent) of the special school pupils. About half of all the teenagers had been given advice by their parents about what to do when they left school. We also asked them which other people had given them vocational advice while still at school. Most of the controls (85 per cent) and handicapped teenagers in ordinary schools (92 per cent) confirmed that there was a careers teacher of some kind in their school. This agrees with the number of ordinary schools who professed to have a designated careers teacher (twenty-seven out of thirty-two schools). Just over half (57 per cent) of the special schools pupils said that someone acted in this capacity in their school, and again that was in general agreement with the schools' reports. However, over half the teenagers who mentioned that there was such a service available in the school (61 per cent of controls, 65 per cent of handicapped in ordinary schools and 53 per cent of special school pupils) claimed that they had *not* talked to this member of staff about their own career, or what they were going to do when they left school.

Most teenagers had heard of the careers officer (only 10 per cent of handicapped pupils and 6 per cent of controls had not), but only one-third of ordinary school pupils (33 per cent of controls and 40 per cent of handicapped) had talked with one. By contrast, over half (57 per cent) of the special school pupils had done so. While this is encouraging, it may in part be an artifact due to the fact that a higher percentage of the special school pupils were rather older at interview. What is important is that two-thirds of the handicapped in ordinary schools and nearly half

(42 per cent) of special school pupils had never seen a careers officer by the time of their fifteenth birthday, just one year before they are eligible to leave school, which does not leave anything like enough time to consider their future and find a placement.

Nearly all of the teenagers in ordinary schools who saw careers officers had made suggestions to them about what they might do when they left school, and most of the careers officers thought the suggestions made by the controls and the handicapped in ordinary schools were suitable. This was true for less than half the special school pupils. In fact one-third of the careers officers were definitely against the suggestions made by special school pupils and thought them unsuitable. A number of teenagers mentioned other people who had advised them or helped them, including relatives, parents' friends, various members of the school staff, social workers and the Spastics Society careers officer. Overall, the findings indicate that for many handicapped pupils in ordinary and special schools no discussion about the post-school future had been initiated one year prior to statutory schools leaving age (many in fact were already over the age of sixteen).

*Parents' perception of school-based career services*

We also asked the parents whom they had talked to about their child's future, and Table 11.1 shows that a high proportion of the parents (70 per cent of the controls and 45 per cent of the handicapped) claimed that they had not been to the school or discussed their child's future with anyone on the staff. Where the parents had discussed this, it was usually with the head or class teacher at open evenings or at a special case conference.

Most of the parents of ordinary school pupils who had been to the school had been only once, whereas one-fifth of the parents of special school pupils said they had been more than twice. Nearly all of these meetings were suggested by the school and very few initiated by the parents themselves. However, most of the parents of the handicapped pupils said that they had received few suggestions from the school staff about their child's career, or that the school was very vague or merely suggested that the handicapped pupil stayed on at school. Few parents reported that they had found anyone at the school particularly helpful – in fact only about one-quarter of the parents who had been to the school.

A number of the parents of handicapped teenagers, especially those in special schools, had discussed their child's future with a specialist from outside the school – 29 per cent of the handicapped pupils' parents in ordinary schools, and 57 per cent of the parents of special school pupils compared with only 19 per cent of the control parents. The person that most of the parents of handicapped children had talked to was the careers officer or a Spastics Society representative. The parents of ordinary

Table 11.1 *Whether parents discussed careers with school staff*

| | No one N (%) | Head N* (%) | Careers teacher N* (%) | Class teacher N* (%) | Other N* (%) |
|---|---|---|---|---|---|
| Handicapped (N = 119) | 54 (45) | 42 (51) | 13 (16) | 20 (24) | 23 (28) |
| Controls (N = 34) | 24 (70) | 1 (2) | 0 (0) | 2 (5) | 2 (5) |

* Some parents are included more than once if they had seen more than one person.

school pupils usually said that they had met a careers officer only once, while over one-third of the parents of special school pupils had met a careers officer on two or more occasions. It is difficult to generalize about how helpful the parents found the careers officer as it varied greatly according to the suggestions that were made and the expertise of each individual. Some said the careers officer had made good suggestions about assessment or possible placement, while others were at a loss to propose anything at all, or made inappropriate suggestions. Suffice to say that half the parents of the special school pupils did not find the careers officer to be helpful at all.

In fact when the parents were asked if they felt they had had as much advice as they needed about their child's future nearly half (47 per cent) were dissatisfied with the advice they had been given, including 23 per cent who were very dissatisfied. Fewer of the parents of the teenagers in ordinary schools were dissatisfied (18 per cent of control parents, and 32 per cent of parents of handicapped teenagers). Most parents didn't know who else they would have liked to discuss their child with, and many simply expressed a general wish to see 'someone who knows what they are talking about'. Some parents mentioned the specialist careers officer or the Spastics Society, and one parent summed up the feelings of most when she said, 'That's the problem. I just don't know what is available or who is available to help.' Most of the parents of the handicapped teenagers were very worried about their child's future when we visited them, and were desperate about whom to turn to for help. Leaving school presents great problems for both the teenagers and their parents, and expert advice is badly needed to help in relieving some of this anxiety. Even if expert advice is not available – or perhaps particularly so in these cases – parents should at least be helped to realize what services exist and which of these are most suitable for their child.

## Section B

### Services provided after leaving school

Surveys of handicapped school leavers, including our own findings described in chapter 8, show that the period after leaving school can be full of great uncertainty and stress. It is well recognized that finding a satisfactory placement or adjusting to life after school can create many problems and anxieties, but it is often impossible at present to identify precisely who has responsibility for supervising a particular leaver. The local education authority, the school services department, the employment services agency or voluntary agencies may all be potential sources of help.

It has earlier been suggested (Anderson and Spain, 1977) that three people should play key roles in the support of school leavers – (i) a member of staff in every special school who should follow up the leavers to provide a continuing link for the leaver with someone he knows well. (This would also give invaluable feedback for each school on exactly what happens to leavers and the problems they face, so that this can be acted on for the benefit of future pupils.); (ii) the local careers officer; and (iii) the local social worker (as recommended in the Tuckey Report) to ensure the emotional, medical and social welfare of all leavers.

Careers officers and teachers must be very careful not to stop giving follow-up surveillance and advice to teenagers once they have been found a placement. It may be that extra support will be needed after leaving school, or that the initial placement will be found to be unsuitable. After all, many able-bodied teenagers change jobs more than once during their first few years after leaving school. It is very important that once a handicapped teenager starts a placement of any description, however hard it is to find, he is not considered as being settled there indefinitely, as this may unnecessarily create a negative view of the placement with the teenager feeling abandoned and doomed.

To this end, we asked how many schools systematically followed up leavers, or had done so in the past, in order to see how placements were working out. Only seven of the ordinary schools said that they had followed up leavers – usually in the form of letters sent by the careers teacher to the teenagers in the year after they had left school to find out what they were doing. The aim was to help in advising future leavers rather than to offer assistance to leavers with difficulties. There was no systematic link kept with leavers so that they would come to school staff for advice or help once they had left school, although some schools said they would offer help in exceptional cases.

Only five special schools had follow-up schemes, two of which were residential schools, where leavers were followed up through the sponsoring authorities concerned to see how the teenagers fared when they returned home. The leavers were followed up via their local social workers or the societies' social workers, but no direct contact was kept by the school itself. One day special school had carried out a postal follow-up survey of thirty-five ex-students (though only eleven replied) and had visited centres where fifteen ex-students were in residence, in day care or working, in order to find out what was happening to them. (The conclusion of this survey was a call for urgent attention to be given to the young severely handicapped leavers in the provision of more suitable day care centres where they could enjoy peer contact and stimulation.) The head of one other day special school said that she made it her business to find out what had happened to school leavers, and certainly encouraged teenagers and their families to continue their relationship with the school. She said that both she and the school nurse kept in close contact with teenagers and their families and the careers service and would help in placing and supporting all leavers if they wanted this. This was the only school where such a service was reportedly available, albeit on an informal and unsystematic basis.

*Schools' perception of the careers service*

The schools themselves raised the problem of support for leavers when we asked about the difficulties they had experienced in connection with careers education. The main and general complaint by the special schools was that there was a great lack of opportunities available for the non-academic leaver, and that, however good the vocational guidance system, this was no good when there was nowhere to send leavers and no prospects for their future. The main complaints were the lack of good work-centres for young leavers, or of colleges or alternatives to work for the severely handicapped or low ability teenagers. One school felt that communication between the different services and the authorities was the biggest problem, whilst another was worried about how emotionally dependent pupils became in the protective atmosphere of their residential special school so that leaving became very traumatic for these young people.

The ordinary schools raised similar problems about what the handicapped pupils could do when they left school. Some also mentioned the small amount of time that was available for careers advice, or the fact that they could not do much because of how few handicapped pupils they had in the school and the staff's lack of specialized knowledge. (However, this would not prevent their using the services of the specialist careers officer and voluntary bodies which we have already mentioned.) One school in particular felt that their handicapped pupil had missed out on individual attention and encouragement as far as careers advice was concerned by being in an ordinary school.

**Section C**

*Teenagers' and parents' perception of careers guidance after leaving school*

We questioned the fifty-one teenagers in the follow-up group and their

parents about the careers advice and practical help with finding a placement that they were given after leaving school.

It is very interesting that the teenagers' and their parents' reports of
whether they found anyone especially helpful in giving advice or
practical help just before and after they left school conform closely.
Roughly two-thirds of the teenagers in ordinary schools (67 per cent) said
that they found no one (or only a member of their family) helpful, while
a similar proportion of their parents also said that they had not found
anyone helpful. This was also the case for over one-third of the teenagers
in special schools (36 per cent) and nearly half (47 per cent) of their
parents. In other words, even though more of the special school pupils
said they had received help or advice from people other than their
families, a large proportion of all the teenagers and their parents had
found no one at all helpful when deciding what they might do when they
left school.

We asked both the teenagers and their parents about whether they
had spoken to specific people in connection with leaving school and
asked if they had found this useful or helpful. We got very similar replies
to those given to us by the teenagers while still at school. All but a few of
the teenagers who could not remember said that they had met a careers
officer, but only one-third said they had found the careers officer
helpful, while another quarter said the careers officer was kind, but
provided no useful help. Over 20 per cent said that they had found the
officer definitely unhelpful.

Again, as in Phase I of the study, not many of the teenagers said they
had talked to a careers teacher. In fact only 17 per cent of the teenagers in
special schools, compared with over half of the ordinary school pupils,
said they had done so, and most of the parents (88 per cent) reported
that they had not talked to a careers teacher at all. Two-thirds of the
special school pupils reported that they had talked to another teacher
(usually the head or class teacher) about leaving school, and just under
half said that they had found this teacher helpful. Their parents were not
so satisfied: only one-quarter said they had found the teachers helpful,
while 18 per cent found the officer definitely unhelpful, and another 18
per cent found the officer pleasant but not any actual help. (The
remainder had not seen a teacher.)

We also asked about professionals from the voluntary organizations,
the Spastics Society and ASBAH. Three pupils who had attended ordinary schools had been in touch with the Spastics Society, compared with
just over one-third of the special school pupils. Most of the teenagers and
their parents who had been in contact had found this helpful, although
about 10 per cent said the contact was friendly but had proved no actual
help. Four of the parents and two of the teenagers said that their contact
with the Spastics Society had definitely been unhelpful.

Not many teenagers (one-third of special school pupils and only one ordinary school pupil) had talked to a social worker, but only f reported they had found this person helpful in relation to the placeme of special school pupils. More of the parents had talked to a social worke in connection with leaving school, and half doing so had found it useful. This is important as most parents said they had not talked to a relative or any family friend about their child leaving school, so the support from a social worker or other professional would be much valued.

Six parents mentioned other people with whom they had discussed careers, including the child's consultant psychiatrist, a Disablement Resettlement Officer, while two teenagers had been assessed by psychologists at further education colleges, which their parents found helpful.

As we mentioned previously, it has been suggested that some handicapped school leavers are inappropriately placed because their potential is inadequately assessed. In our follow-up group three (25 per cent) of the ordinary school pupils had been on an assessment course of some kind compared with sixteen (42 per cent) of the special school pupils, while a further four (11 per cent) special school pupils had been assessed after leaving school as part of their post-school placement. Nearly three-quarters (71 per cent) of the young people who had been on an assessment course thought that this had helped them in some way, though their parents were less certain. In fact, some parents were extremely vociferous in their complaints about these courses, the most usual being that they felt it was a 'waste of time' as they were not told what sort of placement would be best and were not given a recommendation. Other complaints included: 'They didn't tell us the results', '[the Spastics Society] are blinkered – only put you in their places', 'They told him he had done very well and then wrote and said there was nothing he could do', '[gave] only their ideas . . . not told of the possibilities x, y, z, only their opinions', and 'The only thing they said was he'd be wasting his time going to college. They didn't explain what the alternatives were.'

In fact, as can be seen from Table 11.2, two-thirds of the teenagers and an even higher proportion of parents were dissatisfied with the amount of information they were given about what they might do when they left school. Nearly half the parents were 'definitely dissatisfied' and complained bitterly about the dearth of information available to them, or despairingly asked us for advice about what their child could do or to whom they could turn to for help. This is a sad indictment of the careers advice and guidance given to handicapped school leavers and their parents.

One important failure in the professional help and support given to some of the teenagers was mentioned in chapter 7. This was the lack of follow-up support during the months after leaving school, shown by the numbers who were either waiting several months for a placement, or were still at home without any promise of a placement when interviewed. Some of the teenagers, although in contact with the careers

Table 11.2 *Do teenagers and parents think they were given enough information about the different things the teenagers might be able to do when they left school?*

| | No, definitely dissatisfied N (%) | Somewhat dissatisfied N (%) | On the whole satisfied N (%) | Definitely satisfied N (%) | Don't know N (%) | Total N |
|---|---|---|---|---|---|---|
| Teenagers | 17 (36) | 14 (30) | 5 (11) | 10 (21) | 1 (2) | 47 |
| Parents | 23 (46) | 13 (26) | 8 (16) | 4 (8) | 2 (4) | 50 |

officer or other professionals, were left sitting at home getting worried and frustrated, while others sadly slipped through an administrative gap and were not given help or advice by anyone after leaving school. We have already examined the lack of follow-up support provided by the schools and suggested that this crucial changeover period could be jointly borne by the schools and careers service. The school leavers and their parents have a long and established relationship with the school which can be a helpful back-up service during this time of transition. It is important this relationship is not severed totally and abruptly so that the school leaver is given time to make the adjustment to adult life with maximum support.

### Parents' and teenagers' views on improvements required

*School-based services.* While there has been much improvement in recent years, it can be seen from the findings above that the vocational guidance arrangements for handicapped school leavers still leave much to be desired. We should like to make some suggestions about the ways that young people could be better helped, both before and after leaving school, from the comments made by the teenagers and the parents in our follow-up study.

Many of the teenagers (twenty-eight) and their parents were very articulate in making suggestions about things that could or should have been done by their school which would have made life better or easier to cope with after leaving. Most of the teenagers wanted improvements in academic tuition or careers advice. Many complained that they wanted extra help to brush up their English, reading or maths in the last year at school, 'instead of doing nothing' as one girl expressed it. Others wanted the chance to take exams so that they could get qualifications. (These were mainly special school pupils who felt they were not encouraged to attempt exams.) As one girl said, 'At school they pushed you into doing things you didn't want to do and wouldn't let you try something if they thought you couldn't do it'. The majority of the teenagers said they wanted more information about careers, or advice on what they could do when they left, while a number wanted to know about further education. One boy in an ordinary school complained that his school was 'inexperienced to tackle with the problem of my disability – my writing and typing – I needed special advice when it came to leaving school'. Another boy in an ordinary school said, 'They should have given me more confidence to ask questions'. Some of the special school pupils said that they had felt 'too protected. We couldn't go out without an adult'. One girl also said they 'could have told me what a day centre was. I didn't know till after the interview'.

The parents' emphasis on the innovations that were needed in the schools was different. Most of the parents of teenagers who had attended ordinary schools felt that basic academic instruction was lacking, and that their child had not reached his full potential; they complained too that they were not given enough individual attention or instruction in basic skills.

The parents of teenagers who had attended special schools had very different complaints and suggestions. The vast majority of them singled out what they saw as the sheltered atmosphere of the special schools which resulted in a lack of experience of the outside world. They made comments like: 'It was good while she was there, but now, looking back, she doesn't know anything about life.' 'He was still treated as a young child.' 'It was so sheltered she was not encouraged to be independent.' 'They never told her much about life in general – it was too protected.' A number of parents specifically named the encouragement of independence as an important area for improvement within the special schools and also said there was not enough concentration on the social side of education. One mother said, 'It was sadly lacking in instruction on things like writing letters, filling in forms, claiming social security,' and another 'They should go through each pupil when coming up to school leaving to give a guideline and encourage independence – nothing came out of it'. One mother also thought that 'they should have explained his sexual situation to him'.

These comments reiterate the recommendations made in chapter 10 about the need for improvements in the social education programmes in schools for the physically handicapped. Many parents said that they felt that the school curriculum was not sufficiently stimulating and relevant to their child's future potential. It is very sad that a parent summed up her daughter's preparation for school leaving in these words: 'I think she wasted a lot of time in the last year at school – she got very bored.'

The need for more and better assessment was also raised independently by the parents: 'They should have sent him on an assessment before he left school . . . it could have told us more about what he could do. Three years before he left this should have been done – all schools have the same problem.' 'They should have done a lot more for her, assessed her, realized the problems these kids have.' 'They could have had more information on the alternatives available when he had finished school. Those going to a spastics place got lists of places of contact – we didn't . . . feel definitely school should have wanted him to go to Spastics Centre [an assessment centre].'

After asking the general question about what improvements the teenagers and parents would like to see, we made some suggestions about the things which schools, or people working together with schools, could do to make life after school better for young people, and asked the teenagers to rate these ideas. (We mentioned the suggestions that concerned social education in the previous chapter.) Most (60 per cent) thought it a 'very good' idea that their school should give 'more practical help in finding a placement when you leave school'. Only one-quarter of the teenagers said they did not think this was a very good idea for them personally as they were satisfied with the help they were given or did not require it. Over half also thought it a 'very good' idea that their school should 'offer more advice on how to apply for jobs/college etc. and how to handle interviews'. The teenagers overwhelmingly favoured the suggestion that schools should 'give you more information about the sort of jobs or activities a person with your kind of disability could do after leaving'. Three-quarters (73 per cent) thought this was a 'very good' idea and 15 per cent quite a good idea. Two-thirds (68 per cent) of the teenagers also expressed interest in the school giving more actual work experience, although a quarter (27 per cent) did not want this.

We also asked parents if they felt that their son or daughter had left school at the right time. Most of the parents were happy about this, but one-quarter of the parents of pupils from ordinary schools and 14 per cent of those of special school pupils felt they should have left school earlier; very few felt their son or daughter should have stayed on longer.

*Contact with services after leaving school.*　　Very few parents said that they had had any contact at all with their son's or daughter's school after they had left. In fact, none of the parents of teenagers who attended ordinary schools had heard from the school or contacted the school themselves since their child had left, and only a third (34 per cent) had had contact with the special schools. Half of these said that they had not found the school helpful during this encounter.

It is perhaps surprising that most of the parents said they would not have liked any more contact with the school. (In fact, all of the parents of ordinary school pupils and over three-quarters (79 per cent) of special school parents did *not* want more contact with the school.) This was either because their child was satisfactorily placed, or because they felt that the school did not or could not offer them any practical help in finding a placement, or because they found that the school did not offer constructive advice. They also felt that an outside professional with knowledge of the opportunities available would be more help. Only

seven (18 per cent) parents said they would have liked more contac'
the school. This does not mean that the schools need not provid€
follow-up support since parents were commenting on the *status quo*, aพ.
on whether they thought their child's ex-school would be helpful in the
present set-up. In fact, the majority (even those who had initiated
contact with the school themselves) felt that the school had not been, or
could not be, helpful. This should be accepted as a challenge by the
special schools if only in offering a sympathetic ear to post-school leavers
and their parents.

We asked the parents about any other people – apart from the school
staff – they or the teenager had been in touch with (by the telephone and
letter, as well as personal contact) in connection with the teenager's care
since he or she left school. One might expect all of the teenagers and their
parents to have been followed up by the careers service and to have seen a
careers officer at least once in the year after leaving school. However, one-
third (32 per cent) of the special school pupils and their families had not
been in contact with a careers officer *at all* since leaving school. This was
also the case for one of the handicapped pupils from an ordinary school.
Since for many the contact they had had was only at the point of leaving
school, the proportion who had not in fact had any contact with the careers
service *after leaving* was even higher than these figures suggest.

Neither was it the case that teenagers were immediately taken on by
the Disablement Resettlement Officer – less than 20 per cent of teenagers had been in contact with a DRO. However 40 per cent of the
families reported that they had been in contact with a voluntary organization (nearly always the Spastics Society) with regard to an assessment
course or recommendations following on from this. One problem, however, is that the Spastics Society only appears to refer young people to
their own colleges, sheltered workshops and day centres so these are the
only alternatives offered to a teenager after assessment. If none is
suitable, the teenager is merely passed back to the local services which
may not follow through the case adequately, and in consequence the
parents and young people feel very let down.

We also asked parents about contact with services in general, to see
how much help and support the family were offered from any service
since leaving school, for things other than job finding. One third (37 per
cent) of the parents said they had seen a social worker, while nearly half
(48 per cent) had been in contact with the social security office in connection with benefits and allowances. Just under half (42 per cent) had seen
a hospital consultant in the last year, implying that most teenagers had
no medical follow-up after leaving school, though many parents said
they would have liked this. A quarter of the parents mentioned other
people the family had seen since the teenager had left school and this
included a neurologist, physiotherapist, teacher and a church minister.

In total the majority of parents (60 per cent) had seen less than two.

people who could have helped in the care of their son or daughter since leaving school, and over half (54 per cent) of the parents of ordinary school pupils and one-quarter of special school pupils had not had contact with *anyone at all* from any services. A rather higher percentage of teenagers had been in contact with someone, and one-third had seen three or more people; nevertheless, one-quarter of the teenagers had seen no one from any service in the year after they left school.

It is indicative of the poor support offered to these school leavers, both at school and after leaving, that one-quarter of parents said they had found it more difficult to obtain advice and help since their child had left school compared to when he or she was at school, while half said they had *always* found it difficult to get advice and help. Only three parents (8 per cent) said they had found it easier since the teenager had left school.

When asked about how services could be improved after leaving school, the teenagers themselves mostly wanted more help in finding a placement – whether in a college, day centre or job. Their comments included: 'They could have found me something to do so I was occupied'; 'Seeing my careers officer more often. I have only seen her once to say hello . . . Also to see more job centres and factories'; and 'The careers officer could have taken me around to find a job'. One boy said, 'I would like to do something more worthwhile at the day centre . . . and meet people outside'. Another boy wanted 'better facilities . . . and a better understanding of disabled people'.

The parents were presented with a list of the things previously suggested as needing improvement, and were asked if, in their particular case, they felt improvements were needed in these areas. By far the most popular request was for better services to facilitate post-school placement. Three-quarters (76 per cent) of the parents wanted better advice about placements when the teenager was leaving school, and two-thirds (68 per cent) wanted more help in actually finding a job.

There were two other suggestions that produced an enthusiastic response. These were an improvement in clubs and leisure facilities in their own area (70 per cent), (which is not surprising given our findings on the large proportion of teenagers who are socially isolated both at school and after leaving. This was certainly something that worried their parents); and an improvement in the information about benefits and allowances (two-thirds (68 per cent) asked for this).

Although the other suggestions that we made were not so unanimously acclaimed, this does not mean they are unimportant, but only that the problem did not affect all the sample. Over one-third of the parents (including ten with severely handicapped teenagers) wanted improvements on the medical side in the form of check-ups or medical care. We mentioned earlier that when teenagers leave school they often become ineligible to see the paediatric consultant with whom they have always been a patient. Very often this means they are not referred to another consultant or hospital and, for spina bifida teenagers especially, this may mean visiting several different consultants or hospitals for each of their problems as there is no one hospital specializing in all of them.

One-third of the parents (32 per cent) wanted transport to and from social activities; one-third said they would like contact with a social worker to help with problems; and one-quarter said they would like counselling for the teenager about any personal problems. Twelve parents made their own suggestions about how help could be organized for the parents of handicapped teenagers after they have left school, generally to do with more assistance and advice on careers and from the social services. (Someone to 'put us in the picture', 'take it off our shoulders', 'someone to guide us and tell us what is available'.) Some made specific suggestions: 'The careers officer should take teenagers to big firms to see what the possibilities are.' They complained that 'no one involved the parents' and that there was 'no follow up by his school, they simply made suggestions but did not pursue them'. Other suggestions concerned the social services or social workers. They complained that 'the social services are not good enough . . . you need to know what you're entitled to . . . maybe the school should tell you when you leave'. They wanted to know more about both monetary benefits and allowances, and assistance with such matters as transport. One parent summed it up: 'You should have somewhere, for example the social services, or some person who could tell you what you could do, what benefits you can get, where to go to get things. For example, many handicapped children are entitled to mobility allowance and don't know it.' Another said, 'You need someone you can always contact, social workers are always leaving and changing'.

This idea, in fact, is very similar to the Warnock Report's 'named person' proposal. This recommendation was that when a disabled teenager left school they should have one 'named person' who would be responsible for helping them with all problems – social and occupational – to give them advice on which service or which professional to approach for help, and to have as a single point of contact during the transition from school to adult life. Warnock recommended that for young people with special needs the careers officer or specialist careers officer should act as the 'named person'. When we asked the parents and the teenagers in our follow-up group what they thought about this idea, they were overwhelmingly in favour of it (only one parent and three teenagers felt that they did not need this). They felt that the continuity of a single person who could advise them on all matters, or act as a support during this time of change, would be extremely helpful.

## Summary and recommendations

From the evidence of the teenagers that we followed up after leaving school and the schools that we interviewed it is obvious that the facilities for vocational training, as well as opportunities for satisfactory alternatives to work, are inadequate at present. At the time of writing it is difficult for many school leavers, handicapped and able-bodied, to find satisfactory placements. While we cannot effect a change in the economic and political climate, we would re-emphasize the obligation on both schools and careers services to provide good advice, guidance and preparations before leaving school, whatever the teenager's position will be after leaving. What is equally important is support for the teenager once he has actually left school.

The findings of this study indicate that good guidance about the existing possibilities of placements is sadly lacking. While there has been much improvement in recent years, the vocational guidance arrangements for handicapped school leavers still leave much to be desired. What is needed is information and advice on all the possibilities, with preparation for school leaving starting as early as possible. Only by encouraging teenagers to make realistic decisions about the future will they be able to make a satisfactory adjustment to life later.

As we have shown, neither ordinary nor special schools prepare the handicapped for school leaving adequately. None of the ordinary schools we visited had a designated member of staff to take responsibility for handicapped pupils and give them extra support if this was needed, although most had a careers teacher, while most special schools did not even have a teacher responsible for careers. This might not necessarily be a problem if a member of staff has a good relationship with the careers service, which bears the ultimate responsibility for careers guidance. However, vocational guidance is not everything, and special schools still need to concentrate much more on preparing teenagers in general for life after school. We have also shown that special schools rarely set aside periods for careers education and this needs improvement since, while individual guidance can be handled informally, teenagers should also learn about the different aspects of work in order to get a realistic view of the world around them. In addition, special schools should not rely entirely on the careers service to provide advice, since the teenagers may need support from the school staff with whom they have built up a relationship over many years. Furthermore, as shown in chapter 7, many of the teenagers in our follow-up group did not receive sufficient or relevant advice or support from their allotted careers officer. Unfortunately, while a good careers officer can be invaluable, some of the experiences of the teenagers show that many do not provide a good service. In both special and ordinary schools, there seems to be a need to build up a relationship with the careers officer at an earlier age.

Many of the special schools or the careers officers referred the cerebral-palsied pupils to the Spastics Society for assessment. While some of the teenagers and their parents complained about these courses, it must be said that this service does provide an opportunity for assessment which is more thorough than that offered by the schools themselves, and that the lack of a similar service was certainly felt by the spina bifida teenagers. However, many of the teenagers in the study did not know about the Spastics Society assessment, and were not referred to it by their school. In general, the schools did not make very much use of professionals from outside, for example, the Schools' Psychological Service (for assessment or vocational guidance purposes) (SPS), the voluntary societies or medical personnel.

Greater co-operation and liaison with establishments of further education also need to be developed. The ordinary schools in our survey provided numerous linked courses with colleges of further education, but few special schools had similar contacts with either colleges or ordinary schools. Special schools should encourage this as far as possible because not only does it provide an invaluable social experience for the handicapped teenagers, it also gives them a broader insight into the range of options open to them when they leave school. Judging from our study few of the special schools had established formal liaisons with further education colleges, even to take pupils on visits to colleges. As we pointed out in chapter 7, some of the teenagers in the follow-up study who were not satisfactorily placed since they left school could have benefited from further education, and many of the teenagers were not aware of the range of opportunities open to them in further education.

A high proportion of the teenagers and their parents were dissatisfied with the amount of information they were given about what they might do when they left school. Many teenagers asked us, in desperation, what they could do and who they could turn to for help, and when asked what improvements in services might be made many mentioned the need for more information about what they could do after leaving school. The parents similarly wanted more information about the alternatives.

Leaving school is a period of great stress both for the teenagers and their parents and they were very worried. One idea we mentioned earlier, which seems to be overlooked by the special schools, is arranging parents' meetings where parents can talk to each other and members of the staff about their worries and seek some support.

What is desperately needed for all handicapped school leavers is a better system of support during the changeover period after leaving school. Very few of the schools followed up their ex-pupils, while one-third of the teenagers were not seen by their careers officers after leaving school. In fact, one-quarter of those interviewed had seen no one in the year following school. This is not necessarily a criticism of the personnel at present providing services but an indication that the service at present is not organized in such a way as to ensure an adequate follow up of leavers.

Clearly, contact should be initiated after leaving school, even if a placement has been found, to make sure that this has worked out satisfactorily and to deal with any problems that arise. Pupils returning home from colleges of further education also need to be supported in their efforts to gain recognition and to make social contacts. This study emphasizes the need for a 'named person' to be responsible for the handicapped teenager in the year after leaving school, as recommended in the Warnock Report. Parents and teenagers alike were enthusiastic about this idea.

# 12

*Coping with disability: theoretical issues and findings on the role of the family and other informal resources*

Research concerning psychological problems and stress, as well as considering the incidence and nature of the problems, must also attempt to disentangle the factors determining why one individual succumbs to stress when others, apparently equally at risk, cope successfully. Examples of four very different studies which attempt to do this are the Brown and Harris study of the social origins of depression in women (1978); Hewett's study of families with cerebral-palsied children (1970); Burton's *Family Life of Sick Children* (1975); and Cohen and Taylor's study (1972) of long-stay prisoners in a maximum security prison. These studies are all concerned, to some extent, with the reactions of the subjects to major life stresses. In all of them, as in this study, the question arises as to what it is that enables some families or individuals to cope better than others. However, as Brown and Harris state, the honest answer is that we just do not know, and the issue of coping 'remains to be explored adequately'.

Our own study was designed, as most others have been, to focus on the problems of the young people rather than on their coping strategies. The main reason for this emphasis was that so little work has been done on the problems of congenitally disabled adolescents that it was considered only logical to start by establishing the nature and extent of their problems. Nevertheless, we did not entirely neglect the question of coping which was explored in both phases of the study. We shall now look at some of the theoretical issues involved, and in doing so focus on two major questions: first, what is meant by 'coping'; and second, what ideas have been put forward about the ways in which people do cope? As in chapter 8, particular attention has been paid to the theories and models put forward by Lazarus (1966) on stress, by Adams *et al.* (1976) on coping with transition, and by Brown and Harris (1976) on the social origins of depression.

Mattson (1972), in considering children with a chronic illness, looks on successful coping as 'adaptation' or 'effective functioning' in the home, in relation to peers, and in school (or presumably, for those who have left school, at the place of work or its equivalent). The criteria for 'effective functioning' he suggests include age-appropriate dependence on the family, little need for secondary gain from the illness, acceptance of both limitations and responsibilities imposed by the illness, and the ability to find satisfaction in 'a variety of compensatory activities and intellectual pursuits'. He also suggests that 'cognitive flexibility, the appropriate release and control of emotions and the adaptive use of psychological defenses . . . are components in successful adaptation' (quoted in Pless and Pinkerton, 1975).

Burton (1975) considers coping strategies, although she never clearly defines criteria for coping. Coping parents are, it is implied, those who 'surmount the many anxieties and stresses which beset them', and are therefore able to 'function effectively as parents'. In her judgement,

> Despite all the personal distress attendant on their child's handicap, most parents function effectively, curbing their own more negative emotions, mobilizing hope and maintaining a sense of personal worth. Feelings of resentment, depression, isolation and discouragement are rarely allowed to predominate. Rather the reverse. Where they exist, they are usually kept firmly in check.

The most relevant part of the Brown and Harris study to a discussion on coping are their findings on 'vulnerability factors' and their obverse 'protective factors'. They found four main factors which made a woman more likely to break down in the presence of a severe life event or major difficulty, these being absence of a confiding relationship, the presence at home of three or more children under the age of fourteen, loss of her own mother before the age of eleven, and the lack of a full- or part-time job. None of these factors was capable of producing depression, but each increased its risk in the presence of a provoking agent. What the authors call 'protective factors' are simply the reverse of these – women are less likely to become depressed if they do have an intimate, confiding relationship with someone (especially a husband or boyfriend), if they have a full- or part-time job, if they have not lost their mother before eleven, and if they do not have three or more children under the age of fourteen. The question of personality factors is not one about which they collected evidence. All they have to say about this is that 'if they play a role, it is probably substantially related to a dimension of optimism–pessimism'.

The authors suggest that the common feature behind this collection of vulnerability factors is low self-esteem (other almost interchangeable terms which they suggest are low self-worth, a poor sense of mastery, and, a term used by many of the women themselves, 'lack of self-confidence'). However they point out – and this is again very relevant in the case of some severely disabled youngsters – that 'an appraisal of hopelessness is often entirely realistic, the future for many women *is* bleak. But given a particular loss or disappointment, ongoing low self-esteem will increase the chance of a general appraisal of hopelessness'.

It should be clear by now that many disabled young people are likely to be very vulnerable. First, as we showed in chapter 5, they already have low self-esteem (or lack of self-confidence). Secondly, after leaving school many will not have the 'protection' (to self-esteem) of a full- or part-time job, while the alternatives – day or work centre placements – may, completely understandably, not be perceived as worthwhile. Thirdly, they are less likely to have the protection of the sort of intimate confiding relationship with a close friend of the same or the opposite sex which the majority of other adolescents and young people either currently enjoy, or anticipate having in the future. Both these factors are likely to be of considerable importance in influencing whether or not a young person will cope.

The existence of a close confiding relationship with somebody, even if this is not a boyfriend, is likely to be critical according to Brown and Harris's findings. 'Such a relationship is likely to provide some women with a basic sense of self-worth. [But] it also has its more active aspect. The availability of a confidant, a person to whom one can reveal one's weaknesses without risk of rebuff and thus further loss of self-esteem may act as a buttress against the total evaporation of feelings of self-worth following a major loss or disappointment. Furthermore, the ability to talk to someone about one's feelings is a safeguard against some sort of blanket defence mechanism of denial preventing the working through of grief.' The second extremely important factor is whether it is possible to obtain a job or, if this is not desired or possible, an alternative which is *perceived* as acceptable and worthwhile.

While Brown and Harris concentrated on provoking agents and vulnerability factors rather than on coping factors, Lazarus (1966) pays much more attention to coping in his theoretical model. Once a particular situation (for example, the possibility of obtaining a job or finding a boyfriend) has been perceived as a threat, and therefore potentially stressful, the coping processes come into play. Lazarus has attempted to classify the main coping strategies employed by an individual. Some are adaptive and some maladaptive, some will be expressed in direct action and others in inaction. Direct action can include adaptations in behaviour aimed at strengthening the individual's resources – 'attack' (either directly expressed anger which may or may not be adaptive, or anger felt but not expressed), or avoidance of the situation. Coping strategies other than direct action may include inaction or apathy, anxiety reactions, or a reappraisal of the situation (defensive reappraisal) which may be adaptive or maladaptive. For example, a mildly or moderately handicapped teenager who has been highly self-conscious about his hemiplegia for many years might for various reasons (for instance after counselling) 'reappraise' the situation and decide that there is no reason why his disability should make his life essentially any different from that of his peers. He may then act accordingly. This reappraisal may be entirely appropriate. On the other hand he might 'reappraise' by developing inappropriate fantasies about his future, for example, that he will one day be 'cured'.

Adams *et al.* (1976) regard coping as something essentially active. In their chapter on 'human coping processes' they describe coping as 'a series of control activities where a person is attempting to exert influence in such a manner that his various requirements are catered for'. Later they state that 'fairly common criteria for evaluating a person's control activities . . . include . . . whether a person exhibits appropriate types and intensities of emotional arousal, whether he can establish and maintain social relationships and whether he can earn a living by approved methods'. (For young people unable to find work because of disability, the third criterion might be replaced by whether a person can find a way of living without work which has significance for him.)

These authors discuss coping strategies for the effective management of stress which are useful to consider in relation to the young people in our study. One strategy they label 'cognitive shielding' by which they mean controlling the amount of stressful stimulation by disregarding certain stimuli according to some priority scheme – for example by delaying decisions, making rapid and so less thoughtful decisions, or by 'temporary drop-out' (that is, deliberately refusing to make a decision until after a recuperation period). A second strategy is the creation of a personal stability zone, so that there is always someone, somewhere or something to fall back on in time of stress. (This may be one factor underlying some disabled teenager's dislike of even minor physical changes such as the arrangement of the furniture in the home.) A third strategy is situational grouping, that is, meeting for discussion with other people experiencing similar transitions, the purpose of the grouping being to work together on the problems and the opportunities for solution. Crisis counselling, that is, making use of interpersonal or of professional resources, is a fourth strategy, and links with Brown's findings on the importance of a confidant. A fifth strategy is 'anticipatory socialization' that is, the gradual adjustment to a new situation, for example not moving into one's first job or going to college until one has first read about it, visited it, met others who work there and so on. A sixth strategy is for the person to be able to make use of appropriate support systems. This might mean, in the case of a disabled teenager and his family, knowing exactly what statutory and professional support exist, and how best to utilize them.

We have already looked at some of the formal support systems available for the handicapped teenagers and their families (see chapters 10 and 11). However, we have said little directly about the informal resources available from family and friends and it is to these that we now turn.

## Resources available within the family

In this section we look at the ways in which the sibs and parents were providing support to the teenager, especially in their role as people in whom the teenagers could confide.

### Sibs as a source of support

In Phase I of the study the handicapped teenagers and their parents were asked a general question about their relationships with brothers and sisters (see Table 12.1) and then the teenagers were specifically asked about whether they confided in them. Only a small proportion of teenagers had marked difficulties in relationships with sibs, and on the whole the handicapped young people seemed to be on good terms with their brothers and sisters, rather better, if anything, than the controls. Only seven had severe difficulties in their relationships with sibs and there did not appear to be any correlation with severity of handicap.

Table 12.1 *Difficulties in relationship with sib(s) as reported by the teenagers*

| Difficulties | Handicapped | | Controls | |
|---|---|---|---|---|
| | N | (%) | N | (%) |
| None/only trivial | 79 | (80) | 19 | (63) |
| Slight | 15 | (24) | 10 | (33) |
| Marked | 7 | (4) | 1 | (3) |
| Total | 101 | (100) | 30 | (100) |

Those who had none or only trivial problems ranged from young people who made remarks to the effect that they got on as well as brothers and sisters usually do, or of the kind, 'all right . . . sometimes they get on my nerves', to those who were very positive: 'I think we get on very well. If we have an argument we're back to normal in five to ten minutes.' 'Whatever I say to my sister she won't split. She's not my special friend [but] she's my second best.' 'Smashing.'

Teenagers with slight difficulties included those who reported frequent arguments, or who just didn't consider the relationship very good. Here are a few examples: 'I get on better now [but] we argue a lot and she reckons I'm miserable.' 'The others talk too fast and shout at me' (athetoid girl with a marked speech defect). 'I don't get on with my sister. I think she's a bit of a snob. We don't actually quarrel.' 'My sister is always annoying me and we're not the best of friends.'

Only in a few cases did the problem appear to be very serious. A control girl said that she and her sister had constant arguments and fights, including actual fist fights. A cerebral-palsied girl in an ordinary school said she could talk to one of her sibs but she didn't get on with the other two at all, and 'hated' them. A mildly handicapped girl with many emotional problems became very upset indeed at this question; she thought her sister was 'getting at' her all the time. One boy had fights with his sister whom he said frequently got 'very angry' with him, and another had problems in his relationship with his younger sister whom he spoke of contemptuously, and described as constantly irritating him. One wheelchair-bound teenager reported a marked problem in getting on with her brothers, one of whom was mentally handicapped with behaviour problems, and whom the whole family found difficult to cope with.

The teenagers' reports of their relationships with their sibs were confirmed by what their parents said. Here are a few examples of close relationships: 'Chris [the sib] is very fond of him . . . he's the only one John could call a friend . . . it's extraordinary . . . Chris is not at all ashamed or embarrassed' (mother of a hemiplegic boy who was herself somewhat 'embarrassed'). A mother of another boy reported that 'Paul [the handicapped brother] is very orderly and Jim [the sib, two years younger] takes Paul's money and wears his clothes . . . they fight all the time, but they make it up quickly and are very close. Jim has insisted that he wants to look after Paul when we die.' A mother of a severely handicapped girl thought the girl's seventeen year old brother was 'marvellous . . . he'd lay down his life for Anne. For instance, last Monday he took her out with his friends to the pictures and to supper afterwards . . . they may squabble on the surface but deep down they're very close . . . he's not ashamed of her at all.' Later, she added that if Anne had any problems she'd take them to her brother first to discuss, and 'they'd sort it out'. A mother of an athetoid girl said that during the school holidays Mary shared the room with her three sisters. They never seemed to quarrel and 'won't be separated'. The very close relationship between the handicapped girl, the oldest in the family, and the sister next in age was quite clear to the interviewer from observation and discussion.

A smaller proportion of parents than of young people reported marked problems in relationships with sibs. Where problems did exist they seemed to be of four main kinds. One was when the handicapped teenager had marked behavioural or emotional problems which the sibs found difficult to cope with. For example, one mother felt that her teenage daughter, who had epilepsy, severe tantrums and often somewhat bizarre behaviour, simply didn't appreciate the efforts of the two younger sibs to help her. She said the sibs 'tried very hard', the younger sister would love to have her handicapped sister as a 'big sister', but the handicapped teenager was often unkind and inconsiderate and had to be handled by all the family 'with kid gloves'. A second type of problem was where family relationships in general were disturbed, this being reflected in relationships between the sibs. A third type mentioned was where the sibs resented the attention paid to the handicapped teenager. Finally, there were cases where the mother simply felt that the handicapped teenager and his or her sib(s) simply had very difficult personalities, and clashed because of this.

Although the great majority of disabled teenagers got on well with their brothers and sisters, and in fact spent more time with their sibs than did the controls (see chapter 3), most of the young people did not actually confide in them, and this was true for both the handicapped teenagers and the controls. Less than 10 per cent said that they had a close confiding relationship with one of their sibs, while only around 20 per cent confided in them occasionally. A rather higher proportion of girls than boys reported a close confiding relationship, but severity of handicap did not appear to be an important factor. However, the bond of affection described by the teenagers and the parents was often, in itself, a very effective support.

## Parents as a source of support

We have already looked at two aspects of the parent-teenager relationship – in chapter 5 parent-teenager alienation was considered, and the relationship between maternal anxiety and adjustment in the teenager. In this chapter we are much more concerned with the positive side of parent-teenager relationships. Although fathers were not totally neglected, we concentrated on mother-teenager relationships, since other studies (Baldwin, 1976; Wilkin, 1978) have shown that it is, to a great extent, the mother who shoulders the physical burden of caring for a handicapped child, and Philp, in his review of recent research (1978), comments that 'there is litle evidence of fathers radically altering their level of participation in domestic tasks as a result of the presence of a handicapped child'. As the findings presented in the next section will show, it is also the case that disabled teenagers rely predominantly on their mothers rather than their fathers for emotional support, and are much more likely to confide in them.

*Getting on with parents generally.* As a lead into the more detailed question about confiding in parents the teenagers were asked whether they thought they got on with their parents 'about as well as other teenagers', 'not as well as other teenagers', or 'better than other teenagers'. Very few teenagers (four with cerebral palsy, three with spina bifida and one control) thought that they got on worse with their parents than other teenagers did. Of the remainder, about half of those who were disabled said they got on 'about as well as others'. Compared with the disabled teenagers, a slightly lower proportion of controls said they got on better, but the differences were not marked. When asked which parent they got on with better a higher proportion, irrespective of sex, said that relations were better with their mothers. The proportions were similar (about 60 per cent) in both the handicapped and the control groups.

After these introductory questions the teenagers were asked in more detail about their relationships with their parents. This was a difficult area to probe, and it was our impression that many teenagers were very loyal to their parents, and more reluctant to talk freely about their relationships with them than about other issues raised in the interview. As we were particularly interested in whether the teenagers actually confided in their parents, this was asked specifically, and the results are shown in Table 12.2.

Table 12.2 *Relationship with mother according to teenager*

| Relationship | Handicapped N | (%) | Controls N | (%) |
|---|---|---|---|---|
| Poor* or dubious | 17 | (15) | 1 | (3) |
| Good, but doesn't usually confide | 29 | (25) | 12 | (38) |
| Close and confiding | 69 | (60) | 19 | (59) |
| Total | 115 | (100) | 32 | (100) |

* Only two handicapped teenagers had a definitely poor relationship. In the other cases the teenager appeared to have some not very clearly articulated reservations which led to the coding 'dubious'.

The proportion of teenagers who claimed that they confided most in their mothers was high and very similar (about 60 per cent) for both groups. However, more handicapped teenagers than controls described a relationship which was coded as poor or dubious. When sex was looked at as a variable, a slightly higher proportion of the control girls and of the cerebral-palsied girls said they had close confiding relationships, but no sex differences were apparent for those with spina bifida. Degree of handicap did not appear to be important, though there was a tendency for more of those with moderate or severe handicaps to be close to their mothers.

Here are some comments made by those whose relationships seemed to be poor or dubious: 'Things break out . . . we argue about my future. They [parents] can't see me doing anything when I leave school . . . it's only recently been like this. They're very good parents.' 'She doesn't have much sympathy [for me] . . . she favours others . . . for instance the dog . . . she just tolerates me.' 'She tries to help [but] I find it difficult to get on with her.' 'I don't talk to her much . . . I don't like her nagging, and not letting me go out.' (This boy had discussed his relationship with a school counsellor.)

A number of teenagers said that they had a good relationship with their mothers, but didn't usually confide in them. 'We get on very well . . . [but] I wouldn't [confide in] her or anyone else.' 'We're quite close . . . but I don't talk about my problems because she has enough of her own.' 'She understands me and I talk over school worries with her. But not other worries . . . I don't like my parents to worry . . . like if I'm ill, I won't tell them.'

However, as Table 12.2 shows, the majority of teenagers did claim to have a close confiding relationship with their mothers. Many made remarks like, 'Mum understands me', or said that they were 'very close', even though they might voice some criticism. 'She's like a big sister . . . I can talk to her about anything.' 'She understands everything . . . I talk to her all the time. She's my only friend' (cerebral-palsied girl with many emotional problems). 'I'm close to her . . . she annoys me sometimes but I'd talk to her about anything.' 'We talk about everything . . . I only get annoyed when she helps me a lot.' 'I'm really close to her . . . she really is a friend . . . understands most of my problems.'

The mothers' point of view was also obtained, the findings being fairly similar to those of the teenagers themselves. A number of mothers described the relationship as basically a good one but not really close; most saw this as a normal. However, rather more mothers of both controls and the disabled claimed to have a close relationship than did the teenagers themselves, especially where the teenager was handicapped. Conversely, where there was a handicap, fewer parents than teenagers reported any problem in their relationship (3 per cent compared with 15 per cent), but included the mother of a very mildly handicapped cerebral-palsied boy who said that he was constantly quarrelling, stirring things up and refusing to help her, and calling her names such as 'deaf old bag'. On the interviewer's visit to the home the situation was exactly as she had described it. (This was a family in which relationships generally were very disturbed.) Another mother reported that she and her daughter quarrelled the whole time when the daughter was at home in the holidays, while one mother said that things were so bad that she couldn't really be bothered to talk to her daughter and said that this was a 'horrible feeling' and that she felt 'very guilty' about it.

The great majority, however, thought that they had close relationships with their children, despite the disputes which sometimes occurred. 'We argue a lot but we're very close.' 'We've a very close relationship . . . I think J tells me everything that's worrying her . . . but there's also a lot of friction about looking after her [urinary] bag and her clothes.' 'I feel there's nothing she wouldn't tell me.' 'I think [our relationship] pretty marvellous.' 'We have our ups and downs, but if she's any problems she comes to me.' 'We get on very well indeed . . . we sit and have long chats together.' A few mothers spontaneously described the relationship as *too* close: 'We're very close . . . but I'm very protective, I know.' Even mothers of mildly handicapped children in ordinary schools sometimes admitted this. For example: 'We're very close and she's dependent

Table 12.3 *Whether teenager has discussed handicap with mother over past year*

| | Cerebral-palsied | | | | Spina bifida | | | |
|---|---|---|---|---|---|---|---|---|
| | Boys | | Girls | | Boys | | Girls | |
| | N | (%) | N | (%) | N | (%) | N | (%) |
| No | 28 | (60) | 16 | (42) | 7 | (64) | 4 | (21) |
| Yes, once or twice | 6 | (13) | 9 | (24) | 0 | (0) | 1 | (5) |
| Yes, more than twice | 13 | (28) | 13 | (34) | 4 | (36) | 14 | (77) |
| Total | 47 | (100) | 38 | (100) | 11 | (100) | 19 | (100) |

on me. It's not healthy.' 'We're very close . . . very good friends who do everything together . . . he needs to get away from me.'

The mothers were then specifically asked whether the teenager had, during the past year, discussed his or her handicap with them. The results are shown in Table 12.3. The group who had talked most to their mothers were the spina bifida girls, nearly three-quarters of whom had done so on more than two occasions, their problems over incontinence management making this almost inevitable. In general, girls seemed more likely than boys to discuss their handicap, as over 60 per cent of the boys had never done so over the past year. As expected the extent to which teenagers discussed their handicaps was related to the severity of their disability. Only 27 per cent of those who were mildly handicapped had talked with their mothers more than twice about their handicap over the past year, compared with over 40 per cent of those with moderate or severe handicaps, although as noted already many of those with mild handicaps did have worries about their disabilities.

Among the mothers who said that their teenagers had not discussed their handicaps with them over the past year, a few added comments to the effect that there were 'no problems', or 'it doesn't bother her', or that the teenager 'could talk openly about it but just takes it for granted'. Only a few made remarks such as 'he keeps it in' or 'he never talks about it' (implying that there *was* a problem needing discussion). Many mothers, therefore, appeared to be unaware of the extent to which the teenagers did worry about their handicap and their need to discuss this with someone.

Mothers who had talked to the teenagers about their handicaps were asked for details, including who had brought the subject up, and what they had discussed. In almost all instances mothers left it to the teenager to raise the subject. Especially in the case of those with spina bifida the problems discussed were often of a practical kind, for example management of a leaking urinary bag, bowel incontinence, bladder infections, or finding shoes and clothes which fitted but were also fashionable. Much less frequently the teenager's long-term future was discussed, for example whether he or she would ever find a boy- or girlfriend, and what life had to offer them. Here are a few examples: 'We're very open . . . we discuss how he feels about being handicapped and about his being teased' (mildly handicapped boy in an ordinary school). '[She discussed her handicap] when we were out recently . . . talked about other girls and their clothes . . . she gets upset because she doesn't look attractive.' 'She's started . . . since she's been looking for work: she says, "if I wasn't like this I could get a job".' Three mothers of deaf boys reported that their sons had, during the past year, asked for the first time about why they were handicapped. '[We've discussed it] in a very limited way. When I was trying to explain to him that he'd soon be going to hospital for an operation on his nose he made gestures to his ears and legs . . . he seemed to want something done about them too. But when I told him nothing could be done about them he just shrugged his shoulders and went out. He didn't seem very upset.'

Mothers who did talk to their teenage children about their handicap were asked whether they could do this quite easily, or whether they found it quite difficult. Most said that they could discuss the handicap quite freely and only a few mothers admitted that they found it difficult. One said that she still hadn't fully accepted her daughter's handicap and felt very strongly that she need never have been handicapped if she had had better pre-natal care. Another, coping alone extremely well with a very severely handicapped son, still felt 'underneath' that it was her fault that her son was handicapped, and this was why she didn't like discussing it with him, especially as he found it very difficult to accept. A mother of a cerebral-palsied boy who attended an ordinary school and identified strongly with his non-handicapped peers said that her son found it difficult to talk about his condition. He had done so when he was younger but now never brought up the subject.

Those mothers who were able to talk to their sons and daughters about their handicaps clearly have an extremely important counselling role to play, especially as they were often the only person in whom the teenagers confided. However, most teenagers, especially the boys, did not appear to feel it possible or appropriate to discuss their handicaps with their parents, or spoke with them about practical problems only.

*Relationship with the father.* The teenagers were also asked about their relationship with their fathers. Although the majority reported that they had a good relationship with their fathers, a substantial minority (about one-quarter of the disabled teenagers and 14 per cent of the controls) had a relationship which was coded as poor or dubious (see Table 12.4). More disabled than control group teenagers seemed likely to have problems in getting on with their fathers, but it was also true that a higher proportion of disabled than of control group teenagers said that they actually confided in their fathers, this being more likely for disabled boys than girls.

Table 12.4 *Relationship with father – teenagers' report*

| Relationship | Handicapped | | Controls | |
| --- | --- | --- | --- | --- |
| | N | (%) | N | (%) |
| Poor or dubious | 27 | (27) | 4 | (14) |
| Good but doesn't usually confide | 35 | (35) | 20 | (69) |
| Close and confiding | 37 | (38) | 5 | (17) |
| Total | 100 | (100) | 29 | (100) |

Although few teenagers seemed to have very poor relationships with their fathers, there were quite a large number whose relationship with their father was not at all helpful. Here are a few of the comments: 'I don't get on particularly well with him . . . he's not the sort of person you can talk to . . . he's interested in electrical things . . . he doesn't understand me so much.' 'I don't find him sympathetic to talk to . . . he'd laugh [if confided in].' Some of the girls either felt that fathers did not understand them, or said that they were frightened of them: 'He does talk to me about my handicap, but not in the same way as Mum . . . he says things like "Don't worry, everything will turn out all right in the end." He's got a bad temper and that frightens me. He never hits me, but he hits my brothers and sisters.' 'I don't see him a lot . . . he's at work or in the garden. I don't really know him, and I'm not sure if he understands me.' (Girl attending residential school.) 'We get on quite well, but I'm frightened of him. He never goes for me but he goes for my sister.'

Many teenagers – both those who were disabled and those in the control group – had a basically good relationship with their fathers but did not feel very close to them. 'I don't feel I could tell him as much as Mum. I want to, but I don't think I could.' 'At my age it's natural to talk more with my Mum.' 'I don't confide in him but we get on well. Mum's more interested in me.' (Spina bifida girl whose father was very helpful in other ways, for example, arranging for adaptations to the house.)

Finally, here are some comments from the teenagers who did have a close relationship with their fathers: 'Most of the time he'll talk over my worries with me . . . I feel he understands me.' 'We get on well . . . better than with Mum. I can talk to him . . . especially about big problems.' 'We get on very well . . . he's calm, not cross . . . I can talk to him.' 'He's funny and cheers me up . . . if I have a row with Mum he doesn't get annoyed.'

## Resources available from outside the family

### Confiding in a special friend

It was believed that for this age group the opportunity to confide in a special friend might be a particularly helpful resource, and for this

Table 12.5 *Confiding in a special friend (findings from Phase I of the study)*

| | Handicapped | | Controls | |
| | N | (%) | N | (%) |
|---|---|---|---|---|
| No friend in whom to confide | 70 | (61) | 13 | (39) |
| Occasionally confides | 34 | (30) | 13 | (39) |
| Close confiding relationship | 11 | (9) | 7 | (21) |
| Total | 115 | (100) | 33 | (100) |

reason after being asked open-ended questions about what they did when feeling low the young people were asked whether, when they felt low or worried, they ever talked things over with a special friend. The results are given in Table 12.5, and show that a much higher proportion of the controls had a close friend in whom they could confide at least occasionally, compared with the handicapped teenagers. Whether or not a disabled teenager confided in a friend was unrelated to the type or the severity of his handicap, or the type of school attended. In the control group, girls were much more likely to confide in a friend than boys (33 per cent compared with 7 per cent), but no clear sex difference was found among the disabled teenagers. Overall, therefore, peers did not appear to provide a frequent source of support for handicapped teenagers when it came to discussing personal matters.

## Confiding in an adult outside the immediate family

The teenagers were also asked whether there were any adults (apart from their parents and school staff) or any relatives (apart from sibs) in whom they confided or talked over their worries with. A third of the teenagers in each group confided in some adult, but in most cases this was not on a regular basis and only twenty (about one-fifth) of the handicapped teenagers reported a close confiding relationship.

Several saw their grandmother every weekend and sometimes stayed with her. Aunts were also quite important as confidants. One boy, for instance, said there was one aunt of whom he was particularly fond. He saw her nearly every weekend and could tell her anything, for example what to do about his mother not allowing him as much independence as he thought he was capable of. Three teenagers had cousins who were a particularly close source of support. Other people confided in included a godmother, a 'social aunt', two house parents, a next-door neighbour, and a family friend. From the warmth with which the teenagers referred to these adults, it was clear that adults, other than parents, can be a very important potential source of support, especially when teenagers had problems which they did not necessarily want to discuss with their immediate family.

The reports of the parents were very similar indeed to those given by the teenagers themselves. Again, grandmothers, aunts and older cousins were frequently mentioned as confidants. 'She thinks the world of my aunt . . . she's like a grandmother to her.' 'She feels her grandfather [who was disabled] really understands her.' 'She talks to her grandmother . . . she doesn't want to worry me too much.' 'He's very close to his aunty E. who's a nursing sister.' 'He confides in his Dad's niece . . . she's twenty-six he'll talk to her about anything.' 'He confides in his grandmother . . . he's known her all his life. She's very outgoing, and he enjoys her company.' Occasionally teenagers confided in neighbours: 'He talks a lot with a neighbour . . . as man-to-man [though] I'm not sure how much he actually confides in him.' 'Mrs. C along the road . . . he told her he was thinking of ending it all . . . but he hasn't told me.'

## Confiding in adults at school

The teenagers were asked whether, during the past year, they had been to talk individually to any adult at their school about anything which had been worrying them or making them unhappy. Most of the controls (85 per cent), two-thirds of those with cerebral palsy, and half of those with spina bifida had not talked to anyone. If they had it was almost always a teacher. Only four handicapped teenagers and one control had talked to a school counsellor. Others to whom handicapped pupils had turned to occasionally included house parents, ancillary helpers, speech therapists, physiotherapists, the deputy head, a school doctor, a school secretary and the psychiatrist (in a school for maladjusted children). Some teenagers mentioned more than one person. The great majority had found these discussions definitely helpful.

From the point of view of staff training, the finding that one-quarter of the disabled pupils had talked to teachers and only 3 per cent to school counsellors is important, especially since, as we discussed in chapter 10, only one of the twenty-eight special schools and nine of the thirty-four ordinary schools actually had full- or part-time counsellors. Those in residential schools sometimes discussed their worries with house parents or helpers, and this too has implications for the formers' training. In terms of type of school attended, over 40 per cent of those in special schools said that they had talked over something which was worrying them with a member of the school staff during the past year, compared with one-third of handicapped pupils in ordinary schools (a difference less marked than was expected), and 15 per cent of controls.

The young people were asked (but not pressed) what they had discussed. Those who were willing to specify this referred to quite a wide range of problems. Several had discussed problems connected with family relationships, including getting on with their parents, getting their mothers to give them more independence, rows between parents and a bereavement. Others had discussed peer relationships, for example, getting on with other people, finding a girlfriend, coping with teasing (a handicapped and a control boy, both in ordinary schools, had been to see a school counsellor about this). Four handicapped pupils in ordinary schools had been to see a member of staff about particular aspects of their school work. All but one had found them helpful. Only four pupils mentioned discussing physical problems with members of staff. Three were spina bifida pupils who had discussed anxieties about whether they would be able to have a child, while the fourth teenager had discussed obesity and problems arising from an ileostomy.

When asked about the ways in which staff members had been helpful some pupils referred to the fact that they had been able to explain and give information about a problem that was worrying them, while others laid emphasis on the moral support they gained: 'just having someone to talk to.' 'It helped me to look at things in a different light.' 'I feel she [a housemother] is a friend. When I'm upset I feel calm with her.' The main finding was that where teenagers had gone to a member of staff with a problem they had almost always found this definitely helpful. This suggests a strong need for more systematic support of this kind to be made available. In the case of the spina bifida pupils in particular many more opportunities to talk are needed over their anxieties about their physical handicaps, and the implications of these for the future.

### Discussion groups

So far we have looked at the forms of support which non-disabled people can provide to teenagers. We were also interested in whether, by means of discussion groups, disabled young people might be mutually supportive about their problems. Consequently, the teenagers were asked whether they had ever taken part in a discussion group, and if so whether they had found this helpful. Only one-quarter of the cerebral-palsied group and one-fifth of the spina bifida group had done so. In nineteen cases the group had been organized by the school, and in eight cases by a body outside the school, including four courses run by the Spastics Society, three by clubs for the handicapped, and one as part of a PHAB holiday.

Of the twenty-seven teenagers who had taken part in such groups, only two said they had not found them helpful, while eighteen had found them definitely helpful and were most enthusiastic about them. 'We talk about our handicaps and you can see other people's ideas.' '[It helps because] others have the same problems as me.' 'I liked sitting around the table where we're all the same and you can talk without worrying.' 'You can express your feelings and everyone understands and feels the same.' 'We discussed all sorts of things . . . for instance, what your mother and father expect you to do [in this case very protective parents] I found it helpful; it brought it out so that I could talk about it and it wasn't just my problem. I could share it.'

Since so few people had actually had experience of such groups, we asked all the teenagers whether they thought it would be helpful if those with the same sort of handicap could meet together in small groups to discuss shared problems. The great majority (about 75 per cent of the girls and 62 per cent of the boys) thought this would definitely be useful, a small number were unsure, and only one-fifth thought they would not be helpful. It was anticipated that those who were only mildly handicapped might not want this kind of discussion, but this was not the case, the difference between them and the other groups being very small, and very similar proportions of disabled teenagers in ordinary (65 per cent) and special schools (73 per cent) thought such groups would definitely be helpful. This is in line with the findings of the Spastics Society (Carlile, 1979) who have found a great demand for their residential courses (which include discussion groups) for comparatively mildly disabled young people from ordinary schools.

Those teenagers who thought that group discussions would be helpful were asked about the sorts of things they would want to talk about. Their varied replies gave some very interesting insights into the questions with which disabled teenagers are most concerned. Some gave rather global answers, or answers covering a great many aspects of life, for example: 'How to get on in life with a handicap.' 'The same sorts of things *we've* been discussing [in the interview].' 'How I came to be handicapped.' 'How to get on in life, how you can be happy, and get a job, and settle down.' 'Jobs, college, boyfriends, growing up and having a family, and leading normal lives.' 'Family problems, health problems and sexual problems.'

Many teenagers (including, perhaps surprisingly, more girls than boys) specifically mentioned finding jobs and what they were going to do when they left school. These included mildly as well as moderately and severely handicapped young people. Many teenagers also mentioned topics related to their social lives, their friends, and their use of time outside school. The phrases 'how to get out and about', and 'what I can do outside school' were used by several teenagers. Some mentioned specific problems such as 'driving or practical things like that', or 'steps and wide doors', or 'getting to a place of work', but more were concerned with actually meeting people. For instance, one severely handicapped boy said he'd like to discuss 'how to get out of the house and visit friends', while a mildly handicapped girl in an ordinary school said 'how to get out and meet people'. Two cerebral-palsied boys attending ordinary schools wanted to find out what others with cerebral palsy did in their spare time.

A number of young people wanted to discuss personal relationships. Some mentioned family problems, and some boy- or girlfriends, while several young people said they would like to discuss relationships with able-bodied people, for example 'how other people react to handicapped people', or 'how to get more co-operation between the able-bodied and the handicapped so that able-bodied people can understand problems with handicaps'. 'Mixing with ordinary people . . . you might get left out otherwise.' One mildly handicapped boy in an ordinary school (who had attended a special school at primary level) said that he felt discussion groups should have both disabled and non-disabled people in them. He felt that 'children in special schools lead too sheltered an existence in their own circle. And it might benefit Joe Bloggs to be part of such a group . . . the Joe Bloggs of this world would be shattered to meet handicapped people.'

Several young people said they'd like to discuss their handicaps and their feelings about being handicapped: 'What's wrong with us, the way I feel and what worries me.' (Severely handicapped spina bifida girl.) 'Whether there's any chance of walking like normal.' 'How long I'll live.' (Severely handicapped spina bifida girl.) 'My feelings about being handicapped and the restrictions it places on you.' Two cerebral-palsied boys said that they would like the chance to discuss sex in a group with others who were handicapped.

### Contacts with disabled adults

One question which has never been systematically explored is whether it would be helpful for disabled teenagers to meet and/or know about disabled adults who are coping well with their disabilities. The teenagers were therefore asked whether they'd ever met or seen adults with 'the same sort of problem as yours'. Just under half (43 per cent) of the cerebral-palsied group and 60 per cent of those with spina bifida had done so. Ten young people mentioned television and radio programmes as their only source, but others had disabled neighbours or family friends. Several had had contact with disabled adults in institutions or clubs (e.g., PHAB, day centre and hospitals).

No attempt was made to go in detail into the depth or quality of the contact but the teenagers were asked how the contact had affected them, and whether they had found it helpful or depressing, or if it had really made no difference. Just under half had found the contact helpful, while only 12 per cent (seven teenagers) found it definitely depressing and the others had no strong feelings either way. On the whole, the teenagers were not very articulate about how the experience had affected them, but a few gave clear answers. A severely handicapped spina bifida boy, for example, had read about a married couple with spina bifida, and found it helpful to see 'how they manage'. A severely handicapped athetoid boy knew another spastic young man 'who lives round the corner and can't feed himself . . . has poor speech' and said that he felt it 'encouraging' to see how he coped. A diplegic girl who depended mainly on a wheelchair said that she had heard a programme about a woman paralysed from the waist down who was coping well, and had found this encouraging.

What really emerged from our very brief exploration of this issue was that disabled teenagers seldom made contact with disabled adults; if at all, it was by chance, and the contacts were often brief and superficial. There was some evidence that such contacts, if more carefully arranged, could be helpful, and this is something to which special schools (or other organizations for disabled young people) could well give much more careful thought. Certainly when asked about this directly in Phase II of the study, 65 per cent of the teenagers believed that it would be a good idea if disabled adults were invited to special schools to talk about their experiences and how they'd got on in life.

### The importance of a confidant in relation to emotional well-being

As young people begin to embark on adult life and start to face the difficulties of becoming independent and accepting more responsibility for themselves, the need for a confidant of some kind begins to be more important, and in Phase II we thought it would be useful to look at this in relation to the psychological adjustment ratings described in chapter 5.

About half the young people (48 per cent) said that they had a confiding relationship with their mothers, and half of these also named one or more other people in whom they could confide, at least occasionally. Only seven of the teenagers said that they regularly confided in a peer, although thirteen others did so from time to time (a total of 40 per cent), while over one-third mentioned a sib. Nearly 30 per cent spoke of some other adult – usually at their college or day centre – with whom they had been able to discuss some problem over the past year. Nonetheless, about one-third of the sample appeared to have no one at all, adult or peer, in whom they could confide.

The quality of the teenager's relationship with his or her mother appeared to be a most significant variable in relation to ratings of adjustment in that three-quarters of those who had a confiding relationship with their mothers were rated as 'satisfactory adjustment', while only one-fifth had 'marked problems'. Two of these were the young people who had changed their status from 'satisfactory adjustment' to 'marked problems' over the year as a consequence of having no placement, while two had over-close relationships with both their parents, and had little opportunity to mature because of this.

However, there was also some evidence to suggest that even if there wasn't a confiding relationship with the mother, having a peer, sib or other adult as a confidant offered some protection against emotional difficulties. In fact, those without a regular confidant of any kind were twice as likely to be rated as having 'marked problems' as those who confided in somebody on a fairly regular basis.

The importance of families, and mothers especially, in helping the young people to cope was emphasized again when we asked, at the end of the Phase II interview, who or what had helped the teenager most in coping over the previous year. Over 40 per cent mentioned their mother or their parents as being their main source of support, compared with 16 per cent who mentioned peers, and 26 per cent who spoke of an adult either in the statutory or voluntary services (usually the staff at their college or training centre). However, four teenagers (9 per cent) said no one at all had helped them, and that they had had to rely entirely on themselves. One said, 'I learnt a lot of lessons this year . . . things don't always work out well', while another, in spite of some support from his family, said, 'It's yourself really – it's really a matter of pushing yourself through the hard bits'.

*Inner resources*

So far we have considered the coping resources available to the teenagers in terms of other people in whom they could confide and who could offer them either practical advice or at least an outlet for expressing their feelings and regular moral support. Much more difficult to explore are the other sorts of resource available within the teenager himself, which might be broadly described as 'inner resources'. One factor which we would have liked to look at, but which proved too difficult to measure, was personality. In planning the study, we considered using 'personality tests' but none seemed particularly useful for our purposes. Thus all we can really do here is to emphasize that although 'personality' was a variable we could not measure, it is certainly of great importance.

However, we did attempt to look briefly at three other aspects of 'inner resources'. First, we asked the teenagers what action, if any, he or she took when low, and whether this was helpful. Secondly, we examined the data to see whether there was any association between coping (defined as 'satisfactory adjustment' as rated in chapter 5), and two other factors, one being whether or not the teenager had an absorbing interest or hobby, and the other whether he or she was interested in their school work, or if they had definite plans for the future.

*Teenagers' description of ways of coping when 'feeling low'.*   Towards the end of the interview in Phase I of the study all the teenagers were asked: 'We've talked about a lot of things which often affect teenagers – like being lonely or depressed or worried and so on. When you feel that things are getting you down, is there anything you usually do to make yourself feel better?' The findings were very similar irrespective of whether or not the teenager was handicapped, the type of school he attended, and the type of handicap. Many said that they found it best to talk things over with someone. 'I talk to my boyfriend.' 'I ring Mum' (girl at boarding school). 'I ring a friend.' A number of teenagers mentioned an adult whom they found it helpful to talk to. 'If it's something that really bothers me I go to one of my parents and talk it over with them and they help me to sort it out.' 'I 'phone up the next-door neighbour.' 'I have a cry with Mum, talk to her, and go to bed early.' Another very popular way of coping which all teenagers made use of was listening to records, often alone in their rooms, while two kept diaries and two others (one exceptionally able and one of below average ability) did creative writing. Reading, radio and television were seldom mentioned as helpful. Teenagers from all three groups sometimes mentioned the need to be by themselves to think through problems when they were worried or depressed. 'I just go and sit by myself . . . it does help . . . I know it sounds daft, but it does.' 'I've taken up exercises, and I sit and meditate' (control girl). 'I go up to my room and stay there for a long time. I might read or play the record player and that would cheer me up.' The general theme which came from the teenagers' descriptions, and was often stated explicitly, was the need to do something to occupy themselves and to take their minds off their problems; it was only a minority who sat down and tried to think them through.

A significant group, however, had not been able to find effective ways of coping with worries and depression. As one boy who was severely handicapped by cerebral palsy and had had long periods of hospitalization put it, 'I go out when I can [in his wheelchair] but when the weather's bad I usually take it out on Mum . . . it was especially [bad] in hospital . . . that's really fed up, that was [sic] I read, but that's not much good . . . and listen to the radio, but *I've had enough of that radio*.' One function of discussion groups could certainly be to help teenagers exchange ideas with one another about ways of coping when life was particularly difficult.

*Interests and hobbies.*   In chapter 3 the young people's interests were described. We compared those who had an interest or hobby (over 60 per cent of the controls and over 40 per cent of the disabled teenagers) and those who didn't have one to see whether there were any differences in their overall psychological adjustment. We found that disabled teenagers with interests were slightly more likely than those without to be well adjusted, but the difference was very small indeed. However, this is perhaps because few handicapped teenagers appeared to have a really absorbing interest which might protect them from depression.

*Definite interest in school work.*   We also compared those who had expressed a definite interest in their school work (27 per cent of the controls, and 18 per cent of the disabled teenagers) with those who had not, again in terms of their overall adjustment. This did not mean simply those who were examination candidates, but perhaps inevitably it was the more able pupils who were more likely to be interested in school work. In the handicapped group a much higher proportion (almost double) of those who were interested in their school work were well adjusted than those (the majority) who had expressed no definite interest, while twice as high a proportion of those who were not very interested as of those who were fell into the group with marked problems (36 per cent compared with 18 per cent); but this is probably related to the association between adjustment and IQ (see chapter 6). This difference was also true when the cerebral-palsied and spina bifida young people were considered separately. Only three of the spina bifida teenagers (10 per cent) expressed a real interest in their school work, and all three were well adjusted. In the cerebral-palsied group about one-fifth had a real interest in school work, nearly three-quarters of whom were well adjusted compared with only 43 per cent of those with no such interest. In the control group the numbers with a real interest (only nine) were so small that the findings are not very reliable.

*Definite plans for the future to which teenager is looking forward.* Another 'resource' which we considered might affect the teenagers' ability to cope was whether they had definite plans for the future which they were looking forward to. The findings here were very similar to those for an interest in school work. The minority (only one-fifth of the whole sample) who *did* have definite plans for the future were a much better adjusted group than those who did not; this being equally true for those with cerebral palsy and spina bifida. Seventeen per cent of each diagnostic group had definite plans for the future, the great majority of them (73 per cent of those with cerebral palsy and 80 per cent of those with spina bifida) being well adjusted. Comparable figures for adjustment in those with no definite plans was about 40 per cent in both diagnostic groups. However, again the factor of difference in ability level makes this result difficult to interpret.

## Summary

The evidence we have gathered suggests that while some teenagers found much support from their families (especially their mothers, but also from sibs and other relatives) it was by no means the case that close confiding relationships were available to all the teenagers from within the family circle. It appeared that a confiding relationship with a parent did act as a protective factor to depression, except in the case of severe difficulties, and also that where this was lacking, a confiding relationship with some other adult or peer had the same protective effect. However, compared with the control group, the handicapped teenagers were much less likely to have a close relationship with a peer, and about one-third of the sample in Phase II had no one at all in whom they could confide.

Whenever the teenager had approached a member of staff for advice or discussion this had been seen to be very helpful, but it didn't appear to be a common pattern for this kind of relationship to be regularly sought. This was especially regrettable since so few teenagers found their parents to be a source of advice for anything other than purely practical matters. Very few ever discussed issues to do with the handicap itself with parents or with their peers.

When they were asked if they would like the opportunity to have group discussions of mutual problems with their handicapped peers, the majority of teenagers were very keen to do so. Again, few had actually had experience of this but those who had were enthusiastic about the benefits. Another idea which the teenagers responded to positively was the opportunity to make contact with disabled adults, discuss problems with them and to find out how they had managed to cope with the difficulties the teenagers were currently facing.

Whether or not the teenagers had a keen interest in school work or had definite plans for the future were also important factors in protecting them from depression (although these things were probably not independent of intelligence which has frequently been shown to relate to coping skills).

We believe it is useful to view many, and probably the majority, of disabled teenagers as being in a situation which is currently stressful and which has the potential for becoming even more stressful once they leave school, becoming at worst a 'severe life event' of the kind described by Brown and Harris, or at best confronting them with the necessity (which may be postponed for several years after leaving school) for making a stressful 'transition', as defined by Adams *et al*. A major aim of those working with these young people and their families, therefore, should be to take action (preventative where possible) to help them to cope with these stresses, particularly with their social relationships, and also to help them see themselves as self-respecting adult members of society, regardless of whether or not they have paid jobs.

The theoretical models and the research discussed earlier in this chapter suggest at least some strategies by which people do cope. These include (i) developing a close confiding relationship with someone; (ii) having some practice in controlling at least some aspects of one's own environment and thus gaining a sense of mastery (rather than simply playing a passive, dependent role); (iii) having some experience of success, with a consequent development of self-esteem; (iv) having, especially in a period of stress, someone or something in one's life which has personal meaning and significance, and which one knows will remain stable; (v) having the opportunity to discuss the stressful or potentially stressful situation with others facing similar difficulties, and possibly, in addition, having available an adult other than a close relative who can provide advice and support; (vi) having the knowledge of where to go for 'support' to which one is entitled; (vii) and this applies particularly to those who have left school, having the opportunity to engage in activities outside the home which, in some way, confirm the young person's sense of identity as an adult or as someone who is preparing him or herself to be an adult member of society; (viii) finally, having the opportunity to develop 'inner resources'. These will include not only relevant personality traits but, especially important in the case of young people, the development of genuine interests, which may either lead to a job or make leisure time more fulfilling.

# 13
## *Conclusions and recommendations*

This study attempted to survey all young people in the relevant age group with cerebral palsy or spina bifida accompanied by hydrocephalus, living in a defined geographical area. Since between a half and two-thirds of all physically handicapped children suffer from one of these conditions, the problems presented by our sample may be regarded as fairly typical of handicapped young people in general.

The study showed that a very high proportion of the sample had severe and multiple handicaps, complicated further in a substantial number of cases by marked learning difficulties.* We are no longer dealing, as in earlier days when conditions such as poliomyelitis were the most common causes of handicap, with young people whose main problem is a simple locomotor dysfunction and whose intellectual abilities are normal. Although this fact has been recognized in the literature and in government documents for some years, it is clear that the school and post-school services are not yet organized in ways which focus on this reality, accepting it as a central and continuing trend, with the clear implication that open employment will not be available for the majority of school leavers; nor that social outlets will be readily accessible without special intervention of some kind. It is essential that those providing services, both field workers and administrators, recognize these basic facts and devise services accordingly.

In common with other studies of young people with similar handicaps, we showed a very high incidence of psychological problems – three to four times as high as among the controls – and in particular depression, anxiety, lack of self-confidence and fearfulness. Those who were most handicapped were most at risk, but these difficulties were by no means uncommon even in teenagers whose handicaps were relatively mild. Again, there was little evidence that those responsible for providing services had fully recognized the extent of the distress which we encountered, or were aware of the young people's need for help. It is important to remember however that over half of the young people, even among the most handicapped, showed no overt psychological problems, and it is crucial that we discover more about what protects these young people.

* Indeed in that we deliberately excluded (for technical reasons) young people of very low ability (IQs estimated to be below 70) our study does not fully reveal the extent of learning difficulties coupled with physical handicap to be found in a representative population.

## Schooling

A third of the sample were being educated in ordinary schools, and this group were on the whole less physically handicapped and more able, although there was a considerable overlap in degree of handicap and levels of ability between those in ordinary and those in special schools. The teenagers in special schools tended to be in all-age schools, which were usually very small, and about half those in special schools had attended the same school from the primary level.

Most teenagers were said to be happy in school regardless of placement, but while all the young people attending ordinary schools said that they preferred this placement to a special school, one-quarter of those in special schools said that they would have preferred an ordinary school. When asked for their preference 'as far as friends are concerned' an even higher proportion of those in special schools (over 60 per cent) opted for an ordinary school. Most expressed a preference for an ordinary school which other handicapped pupils also attended, rather than a situation where they would be the only disabled pupil. In the main, the parents also expressed satisfaction with whichever type of school their child attended, but although appreciating the special facilities available in physically handicapped schools, many complained about low academic standards, and thought that their children did not receive adequate stimulation.

These findings suggest that there should be a wider choice of schools available for handicapped teenagers, including more special units in ordinary schools, which could offer a wider choice of curricula and general stimulation, and help the handicapped to make contact with the able-bodied, while providing whatever special services and support are needed. At the very least, education authorities should ensure that special school pupils attend at least some classes within the ordinary schools, and have the opportunity to meet with their able-bodied peers.

## Independence, helplessness and depression

Parents saw the majority of the teenagers as striving for independence despite the fact that we showed a very high level of dependence in the basic self-care skills. To some extent differences in degree of independence were related to level of handicap, but this did not entirely account for the differences. The teenagers usually claimed that they wanted to be more independent and often thought that they could have achieved more if their parents had allowed this, something the parents often conceded themselves. The physical conditions within the home were also of importance in determining how much independence the young person could achieve. In terms of helping in the home and the exercise of choice, again there were wide differences, but some very handicapped young people were contributing to the running of the household and exercising a degree of personal choice and responsibility. It was apparent that many could and should have been doing more in this respect.

It seems clear that more attention should be given to helping young handicapped people to gain self-sufficiency. This could be achieved if the necessary home adaptations were provided (often only simple and inexpensive measures were needed) and if parents were helped to realize the importance of giving their child more independence, responsibility and freedom of choice, and were involved in programmes to achieve this. Incontinence management was a particularly difficult area where much more help was needed if the young people were to become fully competent.

It became obvious that not only the parents but also schools and medical services failed to encourage independence. Our study revealed an appalling level of ignorance among the teenagers about the nature and cause of their handicaps – indeed over half of those with cerebral palsy did not even know the name of their condition. Their main source of information had been their parents, and though most wanted to know more, this information was not provided for them within their schools or hospital clinics as a basic right. Their knowledge about the services and allowances they were entitled to was also very poor, and many had no clear idea where they should go to get more information, and this did not seem to be part of the school curriculum. Again, in relation to their ignorance about the facts of life, contraception, the likelihood of producing a handicapped child and their capacity for a sexual life, our interviews demonstrated a need to provide this kind of information in schools and colleges. Very few of the handicapped pupils had ever discussed their fears and doubts about these issues with anyone else (including their peers), although they were eager for knowledge.

A message that came through very clearly from teenagers especially (but also from parents) was their general feeling of lack of control over their own lives and in particular in their choice of college or other post-school placement. Because insufficient time had been spent discussing the possible options with them and the reasons why a particular college or centre was being recommended, they felt that they had taken no part in the decision making and were being treated as problem objects to be 'placed'. This was true even when the parent and the teenager were quite satisfied with the placement recommended, or when the choices were so limited that only one decision was possible. The teenagers greatly resented the implication that their views and their contributions to the debate were not considered important, and they described feelings of impotence and vulnerability. Within their colleges, and more especially in day centres, once more the young people were frequently not involved in decisions about curriculum content or choice of activity, which again they found frustrating and demoralizing. Their often perfectly sound ideas about appropriate activities went unheeded, while unexplored ambitions in terms of jobs or training assumed the status of minor obsessions, paralysing further action. It appeared that the professionals continually underestimated the teenagers' ability to enter into a reasoned appraisal of the options or lack of them. Certainly they showed themselves to be well capable of discussing these issues with us in a realistic way, and of being surprisingly articulate and perceptive about their situation, even including those rated by their teachers to be quite low in ability.

Where they saw that opportunities were given them for increasing independence skills and freedom of choice, as happened in the best of the residential colleges and in one day centre which encouraged client participation, the young people were very appreciative and very quick to respond. Where this happened the parents were also ready to acknowledge the benefits in terms of greater maturity and satisfaction with the placement.

The importance of ensuring greater independence, knowledge about the handicap and the services available, and greater involvement in decision making, is not simply because these things are important in themselves, but because they affect the teenager's general level of maturity and self-confidence and whether he feels in control of his own life.

In Seligman's book *Helplessness* (1975), he emphasizes the importance of ensuring that any individual feels a sense of mastery over his own fate. 'Helplessness', states Seligman, 'is the psychological state that frequently results when events are uncontrollable' when the individual finds that 'an outcome occurs independently of all his voluntary responses'. He cites experimental evidence with animals and a wealth of clinical data to demonstrate that an animal or person who construes himself as 'helpless' in this sense is likely to suffer from apathy and depression, and to fail to recognize solutions to his problems even when these are obvious. Conversely, if an individual 'believes that he has control or mastery, he may out-perform more talented peers who lack such a belief'.

The experience of most handicapped children is likely to continually affirm feelings of helplessness. They are deemed to be unable to carry out for themselves many of the daily activities which their non-handicapped peers undertake as of right, and decisions are continually made about their future by professionals or remote administrators without consulting the young person (or even his family). Even when the restrictions of choice are such that few alternatives exist, it is still unacceptable to the recipient and damaging to his self-esteem if these issues are not fully and openly discussed. In particular, it is impossible to imagine how the disabled person is to avoid feelings of helplessness if he is not given the basic information to enable him to understand or account for his handicap. Knowledge about his handicap and about the services available are essential if the disabled young person is to feel in control. The fact that greater efforts have not been made to provide this information indicates a serious failure in education provision.

On the evidence available, one must conclude that a major problem with current service provision is the failure to recognize the importance of cultivating independence and the capacity for decision making among handicapped young people, both as a way of ensuring they are enabled to lead fuller lives, and as a way of enhancing self-esteem and feelings of worth. To have the opportunity to experiment and to make mistakes is probably an essential part of growing-up, and to be denied this opportunity is likely to inhibit maturation.

To be handicapped need not inevitably lead to feelings of helplessness or depression, since, as we have already noted, over half the young people interviewed were judged not to have overt psychological problems of this kind. However, the high levels of anxiety, depression and fearfulness which we found must be attributable, to some extent, to the constant under-valuing of their worth, implicit in the attitudes of many of the adults the handicapped young people encountered.

### Social isolation

Perhaps the most significant finding in our study was the extent of social isolation among the young people, both in their school years and after. There was a clear relationship between social isolation and the presence of psychological problems, and it is this issue which we should particularly like to draw attention to, since it was our impression that the lack of social intercourse caused more distress and misery than any other factor, particularly for young people whose families were not very supportive.

Whether or not the handicapped teenager had an active social life was related to degree of handicap, in particular with locomotor disability, but the problem could not be accounted for entirely by this factor. Even the more mildly handicapped young people in ordinary schools, although they had more social outlets than those in special schools, were disadvantaged compared with their non-handicapped peers. For example, even those who could use public transport and had friends who were fully mobile were still less likely to visit or to be visited by friends in the holidays than their able-bodied peers. It was apparent from responses made by parents and teachers that many young people had difficulties in social relationships. It was obvious that there was a need for counselling and for social skills training to help the handicapped, both in ordinary and special schools, to overcome feelings of shyness and inadequacy, particularly in relation to the able-bodied. Handicapped children in ordinary schools, while benefiting greatly from the opportunities for social interaction offered them, also needed more help than they were getting in coping with peer relationships. By treating them too firmly as 'normal', their teachers overlooked some very real problems which these young people had, and this supports the Warnock Report's recommendations about the help needed for handicapped pupils and their teachers in ordinary schools.

Pupils within special schools tended to be very severely isolated (and to remain so in the post-school years). Over 60 per cent never saw their friends outside school, and in the month previous to our interview only one-quarter had made a visit or been visited by a friend. Mobility was the major barrier to sociability, and the fact that few had school friends living nearby contributed to this. It also became apparent from our inquiries that the quality of friendships among the handicapped was often different from their peers. Fewer were able to name a special friend, they saw their friends less often in the privacy of their own homes, and were less likely to confide in them – hardly surprising if they had little opportunity for interaction without close adult supervision. Neither parents nor teachers appeared to appreciate the significance of this, or to be aware of the shallowness of many friendships compared with those formed between the non-disabled. After school, friendships begun in residential college were frequently lost when the course finished, and no advice appeared to have been offered to help the young people to find ways of pursuing the contacts made there.

We formed a strong impression that helping pupils to develop more social outlets was not a major objective of special schools, colleges or day centres. It should be the general aim in schools to help foster developing friendships between children, so as to ensure that these are strongly established before leaving and have a chance of continuing once school is over, as well as assisting each child to make use of whatever additional contacts might be possible within his own locality. It is because friend-ships are not well established during school days that the handicapped young people quickly lose contact with each other once they leave school and are therefore unable to provide each other with peer support at this crucial time. Of course able-bodied young people often do not maintain friendships with former school mates either but they are in a better position to replace these friendships with others.

It is important to ensure that parents appreciate the teenager's need to establish friendships, and that they encourage mutual visits between friends and create opportunities for the teenagers to meet together and go out without parental supervision, as far as this is possible. Schools and colleges must recognize this problem and actively take steps to promote developing friendships, discussing with parents from an early age ways of helping friends meet at weekends and in the holidays. Parents need to understand that while clubs are important, they cannot fulfil all the child's friendship needs, and that the development of close intimate relationships ('having best friends') are important too. At adolescence in particular, the companionship and support of friends are essential if the teenager is to attempt new social situations – joining a club, going to a party or simply making an excursion to a local café for a snack.

Close friendships are not simply pleasurable experiences in themselves, important though this may be. They are important in helping an individual to understand himself and to mature and, as we have discussed in chapter 12, confiding relationships are likely to act as a protector against depression and contribute to the enhancement of self-esteem. The lack of opportunity to engage in close relationships with his peers at school is likely to put the handicapped teenager at a disadvantage compared with his able-bodied peers in developing the skills of friendship building.

Our findings show that handicapped pupils were less likely to have a hobby or interest, read newspapers or books, and follow sport than their able-bodied peers, although these are all things which, if developed and encouraged, would facilitate social intercourse. Again, schools and day centres did not appear to be helping pupils to develop interests that could be continued after school, or could be used as a basis for establishing friendships. Pupils need help to discover what leisure and social facilities are available within their own areas in which they might be able to participate, or about the adult education facilities available, and the potential these classes have for social contact. Community service or voluntary work within the pupils' own locality could also be explored with the same objective. Each teenager should be helped to make contact with local secondary schools with the aim of fostering social contacts within their own locality, and they should be encouraged to join local clubs for the same reason. A special project for pupils in the leavers' class might be to investigate, with the help of able-bodied peers from neighbouring schools, what leisure facilities are available in each teenager's area, which are accessible, and how to get there. Handicapped adults could be invited to the school to discuss various aspects of increasing social contacts so that the teenagers have some models of adult behaviour to emulate.

It is important that day centres and sheltered workshops see that helping their young clients to develop social outlets could make a major contribution to their general well-being. In Schlesinger's survey of day work centres (1977) she points out that while it might not be appropriate for work centre staff to organize leisure activities themselves, the role of the centres could be more 'one of encouraging those in the community who are more directly responsible to provide the handicapped with opportunities for leading a fuller social life'. She quotes the example of one centre which invited people to come in and talk to the clients about different leisure interests so that they were able to discover the possibilities open to them, and afterwards were helped to pursue any interest which attracted them. 'Hobby partners were also found, some of them visiting the homes of those with mobility problems.' She found that most clients had 'definite ideas about things they would like to do' and that there was 'a decided interest in sport and in attending classes outside work time'.

Since transport is such a major obstacle to social intercourse it seems important that schools help their pupils to explore all the possibilities. The aim should be to ensure that no child is totally dependent on his parents for transport. His potential for driving should be investigated and lessons begun, if appropriate, before leaving school, even if the prospect of a car is not immediate. The possibility of using public transport should be explored thoroughly and practice given. Other sources of transport need to be explored, such as the Red Cross or other voluntary organizations within the child's local area, and taxi or minicab services that would be sympathetic to his needs. Parents need to participate in these discussions and be helped to realize that the mobility allowance should be used in this way to help the young person achieve independence in transport.

All this would take time and local knowledge, and consequently whoever on the school staff was given the responsibility would have to be allocated space on the timetable in order to assist each child individually. Particularly in view of the poor prospects for working, it seems vital that schools devote the resources necessary to helping pupils extend and enhance their social contacts during school years, and that continuing support is available to teenagers in the post-school years to ensure that opportunities are pursued. Because their day-time occupation was so unsatisfying for many of the school leavers and the prospects for improvement poor, lack of social outlets was even more distressing than it had been in the school years. Young people with unsatisfactory (or no) occupation and few social outlets described very serious depression amounting to despair. Indeed we learned that one boy in our study made a serious attempt to commit suicide when he returned home from his residential college because his life at home was so bleak, in spite of the warmth and support of a caring family.

### Education for living and counselling

The ignorance which the young people showed about the nature of their handicap, the services available and their capacity for parenthood and marriage, together with the need to foster social outlets, all suggest that schools and colleges urgently need to develop 'education for living' courses. The high rate of psychological disturbance revealed indicates a clear need for good counselling services. Good models for such courses can be provided by the best of the further education colleges, and aim at preparing the young handicapped person for maximum personal independence and for an adult life where paid open employment cannot be assumed. Alternatives to work and use of leisure time would form a central feature of this course, discussing all the issues raised in the other sections of this chapter.

Our study also demonstrated, as did the investigations made on behalf of the Warnock Committee, that pastoral care and counselling systems within schools could be greatly improved. Little time was assigned for class teachers to discuss personal and social problems, and it appeared that only severe difficulties were likely to be recognized. In fact only nine of the eighty-two survey pupils in special schools, and three of the thirty-seven in ordinary schools had seen a teacher or counsellor for help or advice with personal problems, in spite of the fact that so many were very distressed and anxious. Little back-up specialist help was used by schools, for example from psychologists, social workers and other professionals with experience in handicap.

Individual counselling for teenagers should be available to those who need it, as well as group discussions. Because it is likely that many teenagers will not have the opportunity to marry or have children, it is most important to spend some time discussing this, emphasizing the value of close and fulfilling friendships, and companionship outside marriage. Schools should ensure that someone from outside is available to talk to the teenagers both about general problems related to handicap and in particular about sex and marriage, making use of organizations like SPOD. The one school in our study which seemed to be meeting the teenagers' needs in this respect had used a marriage guidance counsellor who visited the school regularly to help young people discuss their problems both individually and in a group.

When the suggestion of group discussions was put to the young people, the majority said that they would like this. In addition to discussing feelings and attitudes, self-assertion training to promote self-confidence, as well as social skills training, could usefully be tackled on a group basis. The presence of able-bodied teenagers at least at some of these discussions would help the disabled to see their problems in perspective – for example, by appreciating that most teenagers worry about their physical attractiveness to the opposite sex, and that the problem of finding employment is not confined to those with a handicap. Having handicapped adults along from time to time would both help focus discussion and make it more realistically based.

No one could pretend that the provision of these services will eliminate the problems entirely. However, the lack of such provision at present results in a situation where young people are bereft of support at this most critical period in their lives, and, once again, it is the families who have to provide information and advice as best they can.

## Work and alternatives to work

Eighteen months after leaving school, only one-third of the young people surveyed were in open employment, while one-quarter were attending college. The rest were in day centres or were at home with no occupation. It seemed likely that ultimately the proportion without occupation or in day centres would be even higher, since the majority of young people in special colleges were unlikely to get into open or sheltered employment.

The large proportion of young people without any occupation eighteen months after leaving school is of particular concern, because these young people were very depressed, socially isolated and anxious about their future. It is essential to prevent this kind of inactivity by providing at least some short-term outlets, through college courses and voluntary work, until a long-term solution can be found.

However, those in day centres were not necessarily better-off. Dissatisfaction with the day centres was very high, largely because these are geared primarily to the needs of the elderly who form the majority of attenders. As a rule they neither provided companionship with young people of the same age, nor offered stimulating work activities. As Schlesinger (1977) points out in her survey of day centres, 'in the main the jobs that are undertaken do not allow for the full use of the worker's abilities, learning of new skills or a sense of achievement or progress. In fact nearly half the workers were rated by Managers as under-using their abilities. [The work] rarely reflects the majority interests of those who are doing it, or gives them the opportunity for developing skills such as responsibility and decision making.' However, both in her study and in ours there were a few centres which did offer a greater variety of activities and engaged the interests of the younger members, indicating that this is certainly possible. There is a great need to disseminate information between centres so that good ideas and models of good practice become more widely known. It should be possible to offer centre clients a more varied day, with more opportunities for social interaction with their age peers by making use of existing adult education or further education classes. As Schlesinger goes on to say 'Most centres could have more and stronger links with the community . . . if centres are integrated in the community then those attending them will in a very real way be integrated too, while still having the necessary support that the centre framework gives.' The model developed by the Tuckeys (1979) could be usefully repeated, at least in part, in other areas of the country.

The possibilities for the teenager to engage in some kind of voluntary work within his neighbourhood should also be explored since this would both widen social contacts and enhance self-esteem. The handicapped so frequently experience themselves only on the receiving end of services, and we tend to overlook the contribution which they can make, and which they would take pleasure and satisfaction in doing. The OECD publication *Alternatives to Work for Severely Handicapped People* (1979) cites a number of examples of schemes where the handicapped participate as volunteers. Many handicapped young people have skills which are not competitive commercially but which could be very useful to some local organization, such as a tenants' association, church or club, and which would offer the disabled person an opportunity for increasing his local contacts and sense of achievement.

It seemed to us a major problem that the teenagers were totally unprepared for the possibility of being unemployed. Their self-esteem was closely bound up with having paid employment, and no one had helped them to think through the possibility of not getting a job or how to organize their lives in a meaningful way if a job was not feasible. It is important that discussions about this are begun with the parents and the teenagers while the teenager is still at school, so that he is properly prepared for this and has some ideas about meaningful alternatives to work. The fact that both the teenagers and the parents are not prepared for unemployment is a definite barrier to finding satisfactory alternatives to work. At present, since the counselling and support services for the post-school leaver are so meagre and the social contacts after leaving school so limited, the young people are left to face their disappointments quite alone, or with only the support of their families.

The pre-leaving programme at school should include visits to a wide variety of normal work environments, as well as day centres and sheltered workshops, so that the young people have a realistic idea of the range of options available and can begin to think about what might be possible, as well as what is likely to be out of the question.

In relation to training or further education, we would endorse the Warnock Committee's recommendation that more facilities should be provided within ordinary colleges so that handicapped young people can continue their education while at the same time building up better local contacts. The young people attending special colleges were very isolated socially when they returned home, and had no means of making new friends locally. However, it also seems important that some local colleges be able to offer residential facilities, since the experience of being away from home did help some handicapped young people develop self-reliance and self-confidence. Residences on the campus or close by would also help the young people take a more active part in college social life than disabled attenders of ordinary FE colleges do currently.

What became very apparent was the need to streamline the services existing at present in the post-school phase so that it is made clear to everyone concerned who has responsibility for overseeing the welfare of each young school leaver, in terms of further education, training, employment or social outlets. At the moment, because a number of agencies are involved, no one person is seen by the teenager as responsible, and no one agent need feel that the responsibility is his. Consequently, once having left the sheltered special school or college environment, the teenagers are commonly lacking support, information and guidance just at the point in their lives when the implications of their handicap are becoming more apparent to them and their need for support is greater than it has ever been before. In the absence of professional help, the young people have to rely on their parents more than ever, at a time when they should, like other young people, be weaning themselves emotionally away from the family. For those young people whose families cannot offer this support for whatever reasons, the situation is very bleak indeed.

To overcome this problem, the Warnock Committee recommended that for each school leaver there should be a 'named person' responsible for generally overseeing the young person's welfare. When we asked for their views on this suggestion there was widespread support both from teenagers and parents. The role of the 'named person' should include contact with those in ordinary placements, who, though more satisfied than those in special placements, often had difficulties in their social relationships. Support for those living away from home for the first time is particularly important to help deal with ill-health or homesickness or other settling-in problems. There were a number of instances in this study of serious problems, resulting in crises and the breakdown of the placement, which could have been avoided if such supervision had been available.

## Conclusion

From the wealth of detail concerning the lives, feelings and aspirations of handicapped young people which this study has yielded, four outstanding points emerge. First, the high incidence of dissatisfaction with their social lives both during school years and after, particularly once the post-school training period was complete. Secondly, how little control over their lives the young people felt that they had and how little information they had about their handicaps or about services. Thirdly, the poverty of choice currently available for those unable to find open employment, and especially how limited was the range of activities offered by most of the day centres. Fourthly, how ill-prepared the teenagers seemed to be for the realities of life as handicapped adults, and how inadequate was the help offered in the difficult transition period between school and adult life. What the young people lack is the continued support and guidance which they need throughout the later years in school and in the post-school period, to help them understand what opportunities are in reality available, not so they merely accept passively the low status society often offers, but so they can begin to construct for themselves a satisfactory life, despite the problems posed by the handicap and by society's response to it.

# Appendices

# A

## *The sample: selection procedure and background information*

### Choice of area

Initially, it was decided that the study should include all those young people with either congenital cerebral palsy or spina bifida and accompanying hydrocephalus, whose homes were in the North-West Thames Health Region excluding Bedfordshire, and the North-East Thames Health Region, excluding Essex. (The decision to exclude Bedfordshire and Essex was taken because it was felt if they were included the size of sample would be beyond the resources available for the study.) However, as there was a shortfall in the numbers expected, Bedfordshire (though not Essex) was finally included. The study area thus included two of the home counties and all the outer and inner London boroughs lying north ot the Thames. The North-West Health Region includes the following area health authorities (AHA): Hertfordshire, Bedfordshire, Hillingdon, Brent/Harrow, Barnet, Ealing/Hounslow/Hammersmith, Kensington/Chelsea/Westminster; and the North-East Region (excluding Essex) covers Enfield/Haringey, Redbridge/Waltham Forest, Barking/Havering, City/East London (Newham, Hackney, Tower Hamlets and City of London) and Islington/Camden. All but one (Islington/Camden) of these twelve AHAs agreed to take part in the study, and it was primarily, though not exclusively, through their co-operation that the young people and their families were identified.

### Locating the sample

Children were selected on the basis of where their families lived rather than where they went to school. Children in care who were living in the term-time *and* holidays aways from their families were not included: those attending boarding schools but going home for the holidays were.

(i) The main way in which the young people and their families were found was through the Area Health Authorities – 75 per cent of the sample being traced in this way. An initial letter to the AHA was followed up in most cases by a visit to the AHA to discuss the study in more detail, and the best way of approaching families. The method of doing this varied from one AHA to another, but in most cases AHA staff (in some but not all cases in conjunction with the LEA) identified the children from their records (usually from the handicap register) and then made the initial contact with the families on our behalf. In some cases the AHA letter to the family was worded to the effect that if the family did not object, their name would be passed on to the researchers, and in other cases AHAs sent both a covering explanatory note from the AHA and a letter and reply slip from the researchers to the families. In one area the AHA was agreeable to one of us going through the handicap register and contacting the families directly: in another, one of us went through the registers, and the AHA then approached the families we had selected. Only one AHA (Islington/Camden) was unwilling to co-operate in the search for families, one of the reasons given being that they were 'inundated with surveys'.

(ii) Several other sources of information were used to trace young people who might not appear on the AHA records. These included:

a) contacting by letter or in person the heads of all day and boarding schools for physically handicapped children in the areas (most of these were being visited anyway). A further twenty children were identified in this way (six being from the AHA which felt unable to help).

b) Contacting by letter all heads of schools for delicate children in the area; this produced one further name.

c) Contacting the Spastics Society, who went through all their records for us; this was quite a major exercise, and produced four more children.

d) Writing to the four local Association for Spina Bifida and Hydrocephalus branches covering the study area: this produced a number of possible children, all of whom were ultimately excluded.

e) Although no effort was made to contact all ordinary secondary schools in the study area, as this would have been too complex a task, we did ask all schools visited if there were other teenagers who might be eligible. This produced two more young people, one of whom refused to take part.

f) One more child was found who was the mildly handicapped sib of a study child.

g) One child was included (in the AHA not taking part) who had taken part in an earlier research study.

## Refusals

In addition to the 119 children identified, a further twelve were located who were eligible for the study, but who refused, giving a refusal rate of 9 per cent. In five cases it was the AHA rather than ourselves who contacted the families, so that no information about them was available. The other seven whom we contacted by letter and who refused, included two families who were reported by the school heads as being generally unwilling to co-operate and who gave no reason; two refusals were from teenagers at ordinary schools who did not want to take part; one from a family who had taken part in previous research but whose mildly handicapped son was now doing well in a public school and who felt it would be best that he was not approached; one from a family with an emotionally disturbed daughter who had been placed in an ESN school, and the seventh from a parent who, for personal reasons (bereavement, then remarriage) wanted privacy, but who wrote a most helpful and informative letter. Eight of the twelve who did not take part had cerebral palsy (three being in ordinary schools) and one had spina bifida. No information was available on the other three cases.

### Young people considered for the study but excluded

There were quite large numbers of young people whose names were given to us by the AHAs but about whom there turned out to be some doubt regarding their eligibility for the study in terms of diagnosis, IQ, or school or family circumstances. This meant that quite a large group of families were approached who were finally not included.

### Completeness of sample

An attempt is made below to compare the expected prevalence rates for cerebral palsy and spina bifida and hydrocephalus with the rates for children actually identified for the purpose of the study.

### *Cerebral palsy*

Henderson (1961) suggests the true prevalence rate for cerebral palsy is around 2 per 1000. Of these, approximately 50 per cent (see pp. 288–9 of his book) are likely to have IQs of below 70, so one would expect a true prevalence rate of around 1 per 1000 for those with IQs in the range 70+. These will probably include a number of mildly handicapped hemiplegics attending ordinary schools.

### *Spina bifida*

The incidence of spina bifida varies widely over the UK: in the south-east it is around 1.4 per 1000, and around 25 per cent of these are likely to be children with spina bifida meningocele and no associated hydrocephalus; thus the incidence of birth of those with myelomeningocele

Table A.1 *Comparison of numbers of young people expected with number actually located*

| Area | Number of children in last 2 years at school (approx.)[1] | Cerebral palsy | | Spina bifida | |
|---|---|---|---|---|---|
| | | Number expected | Number known | Number expected | Number known |
| A (Beds) | 14,000 | 14 | 10 (1[2]) | 4 | 2 |
| B (Herts) | 29,000 | 29 | 22 (4) | 2 | 1 |
| C (Hillingdon) | 6,000 | 6 | 2 | 2 | 1 |
| D (Brent/Harrow) | 11,000 | 11 | 7 (1) | 4 | 1 |
| E (Barnet) | 7,000 | 7 | 2 | 2 | 0 |
| F (Enfield/Haringey) | 13,000 | 13 | 7 | 4 | 0 |
| G (Redbridge/ W. Forest) | 11,000 | 11 | 7 (1) | 3 | 4 |
| H (Barking/Havering) | 12,000 | 12 | 8 (1) | 4 | 2 |

[1] Figures derived from *Statistics in Education*.
[2] Figure in brackets indicates those known but unwilling to take part, or excluded for other reasons (e.g., in care).

will be around 1.1 per 1000 of whom probably 80 per cent will also have hydrocephalus. This will give an incidence of about 0.8 per 1000 of babies born in the south-east with spina bifida and associated hydrocephalus. At least 50 per cent of this group will die shortly after birth, and of the survivors another 10 per cent in the first five years of life, reducing the true prevalence for those meeting the criteria of this study to around 0.36 per 1000. 10–15 per cent of those survivors will have IQs of below 70, giving a true prevalence rate of around 0.31 per 1000.

In Table A.1 the numbers expected are worked out on the basis of these figures (1 per 1000 for cerebral palsy and 0.31 for spina bifida) against the most recent figures (approximate only) for non-handicapped pupils in their last two years at school in the areas under consideration for which figures were readily available. (These figures, it should be stressed, provide a *rough* guide only.)

The shortfall in the number of those with cerebral palsy can probably be accounted for mainly by those with a mild degree of cerebral palsy attending ordinary schools. In the case of spina bifida, the shortfall is mainly in the North-East Thames Region: here Essex was excluded and it is likely that some of those born in areas within the study have moved out into overspill areas in Essex, and were therefore just outside the boundaries of the study area.

Table A.2 *Age of children in sample*

|  | N | Mean age (Yrs/mnths) | Age range (Yrs/mnths) |
|---|---|---|---|
| Cerebral palsy |  |  |  |
| Boys | 50 | (15.8) | (15.0–18.11) |
| Girls | 39 | (15.6) | (15.0–17.2) |
| Spina bifida |  |  |  |
| Boys | 11 | (15.6) | (15.0–17.6) |
| Girls | 19 | (15.9) | (15.0–16.11) |
| Controls |  |  |  |
| Boys | 15 | (15.6) | (14.3–17.4) |
| Girls | 18 | (15.2) | (14.1–16.7) |

Table A.3 *Age when interviewed*

| Age | Cerebral palsy | | Spina bifida | | Controls | |
|---|---|---|---|---|---|---|
|  | N | (%) | N | (%) | N | (%) |
| Below 16 | 57 | (64.0) | 21 | (70.0) | 26 | (78.7) |
| 16.0–16.11 | 23 | (25.8) | 7 | (23.3) | 5 | (15.1) |
| 17.0 or over | 9 | (10.1) | 2 | (6.6) | 2 | (6.0) |
| Total (N) | 89 | | 30 | | 33 | |

## The sample: background information

### Nature of handicap, sex and age

The sample included only young people handicapped with cerebral palsy or with spina bifida accompanied by hydrocephalus. All the young people interviewed were born in 1962 or earlier, that is, they were at least fifteen years old at the time of the first interview, and all were still attending school at the time of the first interview (that is, during the school year commencing January 1977).

The final group consisted of 119 young people, nearly three-quarters of whom (89) had cerebral palsy* and one-quarter (30) spina bifida with accompanying hydrocephalus. As expected on the basis of other studies, boys outnumbered girls in the cerebral-palsied group (50 boys – 56.2 per cent – and 39 girls – 43.8 per cent), while the reverse was true for

---

* One of these *also* had spina bifida but was classified as CP as he did not have accompanying hydrocephalus.

the spina bifida group (19 girls – 63.3 per cent – and 11 boys – 36.7 per cent).

The mean age and age range of the teenagers in the different sub-groups are shown in Table A.2, while Table A.3 shows the distribution of ages. There was no relationship between age and severity of handicap.

Age was also looked at in relationship to type of schooling, but no marked differences were found. The handicapped boys and girls in ordinary schools were, on average, three months older than the controls. The average age of handicapped boys in ordinary schools was exactly the same as that of the boys in special schools, while the handicapped girls in ordinary schools were, on average, four months younger than their special school counterparts.

## Social class

The composition of the sample in terms of social class is shown in Table A.4. (Data were not available for four families – three with handicapped children and one control.)

Table A.4 *Composition of sample by social class (%)*

| Social class | Cerebral palsy (N = 86) | Spina bifida (N = 30) | Total handi-capped (N = 116) | Controls (N = 32) | 1964 National Survey |
|---|---|---|---|---|---|
| I and II | 24.7 | 16.7 | 22.6 | 34.3 | 18 |
| III (non-manual) | 24.7 | 10.0 | 21.7 | 3.1 | 11 |
| III (manual) | 34.1 | 43.3 | 36.5 | 40.6 | 48 |
| IV | 9.4 ⎫ 16.4 | 20.0 ⎫ 30.0 | 11.3 ⎫ 19.9 | 21.8 ⎫ 21.8 | 22 |
| V | 7.0 ⎭ | 10.0 ⎭ | 8.6 ⎭ | 0.0 ⎭ | |

In the case of the spina bifida group, the distribution of children according to social class was very close to the National Survey (1964): in the case of the cerebral-palsied children there was a marked over-representation of families from social class III (non-manual) and under-representation for social class IV, manual, while among the controls, children from social classes I and II were over-represented.

# B
## Useful addresses

Association for Spina Bifida and Hydrocephalus, 30 Devonshire Street, London W1N 2EB. Tel. 01-486 6100

Association of Disabled Professionals, 14 Birch Way, Warlingham, Surrey CR3 9DA. Tel. 01-820 3801 (An organization of disabled professional men and women.)

Break (Holidays for handicapped or deprived children), 100 First Avenue, Bush Hill Park, Enfield, Middlesex. Tel. 01-366 0253

British Council for Rehabilitation of the Disabled, Tavistock House (South), Tavistock Square, London WC1H 9LB. Tel. 01-387 4037/8

Central Council for the Disabled, 34 Eccleston Square, London SW1. Tel. 01-834 0747 (Co-ordinating body of voluntary associations bringing pressure to improve conditions for the disabled. Publishes information on holidays, aids, etc.)

Centre on the Environment for the Handicapped, 24 Nutford Place, London W1H 6AN. Tel. 01-262 2641 (Advice and information on the design of the environment for the handicapped.)

The Cheshire Foundation Homes for the Sick, 7 Market Mews, London W1X 8HP. Tel. 01-499 2665 (Provide permanent care for severely disabled people.)

Disabled Drivers' Association, Ashwellthorpe Hall, Ashwellthorpe, Norwich. Tel. 0508-41449

Disabled Drivers' Motor Club Limited, 39 Templewood, Cleaveland, Ealing, London W13 8DV. Tel. 01-998 1226

Disabled Living Foundation, Information Service for the Disabled, 346 Kensington High Street, London W14 8NS. Tel. 01-602 2491

Disablement Income Group, Queens House, 180/182a Tottenham Court Road, London W1P 0BD. Tel. 01-636 1946 (Pressure group aiming to improve conditions, and especially financial provision, for the disabled. Also has information service.)

The Family Fund, Joseph Rowntree Memorial Trust, Beverley House, Shipton Road, York. Tel. 0904-29241 (Offers help to families of handicapped children whose needs are not being met under the NHS.)

Handicapped Adventure Playground Association, 2 Paultons Street, London SW3. Tel. 01-352 6890

Invalid Children's Aid Association, 126 Buckingham Palace Road, London SW1W 95B. Tel. 01-730 9891 (Provides all kinds of support and help to families with a chronically sick or handicapped child.)

The King's Fund, 24 Nutford Place, London W1H 6AN. Tel. 01-262 2641

Lady Hoare Trust for Thalidomide and Other Physically Handicapped Children, 7 North Street, Midhurst, Sussex. Tel. 073081-3696 (Support and practical help to disabled children and their parents.)

National Association for the Welfare of Children in Hospital, Exton House, 7 Exton Street, London SE1 8UE. Tel. 01-261 1738 (Organizes play schemes, transport services; provides information; publishes leaflets etc. to help prepare children for hospital.)

National Bureau for Handicapped Students, Calcutta House, Old Castle Street, London E1. Tel. 01-283 1030, ext. 643

National Fund for Research into Crippling Diseases, Vincent House, 1 Springfield Road, Horsham, West Sussex RH12 2 PN. Tel. 010-403 64101

National Society for Mentally Handicapped Children, Pembridge Hall, 17 Pembridge Square, London W2 4EH. Tel. 01-229 8941

The Open University, P.O. Box 48, Bletchley, Bucks (Degree courses: lack of 'O' and 'A' levels does not disqualify. Write to Registrar.)

Physically Handicapped/Able-Bodied Clubs (PHAB), 30 Devonshire Street, London W1N 2EB. Tel. 01-935 2943 (Runs youth clubs and short residential courses.)

Scottish Council of Social Services, Information for the Disabled, 18/19 Claremont Crescent, Edinburgh EH7 4HX. Tel. 031-556 3882

Scottish Spina Bifida Association, 190 Queensferry Road, Edinburgh EH4 2BW. Tel. 031-332 0743

The Shaftesbury Society, 112 Regency Street, London SW1 4AX. Tel. 01-834 2656 (Provides special residential care and teaching for disabled children, especially those with spina bifida or muscular dystrophy.)

The Spastics Society, 12 Park Crescent, London W1. Tel. 01-636 5020

Spina Bifida Association of America, P.O. Box 266, Newcastle, Delaware 19720, USA

SPOD Committee on Sexual Problems of the Disabled, 183 Queensway, London W2. Tel. 01-727 4426/7

# References

Abercrombie, M. (1964) 'Eye movements, perception and learning', in Smith, V. H. (ed.), *Visual Disorders*, Club Clinics in Developmental Medicine No. 9, Spastics International Medical Publications, London.

Adams, J., Hayes, T. and Hopson, B. (1976) *Transition Managing and Understanding Personal Change*, Martin Robertson, London.

Anderson, E. M. (1973) *The Disabled Schoolchild: A study of integration in primary schools*, Methuen, London.

Anderson, E. M. (1975) 'Cognitive and motor deficits in children with spina bifida and hydrocephalus with special reference to writing difficulties', unpublished Ph.D. thesis, University of London.

Anderson, E. M. and Plewis, I. (1977) 'Impairment of motor skill in children with spina bifida cystica and hydrocephalus: an exploratory study', *British Journal of Psychology* 68, pp. 61–70.

Anderson, E. M. and Spain, B. (1977) *The Child with Spina Bifida*, Methuen, London.

Anderson, E. M. and Tizard, J. (1979) *Alternatives to Work for Severely Handicapped People*, OECD, Paris.

ASBAH (1975) 'Survey of young people with spina bifida', unpublished report from the Education Training and Employment Officer, London.

Ausubel, D. (1961) 'Personality disorder in disease', *American Journal of Psychology* 16, pp. 69–74.

Bagley, C. (1971) *The Social Psychology of the Epileptic Child*, University of Miami Press, Coral Gables, Florida.

Baldwin, S. (1976) 'Some practical consequences of caring for handicapped children at home', *Family Fund* 57/4, 67SB.

Beresford, A. and Laurence, M. (1975) 'Work and spina bifida', *New Society* 32, p. 751.

Bergstrom-Walan, M. B. (1972) 'The problems of sex and handicap in Sweden: an investigation', in Lancaster-Gaye, D. (ed.), *Personal Relationships, the Handicapped and the Community*, Routledge and Kegan Paul, London.

Bleck, E. E. and Nagle, D. A. (eds) (1975) *Physically Handicapped Children. A Medical Atlas for Teachers*, Grune and Stratton, New York.

Bloom, J. L. (1969) 'Sex education for handicapped adolescents', *Journal of School Health* 39, pp. 363–7.

Blos, P. (1962) *On Adolescence: A Psychoanalytic Interpretation*, New York, Free Press.

Bradshaw, J. and Lawton, D. (1978) 'Tracing the causes of stress in families with handicapped children', *British Journal of Social Work* 8(2), pp. 181–92.

Brown, G. W. and Harris, T. (1978) *The Social Origins of Depression. A Study of Psychiatric Disorders in Women*, Tavistock, London.

Burton, L. (1975) *The Family Life of Sick Children*, Routledge and Kegan Paul, London.

Carlile, G. (1979) *Llanlivery Courses 1976–1977. The report of a follow-up study*, Spastics Society, London.

Carter, C. O. (1969) 'Spina bifida and ancephaly: a problem in generic-environmental interaction', *Journal of Biosocial Science* 1, pp. 71–83.

Cochrane, R. (1979) 'Psychological and behavioural disturbance in West Indians, Indians and Pakistanis in Britain: a comparison of rates among children and adults', *British Journal of Psychiatry* 134, pp. 201–10.

Cohen, S. and Taylor, L. (1978) *Escape Attempts*, Penguin, Harmondsworth.

Cole, T. M. (1975) 'Sexuality and the physically handicapped', in Green, R. (ed.), *Human Sexuality. A Health Practitioner's Text*, Williams and Wilkins, Baltimore.

Cole, T. M., Chilgren, R. and Rosenberg, P. (1973) 'A new programme of sex education and counselling for spinal cord injured adults and health care professionals', *Paraplegic* ii, pp. 111–24.

Coleman, J. C. (1974) *Relationships in Adolescence*, Routledge and Kegan Paul, London.

Cope, C. and Anderson, E. M. (1975) *Special Units in Ordinary Schools, Studies in Education*, University of London Institute of Education, NFER, Windsor.

Donvan, E. and Adelson, J. (1966) *The Adolescent Experience*, John Wiley, London.

Dorner, S. (1975) 'The relationships of physical handicap to stress in families with an adolescent with spina bifida', *Developmental Medicine and Child Neurology* 17(6), pp. 767–76.

Dorner, S. (1976a) 'Psychological and social problems of families of adolescent spina bifida parents: a preliminary report', *Developmental Medicine and Child Neurology* 15, Suppl. 29, pp. 24–7.

Dorner, S. (1976b) 'Adolescents with spina bifida – how they see their situation', *Archives of Diseases in Childhood* 51, pp. 439–44

Dorner, S. (1977) 'Sexual interest and activity in adolescents with spina bifida', *Journal of Child Psychology and Psychiatry* 18, pp. 229–37.

Education, Ministry of (1945) *Handicapped Pupils and School Health Service Regulations*, SR&O 1076, HMSO, London.

Education, Ministry of (1955) *Report of the Committee of Maladjusted Children* (Underwood Report), HMSO, London.

Education, Ministry of (1963) *Half our Future. A report of the Central Advisory Council for Education* (Newsom Report), HMSO, London.

Education and Science, Department of (1973) 'Careers education in ordinary schools', *DES Survey 18*, HMSO, London.

Education and Science, Department of (1978) *Special Education Needs. Report of the Committee of Enquiry into the Education of Handicapped Children and Young People* (Warnock Report), Cmnd 7212, HMSO, London.

Elder, G. H. (1968) 'Adolescent socialisation and development', in Borgatta, F. and Lambert, W. (eds), *Handbook of Personality Theory and Research*, Rand McNally, Chicago.

Elkind, F. (1967) 'Egocentricism in adolescence', *Child Development* 38, pp. 1025–34.

Erikson, E. H. (1968) *Identity, Youth and Crisis*, Norton, New York.

Evans, K. (1977) personal communication.

Evans, K. Hickman, V. and Carter, C. O. (1974) 'Handicap and social status of adults with spina bifida cystica', *British Journal of Preventive and Social Medicine* 28, pp. 85–92.

Feinberg, T., Lattimer, J. K., Jetar, K., Langford, W. and Beck, L. (1974) 'Questions that worry children with exstrophy', *Paediatrics* 53, pp. 242–7.

Framrose, R. (1977) 'A framework for adolescent disorder: some clinical presentations', *British Journal of Psychiatry* 131, pp. 281–8.

Freeman, R. D. (1970) 'Psychiatric problems in adolescents with cerebral palsy', *Developmental Medicine and Child Neurology* 12, p. 64.

Fulthorpe, D. (1974) 'Spina bifida: some psychological aspects', *Special Education* 1(4), pp. 17–20.

Gath, A. (1977) 'The impact of an abnormal child upon the parents', *British Journal of Psychiatry* 130, pp. 405–10.

Goffman, E. (1963) *Stigma: Notes on the Management of Spoiled Identity*, Prentice-Hall, New Jersey.

Goldin, G. J., Perry, S. L., Mongolon, R. J., Stotsky, B. A. and Foster, J. C. (1971) 'The rehabilitation of the young epileptic', *Health*, Lexington, Mass.

Gordon, N. (1976) *Paediatric Neurology for the Clinician*, Heinemann, London.

Greaves, M. (1972) 'Employment of disabled people', *British Hospital Journal and Social Services Review*, pp. 135–6

Greengross, W. (1976) *Entitled to Love*, National Marriage Guidance Council, Rugby.

Halliwell, M. and Spain, B. (1977) 'Spina bifida children in ordinary schools', *Child Care, Health and Development*.

Havinghurst, R. J. (1951) *Developmental Tasks and Education*, Longmans, Green and Co., New York.

Henderson, A. S., Krupinski, J. and Stather, A. (1971) 'Epidemiological aspects of adolescent psychiatry', in Howells, J. G. (ed.), *Modern Perspectives in Adolescent Psychiatry*, Oliver and Boyd, Edinburgh, pp. 183–208.

Hewett, S. (1970) *The Family and the Handicapped Child*, Allen and Unwin, London.

Hunt, P. (ed.) (1960) *Stigma: The Experience of Disability*, Geoffrey Chapman, London.

Hutchinson, D. and Clegg, N. (1975) 'Orientated towards work', *Special Education* 2(1), pp. 22–5.

Jeffree, D. (1977) personal communication.

Kogan, K. L. and Tyler, N. (1973) 'Mother–child interaction in young physically handicapped children', *American Journal of Mental Deficiency* 77(5), pp. 492–7.

Krupinski, J., Baikie, A. B., Stoller, A., Graves, J., O'Day, D. M. and Poke, P. (1967) 'Community mental health survey of Hayfield, Victoria', *American Journal of Orthopsychiatry* 24, pp. 223–37.

Lazarus, R. S. (1966) *Psychological Stress and the Coping Process*, McGraw-Hill, New York.

Leslie, S. A. (1974) 'Psychiatric disorders in the young adolescents of an industrial town', *British Journal of Psychiatry* 125, pp. 113–24.

Lindon, R. L. (1963) 'The Pultibec system for the medical assessment of physically handicapped children', *Developmental Medicine and Child Neurology* 5, pp. 125–45.

Lorber, J. and Schloss, A. L. (1973) 'The adolescent with myelomeningocele', *Developmental Medicine and Child Neurology* 15, Suppl. 2a, p. 113.

Lowe, P. B. (1973) 'Two years at Hereward College', *Special Education* 62(3), pp. 12–14.

McAndrew, I. (1978) *Adolescents and Young People with Spina Bifida*, Ability Press, Royal Children's Hospital, Melbourne, Australia.

McKay, D. (1975) *Clinical Psychology: Theory and Therapy*, Methuen, London.

Maslow, A. H. (1970) *Motivation and Personality* (2nd edn), Harper and Row, New York.

Masterson, J. F. (1967) *The Psychiatric Dilemma of Adolescence*, Churchill, London.

Mattson, A. (1972) 'Long-term physical illness in childhood: a challenge to psychosocial adaptation', *Paediatrics* 50, p. 801.

Miller, S. (1979) personal communication.

Mitchell, S. and Shepherd, M. (1966) 'A comparative study of children's behaviour at home and at school', *British Journal of Educational Psychology* 36, pp. 248–52.

Mooney, T. O., Cole, T. M. and Chilgren, R. (1975) *Sexual Options for Paraplegics and Quadriplegics*, Little, Brown, Boston.

Morgan, M. (1975) 'Follow-up studies of the Spastics Society's school leavers, 1966–1973', unpublished report, London.

Moss, P. and Silver, O. (1972) 'Mentally handicapped school children and their families', *Clearing House for Local Authority Social Services Research* 4, University of Birmingham.

Mott, J. (1973) 'Miners, weavers and pigeon racing', in Smith, M. A. *et al.* (eds), *Leisure and Society in Britain*, Allen Lane, London.

National Development Group for the Mentally Handicapped (1977) *Day Services for Mentally Handicapped Adults*, Pamphlet 5, HMSO, London.

NEDC (1978) Central Policy Review Staff, *Social and Economic Implication of Microelectronics*, NEDC (78) 76, London.

Newbury, K. (1979) 'Survey of special schools', unpublished report for PHAB.

Newsom Report, see Education, Ministry of (1963).

Nordqvist, I. (ed.) (1972a) *Life Together – the Situation of the Handicapped*, Swedish Central Committee for Rehabilitation, Bromma 3, Sweden.

Nordqvist, I. (1972b) 'Sexual problems of the handicapped: the work of the Swedish Central Committee for Rehabilitation', in Lancaster-Gaye, D. (ed.), *Personal Relationships, the Handicapped and the Community*, Routledge and Kegan Paul, London.

OECD report, see Rowan, P., also Anderson, E. M. and Tizard, J.

Parker, S. (1975) 'The sociology of leisure: progress and problems', *British Journal of Sociology* 26, pp. 91–101.

Philp, M. (1978) 'Physically handicapped children and their families. A summary review and critique of recent research', unpublished manuscript, Department of Applied Social Studies, University of Bradford.

Pless, B. and Pinkerton, P. (1975) *Chronic Childhood Disorder. Promoting patterns of adjustment*, Henry Kimpton, London.

Reivich, R. S. and Rothrock, I. A. (1972) 'Behaviour problems of deaf children and adolescents: a factor-analytic study', *Journal of Speech and Hearing Research* 15, p. 93.

Richardson (1977) personal communication.

Richardson, D. and Friedman, S. (1974) 'Psychosocial problems of the adolescent patient with epilepsy', *Clinical Pediatrics* 13, p. 121.

Rodda, M. (1970) *The Hearing-impaired School Leaver*, University of London Press, London.

Rodgers, B. (1979) 'The prediction of occupational adjustment for boys leaving ESN(M) schools', unpublished thesis submitted as part requirement for the M.Sc. Psychology of Education Degree, University of London Institute of Education.

Rogers, C. (1942) *Counselling in Psychotherapy*, Houghton Mifflin, Boston.

Rowan, P. (1980) 'What sort of life?', a paper for the OECD project, *The Handicapped Adolescent*, NFER, Windsor.

Rowe, B. (1973 'A study of social adjustment in young adults with cerebral palsy', unpublished B.M.Sc. dissertation, University of Newcastle-on-Tyne.

Royal Commission on the Distribution of Income and Wealth (1978) *The Causes of Poverty, Background paper to Report No. 6, Lower Incomes*, HMSO, London.

Rutter, M. (1966) 'Children of sick parents; an environmental and psychiatric study', *Maudsley Monograph* 16, Oxford University Press, Oxford.

Rutter, M. (1967) 'A children's behaviour questionnaire for completion by teachers: preliminary findings', *Journal of Child Psychology and Psychiatry* 8, pp. 1–11.

Rutter, M. (1979) *Changing Youth in a Changing Society*, Nuffield Provincial Hospitals Trust, London.

Rutter, M., Cox, A., Tupling, C., Berger, M. and Yule, W. (1975) 'Attainment and adjustment in two geographical areas: I. The prevalence of psychiatric disorder', *British Journal of Psychiatry* 126, pp. 493–509.

Rutter, M. and Graham, P. (1966) 'Psychiatric disorder in 10 and 11 year old children', *Proceedings of the Royal Society of Medicine* 59, pp. 382–7.

Rutter, M., Graham, P., Chadwick, O. F. D. and Yule, W. (1976) 'Adolescent turmoil: fact or fiction?', *Journal of Child Psychology and Psychiatry* 17, pp. 35–56.

Rutter, M., Graham, P. and Yule, W. (1970) 'A neuropsychiatric study in childhood', *Clinics in Developmental Medicine* 35–6, Spastics Society/Heinemann, London.

Rutter, M., Maughan, B., Mortimore, P., Oustan, J. with Smith, A. (1979) *Fifteen Thousand Hours: Secondary Schools and their Effects on Children*, Open Books, London.

Rutter, M., Tizzard, J. and Whitmore, K. (1970) *Education Health and Behaviour*, Longman, London.

Rutter, M., Yule, W., Berger, M., Yule, B., Morton, J. and Bagley, C. (1974) 'Children of West Indian immigrants – 1 Rates of behavioural deviance and psychiatric disorder', *Journal of Child Psychology and Psychiatry* 15, pp. 241–62.

Rutter, M., Yule, B., Quinton, D., Rowlands, O., Yule, W. and Berger, M. (1975) 'Attainment and adjustment in two geographical areas: III. Some factors accounting for area differences', *British Journal of Psychiatry* 126, pp. 520–33.

Schlesinger, S. (1977) *Industry and Effort, a survey of day work centres in England, Wales and Northern Ireland*, The Spastics Society, London.

Scott, M., Roberts, M. C. C. and Tew, B. J. (1975) 'Psychosexual problems in adolescent spina bifida patients with special reference to the effect of urinary diversion on patient attitudes', paper given at the annual meeting of the Society for Research into Spina Bifida and Hydrocephalus, 25–28 June 1975, Glasgow.

Scottish Education Department (1964) *Ascertainment of Maladjusted Children*, Report of Working Party, HMSO, Edinburgh.

Scottish Education Department (1975) *The Secondary Education of Physically Handicapped Children in Scotland*, HMSO, Edinburgh.

Seidal, U. P., Chadwick, O. F. D. and Rutter, M. (1975) 'Psychological disorders in crippled children. A comparative study of children with and without brain damage', *Developmental Medicine and Child Neurology* 17, pp. 563–73.

Seligman, M. E. P. (1975) *Helplessness*, W. H. Freeman, San Francisco.

Shearer, A. (1972) *A Right to Love?*, Spastics Society/National Association for Mental Health, London.

Shearer, A. (1974) 'Sex and handicap', in Boswell, D. M. and Wingrove, J. M. (eds), *The Handicapped Person in the Community*, pp. 225–33, Tavistock, London.

Siegelman, E., Block, J. and vonder Lippe, A. (1970) 'Antecedents of optimal psychological adjustment', *Journal of Consulting and Clinical Psychology* 33(3), pp. 283–9.

Snowdon Report (1976) *Integrating the Disabled*, National Fund for Research into Crippling Diseases, Springfield Road, Horsham.

Spastics Society (1971) *The Spastics Society School Leavers 1966–1970*, Spastics Society Careers Advisory Service, London.

Spastics Society (1978) 'The special needs of handicapped adolescents. Report of a working party', unpublished report, London.

Spastics Society (1979) 'Beaumont College of Further Education: a social learning curriculum', unpublished report, London.

Stewart, W. F. R. (1975) *Sex and the Physically Handicapped*, National Fund for Research into Crippling Diseases, Springfield Road, Horsham.

Szasz, T. (1960) 'The myth of mental illness', *American Psychologist* 15, pp. 113–18.

Tanner, J. (1962) *Growth at Adolescence*, Blackwell, Oxford.

Tew, B. and Laurence, K. M. (1973) 'Mothers, brothers and sisters of patients with spina bifida', *Developmental Medicine and Child Neurology* 15, Suppl. 29, pp. 69–76.

Tew, B. and Laurence, K. (1975) 'Some sources of stress found in mothers of spina bifida children', *British Journal of Preventive and Social Medicine* 29, p. 27.

Thomas, A., Chess, S. and Birch, H. G. (1968) *Temperament and Behaviour Disorders in Children*, University of London Press, London.

Tizard, J. and Anderson, E. M. (1979) *The Education of the Handicapped Adolescent: Alternatives to work for severely handicapped adolescents*, OECD, Paris.

Townsend, P. (1973) 'Sociological explanations of the lonely', in *The Social Minority*, pp. 240–65, Allen Lane, London.

Training Services Agency (1975) *Vocational Preparation for Young People, A Discussion Paper*, TSA, London.

Tuckey, L., Parfit, J. and Tuckey, B. (1973) *Handicapped School Leavers*, NFER, Windsor.

Tuckey, L. and Tuckey, B. (1979) 'An ordinary place. The Stone House, a community work approach to disabled people', unpublished manuscript.

Tyson, M. (1964), in Abercrombie *et al.* (ed.), *Visual, Perceptual and Visuo-motor Impairment in Physically Handicapped Children*, Suppl. 3, 18, pp. 561–625.

Volpe, R. (1976) 'Orthopaedic disability, restriction and role-taking activity', *Journal of Special Education* 10(4), pp. 371–81.

Walker, A. and Lewis, P. (1977) 'Career advice and employment experience of a small group of school leavers', *Careers Quarterly* 29, Vol. 1, pp. 5–14.

Wall, W. D. (1968) *Adolescents in School and Society*, NFER, Windsor.

Warnock Report, see Education and Science, Department of (1978).

Wedell, K. (1960) 'The visual perception of cerebral-palsied children', *Journal of Child Psychology and Psychiatry* 1, pp. 215–27.

Wedell, K. (1961) 'Follow-up study of perceptual ability in children with hemiplegia', in *Hemiplegic Cerebral Palsy in Children and Adults*, report of an international study group in Bristol, Spastics Society/Heinemann, London.

Wedell, K. (1973) *Learning and Perceptions – Motor Disabilities in Children*, John Wiley, New York.

Weiner, I. (1970) *Psychological Disturbance in Adolescence*, John Wiley, New York.

Wilkin, D. (1978) 'Community care of the mentally handicapped: family support', *Nursing Mirror*, 27 April, pp. 39–40.

Woodburn, M. (1975) *Social Implications of Spina Bifida – A Study in S. E. Scotland*, Eastern Branch of Scottish Spina Bifida Association, Edinburgh.

Wright, B. (1960) *Physical Disability – A Psychological Approach*, Harper and Row, New York.

Young, M. and Wilmott, P. (1973) *The Symmetrical Family*, Routlegde, London.

Younghusband, E., Birchall, D., Davie, R. and Pringle, M. I. Kellmer (eds) (1970) *Living with Handicap*, National Bureau for Co-operation in Child Care, London.

Yule, W. (1968) 'Identifying maladjusted children', paper read to the Association for Special Education, 29th National Biennial Conference, August 1968, Coventry.

# Index